Autoimmune Thrombocytopenia

Yoji Ishida • Yoshiaki Tomiyama
Editors

Autoimmune Thrombocytopenia

Springer

Editors
Yoji Ishida
Division of Hematology and Oncology
Department of Internal Medicine
Iwate Medical University School
of Medicine
Morioka
Iwate
Japan

Yoshiaki Tomiyama
Department of Blood Transfusion
Osaka University Hospital
Suita
Osaka
Japan

ISBN 978-981-10-4141-9 ISBN 978-981-10-4142-6 (eBook)
DOI 10.1007/978-981-10-4142-6

Library of Congress Control Number: 2017943031

Printed on acid-free paper

This Springer imprint is published by Springer Nature
The registered company is Springer Nature Singapore Pte Ltd.
The registered company address is: 152 Beach Road, #21-01/04 Gateway East, Singapore 189721, Singapore

Preface

Besides anemia, thrombocytopenia is the most common hematological abnormality encountered in daily clinical practice by general physicians as well as hematologists. The pathophysiology of thrombocytopenia is classified into at least three categories: (1) decreased platelet production, (2) increased platelet destruction or consumption, and (3) abnormal platelet distribution or pooling. Among them, autoimmune thrombocytopenia (ITP), the theme of this book, is a common disease caused by increased platelet destruction due to antiplatelet autoantibodies. However, its diagnosis is still difficult because of the lack of specific diagnostic tests. So far, its diagnosis is still based on differential diagnosis in daily practice. However, recent basic and clinical research has made a great progress in the pathophysiology and management of ITP as well as platelet/megakaryocyte biology.

One of the major advances in the management of ITP is that the development of thrombopoietin receptor (TPO-R) agonists has induced better QOL for ITP patients by preventing pathological bleeding. In the era of TPO-R agonists for ITP, general hematologists should update their knowledge regarding the following: goal of ITP management, who and when should be treated, efficacy and safety of TPO-R agonists, etc.

Here, we propose a book, *Autoimmune Thrombocytopenia*, which updates recent advances in platelet/megakaryocyte biology from basic viewpoints as well as clinical viewpoints. This book includes the history and basic aspects of platelet biology, epidemiology, pathophysiology, and adult and child ITP including clinical manifestations, diagnosis, and treatment. Therefore, this book is for interns, residents, clinicians, and hematologists who are curious about recent information on ITP. Finally, we wish that our book would greatly contribute to the readers for their better understanding of pathophysiology and management of thrombocytopenia.

February, 2017

Yoji Ishida, M.D.
Yoshiaki Tomiyama, M.D.

Acknowledgments

This work was supported, at least in part, by Grant-in Aid for Scientific Research from the Ministry of Education, Culture, Sports, Science and Technology in Japan and the Ministry of Health, Labor and Welfare in Japan.

Contents

Part VI Diagnosis

Part VII Treatment of Adult ITP

Part VIII Child ITP

Part I
Introduction

History of Immune Thrombocytopenia

Yoji Ishida

Abstract The term "platelet" whose function was the adhesive characteristic was first used by Bizzozero in 1882. The word "purpura" is the Latin derivative of the Greek word "porphyra," which is used to designate purple fish. The pathophysiology of this disease had not been unknown until 1951. This chapter describes the history of immune thrombocytopenia.

1 Platelets [1]

Extremely minute corpuscles were described in clotting blood by Addison in 1841 [2]. Since then, discussions about the existence of a third morphological constituent of blood continued for approximately 40 years. The term "platelet" was first used by Bizzozero in 1882 [3]. He also demonstrated the adhesive characteristic of platelets. However, several papers were published before his discovery, including one by Donné in 1844 [4], in which he described elements called globulins. In 1865, Schultze [5] described the third morphological blood element, namely, granular masses, and Osler [6] noted their presence in the venules of rats in 1874. Then, Osler and Schäfer [7] identified the same elements in blood smears by microscopy and correlated these elements with the formation of granular aggregates in the presence of bacteria. In 1878, a Frenchman named Hayem [8] described that the granular aggregates consisted of the product of altered discoid elements called "hematoblasts" in fresh blood. He believed that hematoblasts were transformed into red blood cells. To this day, French hematologists call platelets by this name.

Y. Ishida, M.D., Ph.D.
Division of Hematology and Oncology, Department of Internal Medicine, Iwate Medical University School of Medicine, 19-1 Uchimaru, Morioka, Iwate Prefectire 020-8505, Japan
e-mail: yoji.ishida@gmail.com

Y. Ishida, Y. Tomiyama (eds.), *Autoimmune Thrombocytopenia*,
DOI 10.1007/978-981-10-4142-6_1

2 Megakaryocytes

Megakaryocytes are rare, polypoid, large cells in the bone marrow. In 1980, Howell [9] coined these cells megakaryocytes. James Homer Wright [10, 11] reported that blood platelets are derived from the cytoplasm of megakaryocytes [6, 7].

3 Purpura [12]

According to Dedekind [13], the word purpura is the Latin derivative of the Greek word porphyra, which is used to designate purple fish. It was not used generally until the sixteenth century when the term "purpura" was used to describe a purple-colored eruption. At the same time, Hippocrates [14] observed petechia and described it as a condition that resembles purpura. The reported characteristics were fetid breath, swelling of the gums, and large bleeding ulcers in the lower extremities, suggestive of scurvy. Until the sixteenth century, purpura was often associated with the manifestation of fever, which was called "petechial fever."

A case of purpura independent of fever was reported in 1557 by Amatus Lusitanus [15], who described it as "morbus pulicaris adsque febre." Eugalenus [16] clearly described purpura in 1658 including several distinct cases in which the purpura eruption was related with hemorrhage. In 1734, Hornung [17] divided purpura into the following three categories: simplex, febrile, and scorbutic. The next year, Werlhof [18] called purpura "morbus maculosus hemorrhagicus" and described a case of a girl who suddenly developed epistaxis and large purpura blotches on the neck, back, and arm during menstruation. In 1829, Schönlein [19] described several cases of purpura with acute arthritic manifestations. Later, Henoch [20] described five cases of purpura in children who experienced vomiting, abdominal pain, intestinal hemorrhage, and no fever. This type of purpura is now called Schönlein and Henoch purpura. However, what induced purpura was not known until 1883. Diminution in platelets, which is induced by purpura, was recognized by Krauss [21] in 1883 and by Denys [22] in 1887; the existence of platelets was in doubt, and an actual count of platelets was not conducted until 1890.

Based on blood extravasation after intravenous injection of putrefactive matter, Magendi [23] concluded that purpura is the result of poisoning of the blood. Cole [24], in 1907, and Lee and Robertson [25], in 1916, produced "purpura hemorrhagica" in animals by independently injecting serum specifically against human platelets or antiplatelet serum.

In 1915, Frank [26] described "essentielle thrombopenia" and postulated that there would be marked diminution in platelet production by megakaryocytes. The following year, Kaznelson [27] performed splenectomy in a chronic relapsing case of the disease, because he assumed the spleen has an unusual thrombolytic function. The first case improved after splenectomy. Since then, several investigators have tried to inject the splenic extracts from patients into experimental animals, resulting in thrombocytopenia in the 1940s [28].

In 1951, Harrington et al. [29] first reported that injection of plasma from patients with idiopathic thrombocytopenic purpura into healthy recipients predictably resulted in thrombocytopenia. The factor that induced thrombocytopenia was found in the globulin fraction. Then, Shulman et al. [30] demonstrated that the factor that induced thrombocytopenia was an immunoglobulin that specifically binds to platelets and could be removed from serum by absorption of normal human platelets. Immunoglobulin G antibody against platelets binds to platelet-associated antigen, resulting in phagocytosis by macrophages in the reticuloendothelial system through macrophage Fc receptors.

In 2000, platelet production and megakaryocytes in the bone marrow were evaluated in patients with idiopathic thrombocytopenic purpura. Chang et al. [31] and McMillan et al. [32] demonstrated that antiplatelet autoantibodies from adult patients with idiopathic thrombocytopenic purpura independently suppress in vitro megakaryocytopoiesis in the bone marrow. Later, it was discovered that thrombocytopoiesis is also impaired as a result of either destruction of antibody-coated platelets in the bone marrow by marrow macrophage or the inhibition of proplatelet formation.

These results strongly suggest that idiopathic thrombocytopenic purpura is an autoimmune disease caused by antiplatelet antibodies. Therefore, the term immune thrombocytopenia has been used until today.

References

1. de Gaetano G. A new blood corpuscle. An impossible interview with Giulio Bizzozero. Thromb Haemast. 2001;86:973–9.
2. Addison W. On the colourless corpuscles and on the molecules and cytoblasts in the blood. London Med Gaz. 1841;NS30:144–52.
3. Bizzozero G. Su di un nuovo elemento morfologico del sangue dei mammiferí e della sua importanza nella thrombosí e nella coagulazione. L'Osservatore–Gazzetta delle Cliniche. 1881;17:785–7.
4. Donné A. Cours de microscopie. Paris; 1844, 85 p.
5. Schultze M. Ein heizbarer Objecttisch und seine Verwendung bei Untersuchungen des Blutes. Arch Mikroskop Anat. 1865;1:1–4.
6. Osler W. An account of certain organisms occurring in liquor sanguinis. Proc R Soc Med, London. 1874;22:391.
7. Osler W, Schäfer EA. über einige im Blute vorhandene bacterienbildende Massen. Centralbl Med Wissensch. 1873;11:577–8.
8. Hayem G. Recherches sur l'évolution des hématies dans le sang de l'homme, et des vertébrés. Arch Physiol (decuxième série). 1878;5:692–734.
9. Howell WH. Observations upon the occurrence, structure, and function of the giant cells of the marrow. J Morphol. 1890;4:117–30.
10. Wright JH. The origin and nature of the blood paltes. Boston Med Surg J. 1906;23:643–5.
11. Wright JH. The histogenesis of blood platelets. J Morphol. 1910;21:263–78.
12. Jones HW, Tocantins LM. The history of purpura hemorrhagica. Ann Med Hist. 1933;5:349–59.
13. For a complete discussion of the origin of the word Purpura consult: Dedekind A. L'étymologie du mot pourpre expliquée par les sciences naturelles. Arch. de zool. experim. et génerale bist. natur. Paris. 1896;4(1):481.

14. Hippocrates. De intern. Affectionibus. Sect. V, p. 558.
15. Lusitanus A. Curationum medicinalum Centuriae quatuor. Basileae. 1556;Cent. III, Curat. 70:286.
16. Eugalenus S. De morbo scorbuto liber. Hagae. 1658;Obs. 2:62, 68.
17. Hornung ALF. De purpura sive febre miliari. Jenae; 1734.
18. Werlhof PG. In: Wichmann JE, editor. Opera medica; 1775. p. 748.
19. Schönlein JL. Allegemeine und specielle Pathologie und Therapie. St Gallen. 1837;2:42.
20. Henoch E. Zusammenhang von Purpura und Intestinalstorungen. Berl klin Wchnschr. 1868;5:517.
21. Krauss E. Uber purpura: Inaug [Dissertation]. Heidelberg; 1883.
22. Denys J. Etudes sur la coagulation du sang. La cellule. 1887;3:445.
23. Magendi F. Précis élementaire de physiologie. 3rd ed, vol 2. Paris; 1833. p. 417.
24. Cole RI. Note on the production of an agglutin. Serum for blood platelets. Bull Johns Hopkins Hosp. 1907;18:261.
25. Lee RI, Robertson OH. The effect of anti-platelet serum on the blood platelets and the experimental production of purpura. J Med Res. 1916;33:323.
26. Frank E. Die essentielle Thrombopenie. (Konstitutionellle Purpura-Pseudo-Hämophilie) I. Klinisches Bild. Beri. klin. Wchnschr. 52: 454–58, 1915. II. Pathogenese. J Med Res. 1915;52:490–4.
27. Kaznelson P. Verschwinden der hämorrhagischen Diathese bei einem Falle von "essentieller Thrombopenie" (Frank) nach Milzexstirpation. Splenogene thrombolytische Purpura. Wien, kiln. Wchnschr. 1916;29:1451–4.
28. Troland CE, Lee FC. Thrombocytopenia. A substance in the extracts from spleen of patients with idiopathic thrombocytopenic purpura that reduces the number of blood platelets. JAMA. 1938;111:221–6.
29. Harrington WJ, Minnich V, Hollingsworth JW, Moore CV. Demonstration of a thrombocytopenic factor in the blood of patients with thrombocytopenic purpura. J Lab Clin Med. 1951;38(1):1–10.
30. Shulman R, Marder VJ, Weinrach SW. Similarities between known antiplatelet antibodies and the factor responsible for thrombocytopenia in idiopathic purpura. Physiologic, serologic and isotopic studies. Ann N Y Acad Sci. 1965;124:499–542.
31. Chang M, Nakagawa PA, Williams SA, Schwartz MR, Imfeld KL, Buzby JS, Nugent DJ. Immune thrombocytopenic purpura (ITP) plasma and purified ITP monoclonal autoantibodies inhibit megakaryocytopoiesis in vitro. Blood. 2003;102(3):887–95.
32. McMillan R, Wang L, Tomer A, Nichol J, Pistillo J. Suppression of in vitro megakaryocyte production by antiplatelet autoantibodies from adult patients with chronic ITP. Blood. 2004;103(4):1364–9.

Part II
Basic Aspects of Platelet Biology

Megakaryopoiesis and Thrombopoiesis

Shugo Kowata and Yoji Ishida

Abstract Platelets are formed from the cytoplasm of megakaryocytes (MKs) that reside in the bone marrow (BM). MKs arise from hematopoietic stem cells in the osteoblastic niche in BM. The primary regulator of megakaryopoiesis is thrombopoietin. It is generally accepted that MKs migrate into the vascular niche and produce platelets; however, the mechanism by which platelets are formed and released from MKs remains controversial. The most prevalent proposed mechanism regarding platelet formation is the proplatelet model; in this model, MKs form long extensions (proplatelets) by remodeling their cytoplasm and release cell fragments into sinusoid vessels. Detached cell fragments in the circulating blood are heterogeneous population of cells in regard to size, shape, or structure. Large fragments (platelet progenitors) are believed to have the ability to convert into mature platelets. After leaving BM sinusoids, these platelet progenitors may convert into individual mature platelets in the bloodstream.

1 Megakaryopoiesis

1.1 Megakaryocyte Development

Megakaryocytes (MKs) develop from hematopoietic stem cells (HSC), which give rise to progeny that progressively lose self-renewal capacity and become restricted to one lineage (Fig. 1). In the case of MK development, this is accomplished via several consecutive stages, including MK lineage commitment and progenitor proliferation, differentiation, and maturation. In the classical hierarchical model of hematopoiesis, a major bifurcation occurs between the myeloid and lymphoid branches [1–3]. Restricted myeloid progenitors undergo another bifurcation into bipotent granulocyte-macrophage progenitors or MK-erythrocyte progenitors (MEPs). This hierarchical model suggests that all MKs arise from intermediate

S. Kowata (✉) • Y. Ishida
Division of Hematology and Oncology, Department of Internal Medicine,
Iwate Medical University School of Medicine, Morioka, Japan
e-mail: skowata@iwate-med.ac.jp; yoji.ishida@gmail.com

Y. Ishida, Y. Tomiyama (eds.), *Autoimmune Thrombocytopenia*,
DOI 10.1007/978-981-10-4142-6_2

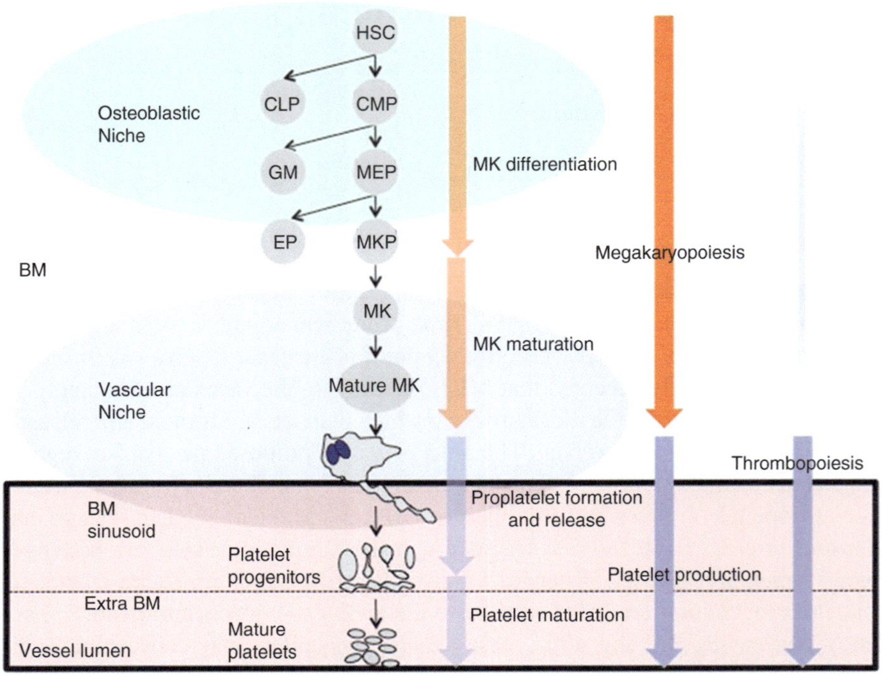

Fig. 1 Megakaryopoiesis and thrombopoiesis. Differentiation from hematopoietic stem cells (HSCs) to platelets proceeds by a number of intermediate stages. Megakaryopoiesis contains stages from HSC to mature MKs in the bone marrow. Thrombopoiesis contains stages in which mature MKs form cytoplasmic protrusion, called proplatelets, into a vascular lumen to produce platelet progenitors and mature platelets. Abbreviations: *BM* bone marrow, *HSC* hematopoietic stem cell, *CMP* common myeloid progenitor, *MEP* megakaryocyte-erythroid progenitor, *MKP* megakaryocyte progenitor, *MK* megakaryocyte, *CLP* common lymphoid progenitor, *GMP* granulocyte-macrophage progenitor, *EP* erythroid progenitor

progenitors, including MEPs (Fig. 1). In addition, it has become increasingly clear that HSCs and MKs exhibit numerous similarities and that MKs arise directly from HSCs as well as from intermediate progenitors [4–6].

1.2 Thrombopoietin

Nearly 1×10^{12} platelets, with a typical average life span of 7–9 days, circulate in the adult human bloodstream [7]. Nevertheless, the platelet number is tightly controlled within narrow physiological ranges [8]. The interaction between thrombopoietin (TPO) and its receptor, myeloproliferative leukemia virus protein (Mpl), is implicated in the proliferation and differentiation of normal HSCs and the bipotential MK precursors [7]. Mice lacking Mpl or JAK2 expression in platelets and MKs show expansion of MK and thrombocytosis, suggesting that TPO/Mpl signaling in MKs is dispensable for platelet production [9, 10]. TPO is produced in the liver hepatocytes [11].

MKs and platelets regulate TPO homeostasis by Mpl receptor-mediated internalization and degradation. Recently, a new feedback mechanism regulating TPO homeostasis was proposed in which the following occur: (1) as platelets age in the circulation, they become desialylated (lose of surface sialic acid); (2) hepatocytes recognize desialylated platelets via the Ashwell-Morell receptor (AMR); and (3) in hepatocytes, AMR signaling leads to JAK2-STAT5 phosphorylation, which leads to upregulation of TPO mRNA expression and subsequent TPO production [12].

1.3 Regulation of Transcription Factors

It has been reported that several transcriptional factors regulate the fate of MK development from HSCs. RUNX-1 functions as a master regulator of hematopoiesis and plays a role in lineage decisions in MEPs by repressing erythroid gene expression via epigenetic repression of the erythroid master regulator KFL-1 [13]. Moreover, mice lacking the transcription factors GATA-1 [14], AML-1 [15], or Fli-1 [16] show markedly reduced platelet numbers, associated with deregulated proliferation and severely impaired cytoplasmic maturation. These transcription factors are thus required for MK maturation in adult hematopoiesis. In addition, GATA-1 is required to cooperate with p45 for normal megakaryopoiesis [17]. Furthermore, NF-E2 is a heterodimeric transcription factor consisting of p45 and small Maf subunits [18–20]. Mice lacking NF-E2 show profound thrombocytopenia and fail to produce proplatelets, the microtubule-based precursors of blood platelets, from MKs [18–20]. The expression of beta1 tubulin is exquisitely restricted to platelets and MKs, where it appears late in differentiation and localizes to microtubule shafts and coils within proplatelets. Restoring NF-E2 activity in NF-E2-deficient MKs rescues the expression of beta1 tubulin [21]. These data suggest that NF-E2 determines the quantity and quality of platelets by activating genes in MKs that mediate platelet production and function [22, 23].

1.4 MK Maturation

One characteristic cellular feature of MK development is endomitosis, a unique form of mitosis in which DNA is repeatedly replicated in the absence of nuclear and cytoplasmic division [24, 25]. Polyploidization, which is considered as incomplete mitosis that is aborted in anaphase, occurs via endomitosis [25]. MKs with polyploidization enable functional gene amplification and experience an increase in protein and lipid synthesis in parallel with cell enlargement [26]. MKs generate a variety of secretory granules, including α-granule, which acquire their molecular contents both from endogenous protein synthesis and by uptake and packing of plasma proteins [27]. Moreover, a demarcation membrane system (DMS) begins as invaginations of plasma membrane that develop into an extensive complex of cisternae and tubules distributed throughout the MK cytoplasm [28]. The DMS is thought to exist as a membrane reservoir for proplatelet and platelet membranes, and it has been proposed that the term "invagination system" may be more appropriate [29, 30] (Fig. 2c, e).

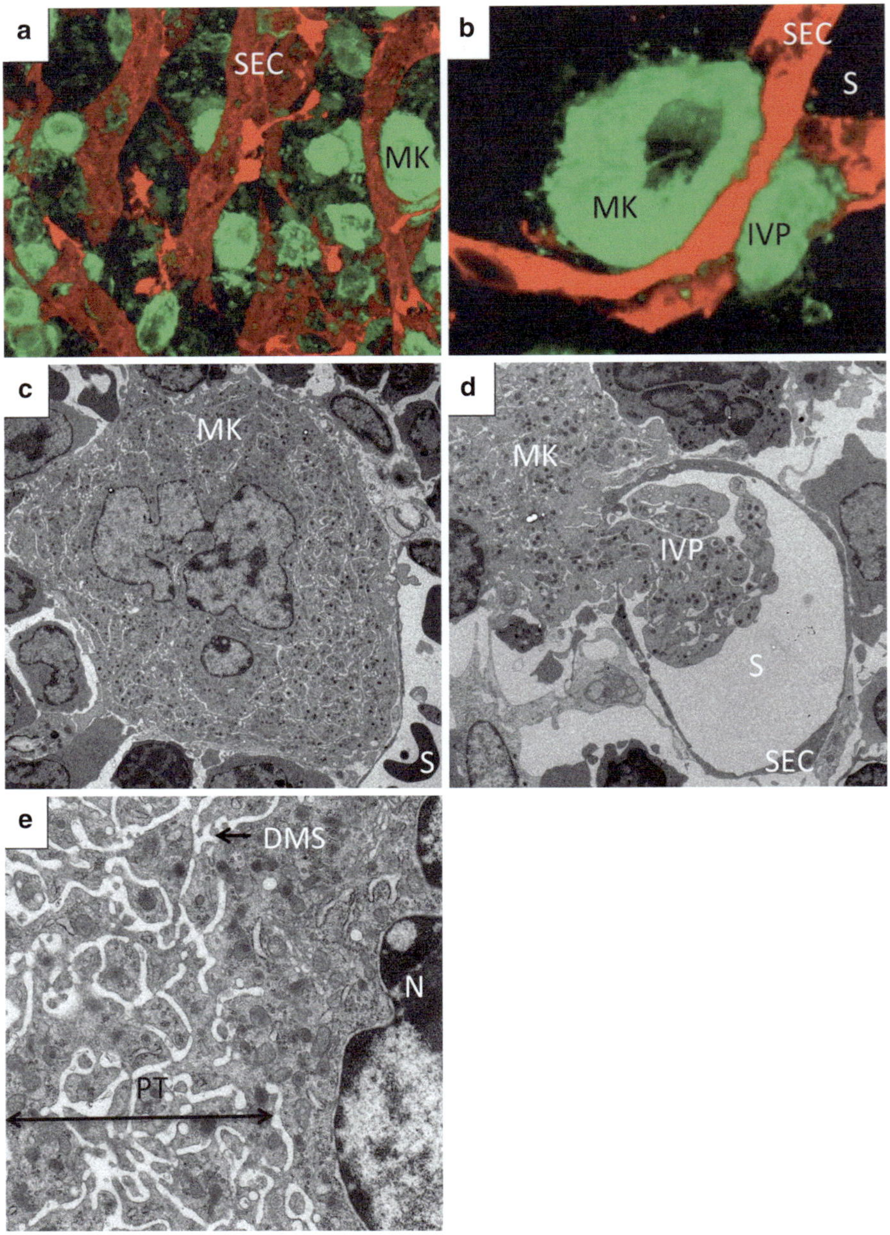

Fig. 2 Megakaryocytes in bone marrow niche. (**a**, **b**) Reconstructed 3D image of BM from FLK-1-EGFP mice stained with anti-GP1b. *Green*, megakaryocytes; *red*, sinusoid endothelial cells. (**c**, **d**, **e**) Transmission electron microscopy of BM from wild-type mice. Abbreviations: *DMS* demarcation membrane system, *IVP* intravascular protrusion, *MK* megakaryocyte, *PT* platelet territory, *S* sinusoid lumen, *SEC* sinusoid endothelial cell

2 Platelet Formation

2.1 *Genesis of the Basic Concept*

After commitment, differentiation, and maturation, MKs migrate from the osteoblastic niche to the vascular niche (Fig. 2a), where they mature and eventually form individual platelets in the bloodstream (Fig. 2b, d) [31]. Although knowledge has accumulated for over a century, the mechanism by which platelets form and are released from MKs remains controversial.

In 1906, Wright first suggested that platelets arise from bone marrow (BM) MKs on the basis of histological sections of BM; he further described the formation of platelets by the "pinching off" of small projections from MK protrusions or of longer segments of MK protrusions in the sinusoid vascular lumen [32]. After this discovery, there have been several aspects of platelet formation that have been studied (Fig. 3).

In the 1950s, the platelet territory (PT) model was developed using transmission electron microscopy (TEM); in this model, MK cytoplasm is divided by the DMS into future platelets, fracturing into platelets in the BM parenchyma [28, 33, 34]. This model is based on the notion that individual platelets are already delineated by DMS in the PT (Fig. 3b). Because MKs reside within the platelet agonist-rich extracellular matrix (ECM) [35], MKs are required to release nascent platelets into the sinusoid vascular lumen without activation by the ECM (Fig. 3a). However, the transport of nascent platelets from the extravascular site through the sinusoid endothelial cells to the vessel lumen has not been elucidated in the PT model [28, 33, 34]. In addition, there are no reports regarding existence of the marginal band composed of microtubule bundles, the cytoskeletal hallmark of definitive platelets [36, 37], in the territories of MK cytoplasm.

2.2 *Proplatelet Theory*

From the 1970s, morphological studies using scanning electron microscopy (SEM) have predicted that platelets or segments of proplatelets are released from MKs via proplatelets, which have a tandem array of platelet-sized swellings with a beaded appearance at the distal end [38, 39]. At that time, it was thought that proplatelet extensions were already delineated by the DMS in the PT and that proplatelet morphogenesis was accomplished in the PT (Fig. 3c).

In the 1980s, it was suggested that microtubules running parallel with the long axis of proplatelets (a cytoskeletal feature of proplatelets) have a role in either the formation or maintenance of proplatelets [40, 41]. In addition, it was proposed that the DMS functions as a reservoir to supply membrane elements to extend the proplatelet in what is known as the synonymized flow model [29]. After the discovery of TPO in the 1990s, studies using cultured MKs in vitro successfully demonstrated

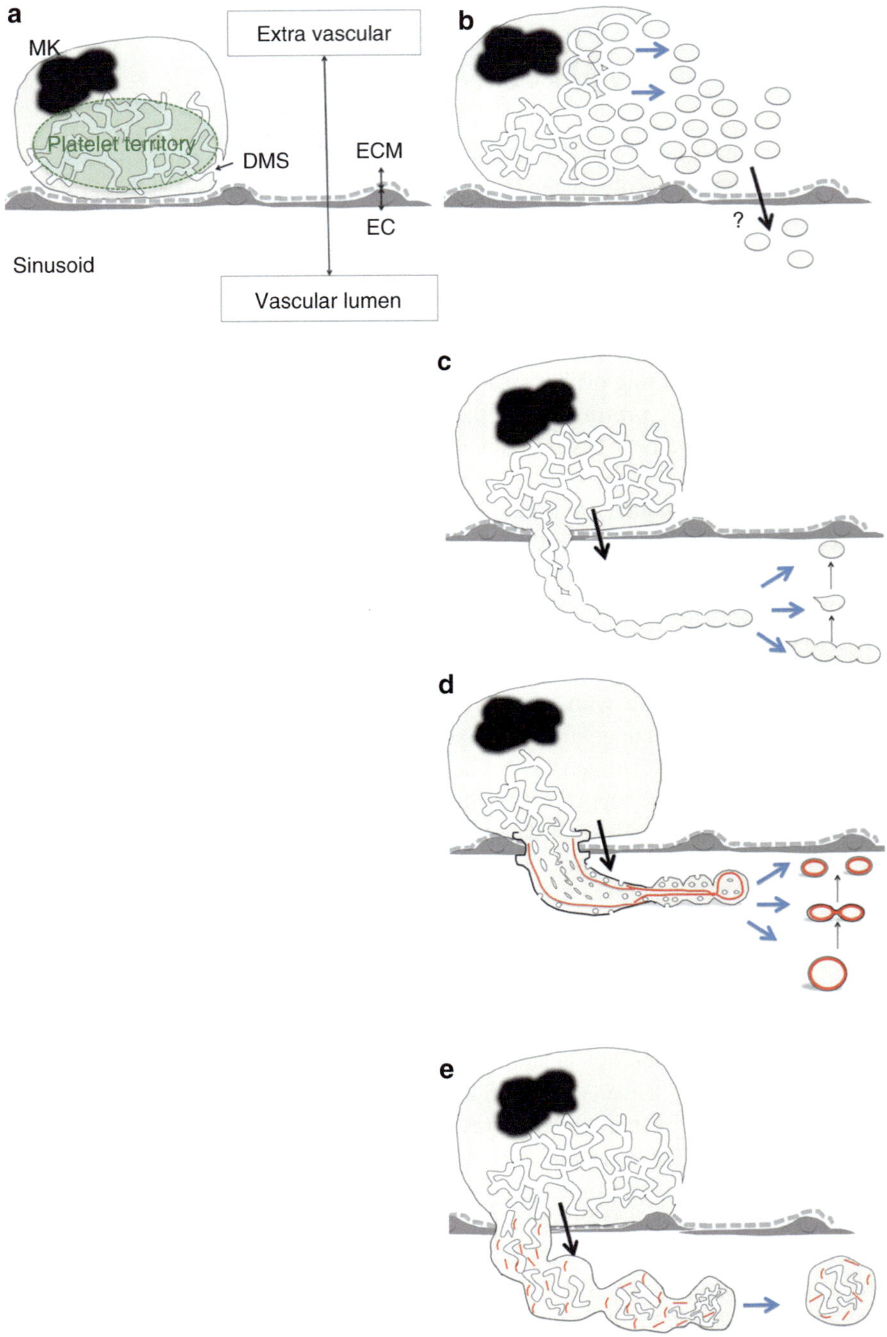

Fig. 3 Schematic view of platelet formation in each model. (**a**) Schema of MK in vascular niche. (**b**) PT model. (**c**) Early proplatelet model. (**d**) Recent proplatelet model. (**e**) Immature large fragment. Abbreviations: *DMS* demarcation membrane system, *EC* sinusoid endothelial cell, *ECM* extracellular matrix, *MK* megakaryocyte. Red line indicates microtubules

the cytoskeletal hallmark, i.e., the marginal band-like structure at the distal end of proplatelets [42–44]. These findings suggest that MKs remodel their cytoplasm into proplatelets that transport products and organelles in the appropriate abundance into the vasculature and release fragments of proplatelets (Fig. 3d). Thus, this has led to the proplatelet theory becoming the unifying and accepted model.

2.3 Dynamic Analysis of Platelet Formation in Native BM

There have been reports of many unclassified snapshots of proplatelet and nascent platelet morphogenesis in BM. For example, intravascular thick protrusions and fragments were reported in early histological studies [32, 45, 46], and they were considered as a sequential stage of proplatelet formation without further dynamic evaluation [29]. However, there were technical limitations regarding performance of temporal and spatial analysis of the sequential stages of platelet formation in living BM tissue.

In contrast, recent studies using multiphoton microscopy, which can visualize platelet formation from MKs in BM of living mice, necessitate a revision of these prior concepts. For instance, Junt et al. captured images of MKs forming large "proplatelet-like protrusions" which routinely released heterogeneous large particles into the sinusoids [47]. They concluded that these large particles might represent multiple intertwined or single immature proplatelets. However, it remained unclear whether all intravascular protrusions translate into proplatelets or whether MKs release cytoplasmic particles without proplatelet formation.

Our group analyzed MKs forming intravascular protrusions using intravital imaging, TEM, and SEM [48]. In analysis of intravital imaging, MKs formed proplatelet processes and released proplatelet fragments that were originally defined as thin cytoplasmic extensions forming a tandem array of platelet-sized swellings with a beaded appearance at the distal end [29, 38–41]. In addition, MKs formed a "thick protrusion," released the cell fragments that preserve the abundant DMS and ER, and randomly organized microtubules; this implies that the fragments have not yet accomplished the intracellular remodeling that was seen in proplatelets. These data suggest that MKs have an ability to release contents of nascent platelets without proplatelet formation (Fig. 3e). Notably, this immature type of MK fragment release may be regulated by platelet demand.

Recently, Nishimura et al. reported rapid platelet release from the MK cytoplasm which they termed "MK rupture" [49]; in intravital images, this seems to represent platelet release as per both the PT model (Fig. 3b) and early proplatelet model (Fig. 3c); however, ultrastructural verification by TEM was not reported. MK rupture also seems to be associated with sinusoid vessel damage, because soon after this event, vascular tracer signals leaked into BM parenchyma. Interestingly, as the mechanism appears to be regulated by elevated levels of interleukin-1α, the authors proposed the importance of balance between TPO and interleukin-1α levels, which determines platelet production mechanism used by MKs.

2.4 Direct Stimulation of Proplatelet Formation

TPO stimulates MK precursors, but suppresses proplatelet formation from MKs in vitro [50–52]. In addition, TPO signaling in MKs is dispensable for platelet production in vivo [9, 10]. These findings indicate that other factors, including interleukin-1α, regulate platelet production from BM MKs. It has been reported that one of the direct regulators of platelet production via proplatelet formation is the thrombin/antithrombin complex included in high-density lipoprotein [53]. Notably, both thrombin and antithrombin are included in the coagulation cascade associated with platelet consumption. Recently, CCL5, a member of the interleukin-8 cytokine superfamily, may have a direct stimulatory effect on platelet production by MKs by inducing more rapid platelet production than that accomplished through steady-state regulation via TPO [54, 55].

3 Platelet Progenitors and Nascent Platelets

Detached cell fragments from MKs are heterogeneous population of cells in regard to their size, shape, or structure in the circulating blood. Large fragments are regarded as platelet progenitors which have the ability to convert into mature platelets. Platelet progenitors are described in terms of barbell-shaped proplatelets [42, 56, 57], preplatelets [56, 58], and giant platelets [48]. After leaving the BM sinusoids, these platelet progenitors may convert into individual platelets in the bloodstream, especially in microcapillaries in the lung, which is the first capillary bed to be encountered [56–59].

In summary, megakaryopoiesis depends on the proliferation and differentiation of HSCs to be committed to the MK lineage and their maturation to large MKs. These processes are regulated by many different factors including cytokines, chemokines, and BM microenvironments. Platelets are formed from MK cytoplasm via their protrusions and fragments into the vessel lumen. Although these processes are biologically complex phenomenon, it has been becoming clear how individual platelets are formed and eliminated in the vessel lumen by recent researches.

References

1. Akashi K, Traver D, Miyamoto T, Weissman IL. A clonogenic common myeloid progenitor that gives rise to all myeloid lineages. Nature. 2000;404(6774):193–7.
2. Debili N, Coulombel L, Croisille L, Katz A, Guichard J, Breton-Gorius J, Vainchenker W. Characterization of a bipotent erythro-megakaryocytic progenitor in human bone marrow. Blood. 1996;88(4):1284–96.
3. Manz MG, Miyamoto T, Akashi K, Weissman IL. Prospective isolation of human clonogenic common myeloid progenitors. Proc Natl Acad Sci U S A. 2002;99(18):11872–7.

4. Yamamoto R, Morita Y, Ooehara J, et al. Clonal analysis unveils self-renewing lineage-restricted progenitors generated directly from hematopoietic stem cells. Cell. 2013;154(5):1112–26.
5. Nishikii H, Kanazawa Y, Umemoto T, et al. Unipotent megakaryopoietic pathway bridging hematopoietic stem cells and mature megakaryocytes. Stem Cells. 2015;33(7):2196–207.
6. Woolthuis CM, Park CY. Hematopoietic stem/progenitor cell commitment to the megakaryocyte lineage. Blood. 2016;127(10):1242–8.
7. Kaushansky K. Determinants of platelet number and regulation of thrombopoiesis. Hematology Am Soc Hematol Educ Program. 2009:147–52.
8. Aster RH. Pooling of platelets in the spleen: role in the pathogenesis of "hypersplenic" thrombocytopenia. J Clin Invest. 1966;45:645–57.
9. Ng AP, Kauppi M, Metcalf D, Hyland CD, Josefsson EC, Lebois M, Zhang JG, Baldwin TM, Di Rago L, Hilton DJ, Alexander WS. Mpl expression on megakaryocytes and platelets is dispensable for thrombopoiesis but essential to prevent myeloproliferation. Proc Natl Acad Sci U S A. 2014;111(16):5884–9.
10. Meyer SC, Keller MD, Woods BA, LaFave LM, Bastian L, Kleppe M, Bhagwat N, Marubayashi S, Levine RL. Genetic studies reveal an unexpected negative regulatory role for Jak2 in thrombopoiesis. Blood. 2014;124(14):2280–4.
11. Shimada Y, Kato T, Ogami K, Horie K, Kokubo A, Kudo Y, Maeda E, Sohma Y, Akahori H, Kawamura K, et al. Production of thrombopoietin (TPO) by rat hepatocytes and hepatoma cell lines. Exp Hematol. 1995;23(13):1388–96.
12. Grozovsky R, Begonja AJ, Liu K, Visner G, Hartwig JH, Falet H, Hoffmeister KM. The Ashwell-Morell receptor regulates hepatic thrombopoietin production via JAK2-STAT3 signaling. Nat Med. 2015;21(1):47–54.
13. Kuvardina ON, Herglotz J, Kolodziej S, Kohrs N, Herkt S, Wojcik B, Oellerich T, Corso J, Behrens K, Kumar A, Hussong H, Urlaub H, Koch J, Serve H, Bonig H, Stocking C, Rieger MA, Lausen J. RUNX1 represses the erythroid gene expression program during megakaryocytic differentiation. Blood. 2015;125(23):3570–9.
14. Shivdasani RA, Fujiwara Y, McDevitt MA, Orkin SH. A lineage-selective knockout establishes the critical role of transcription factor GATA-1 in megakaryocyte growth and platelet development. EMBO J. 1997;16(13):3965–73.
15. Ichikawa M, Asai T, Saito T, Seo S, Yamazaki I, Yamagata T, Mitani K, Chiba S, Ogawa S, Kurokawa M, Hirai H. AML-1 is required for megakaryocytic maturation and lymphocytic differentiation, but not for maintenance of hematopoietic stem cells in adult hematopoiesis. Nat Med. 2004;10(3):299–304.
16. Hart A, Melet F, Grossfeld P, Chien K, Jones C, Tunnacliffe A, Favier R, Bernstein A. Fli-1 is required for murine vascular and megakaryocytic development and is hemizygously deleted in patients with thrombocytopenia. Immunity. 2000;13(2):167–77.
17. Takayama M, Fujita R, Suzuki M, Okuyama R, Aiba S, Motohashi H, Yamamoto M. Genetic analysis of hierarchical regulation for Gata1 and NF-E2 p45 gene expression in megakaryopoiesis. Mol Cell Biol. 2010;30(11):2668–80.
18. Shivdasani RA, Rosenblatt MF, Zucker-Franklin D, Jackson CW, Hunt P, Saris CJ, Orkin SH. Transcription factor NF-E2 is required for platelet formation independent of the actions of thrombopoietin/MGDF in megakaryocyte development. Cell. 1995;81(5):695–704.
19. Shavit JA, Motohashi H, Onodera K, Akasaka J, Yamamoto M, Engel JD. Impaired megakaryopoiesis and behavioral defects in mafG-null mutant mice. Genes Dev. 1998;12(14):2164–74.
20. Onodera K, Shavit JA, Motohashi H, Yamamoto M, Engel JD. Perinatal synthetic lethality and hematopoietic defects in compound mafG::mafK mutant mice. EMBO J. 2000;19(6):1335–45.
21. Lecine P, Italiano Jr JE, Kim SW, Villeval JL, Shivdasani RA. Hematopoietic-specific beta 1 tubulin participates in a pathway of platelet biogenesis dependent on the transcription factor NF-E2. Blood. 2000;96(4):1366–73.
22. Tiwari S, Italiano Jr JE, Barral DC, Mules EH, Novak EK, Swank RT, Seabra MC, Shivdasani RA. A role for Rab27b in NF-E2-dependent pathways of platelet formation. Blood. 2003;102(12):3970–9.

23. Fujita R, Takayama-Tsujimoto M, Satoh H, Gutiérrez L, Aburatani H, Fujii S, Sarai A, Bresnick EH, Yamamoto M, Motohashi H. NF-E2 p45 is important for establishing normal function of platelets. Mol Cell Biol. 2013;33(14):2659–70.
24. Lordier L, Jalil A, Aurade F, Larbret F, Larghero J, Debili N, Vainchenker W, Chang Y. Megakaryocyte endomitosis is a failure of late cytokinesis related to defects in the contractile ring and Rho/Rock signaling. Blood. 2008;112(8):3164–74.
25. Nagata Y, Muro Y, Todokoro K. Thrombopoietin-induced polyploidization of bone marrow megakaryocytes is due to a unique regulatory mechanism in late mitosis. J Cell Biol. 1997;139(2):449–57.
26. Raslova H, Roy L, Vourc'h C, Le Couedic JP, Brison O, Metivier D, Feunteun J, Kroemer G, Debili N, Vainchenker W. Megakaryocyte polyploidization is associated with a functional gene amplification. Blood. 2003;101(2):541–4.
27. Prendes MJ, Bielek E, Zechmeister-Machhart M, Vanyek-Zavadil E, Carroll VA, Breuss J, Binder BR, Geiger M. Synthesis and ultrastructural localization of protein C inhibitor in human platelets and megakaryocytes. Blood. 1999;94(4):1300–12.
28. Yamada E. The fine structure of the megakaryocyte in the mouse spleen. Acta Anat (Basel). 1957;29:267–90.
29. Radley JM, Haller CJ. The demarcation membrane system of the megakaryocyte: a misnomer? Blood. 1982;60:213–9.
30. Schulze H, Korpal M, Hurov J, et al. Characterization of the megakaryocyte demarcation membrane system and its role in thrombopoiesis. Blood. 2006;107:3868–75.
31. Avecilla ST, Hattori K, Heissig B, Tejada R, Liao F, Shido K, Jin DK, Dias S, Zhang F, Hartman TE, Hackett NR, Crystal RG, Witte L, Hicklin DJ, Bohlen P, Eaton D, Lyden D, de Sauvage F, Rafii S. Chemokine-mediated interaction of hematopoietic progenitors with the bone marrow vascular niche is required for thrombopoiesis. Nat Med. 2004;10(1):64–71.
32. Wright JH. Die Entstehung der Blutplättchen. Virchows Arch. 1906;186:55–63.
33. Behnke O. An electron microscope study of the rat megakaryocyte. II. Some aspects of platelet release and microtubules. J Ultrastruct Res. 1969;26:111–29.
34. Kosaki G. In vivo platelet production from mature megakaryocytes: does platelet release occur via proplatelets? Int J Hematol. 2005;81:208–19.
35. Caine YG, Vlodavsky I, Hersh M, Polliack A, Gurfel D, Or R, Levine RF, Eldor A. Adhesion, spreading and fragmentation of human megakaryocytes exposed to subendothelial extracellular matrix: a scanning electron microscopy study. Scan Electron Microsc. 1986;(Pt 3):1087–94.
36. Behnke O. Microtubules in disk-shaped blood cells. Int Rev Exp Pathol. 1970;9:1–92.
37. White JG, Rao GH. Microtubule coils versus the surface membrane cytoskeleton in maintenance and restoration of platelet discoid shape. Am J Pathol. 1998;152:597–609.
38. Becker RP, De Bruyn PP. The transmural passage of blood cells into myeloid sinusoids and the entry of platelets into the sinusoidal circulation; a scanning electron microscopic investigation. Am J Anat. 1976;145:183–205.
39. Muto M. A scanning and transmission electron microscopic study on rat bone marrow sinuses and transmural migration of blood cells. Arch Histol Jpn. 1976;39:51–66.
40. Radley JM, Scurfield G. The mechanism of platelet release. Blood. 1980;56:996–9.
41. Scurfield G, Radley JM. Aspects of platelet formation and release. Am J Hematol. 1981;10(3):285–96.
42. Italiano Jr JE, Lecine P, Shivdasani RA, et al. Blood platelets are assembled principally at the ends of proplatelet processes produced by differentiated megakaryocytes. J Cell Biol. 1999;147:1299–312.
43. Richardson JL, Shivdasani RA, Boers C, et al. Mechanisms of organelle transport and capture along proplatelets during platelet production. Blood. 2005;106:4066–75.
44. Patel SR, et al. Differential roles of microtubule assembly and sliding in proplatelet formation by megakaryocytes. Blood. 2005;106:4076–85.
45. Breton-Gorius J, Reyes F. Ultrastructure of human bone marrow cell maturation. Int Rev Cytol. 1976;46:251–321.

46. Lichtman MA, Chamberlain JK, Simon W, et al. The parasinusoidal location of megakaryocytes in marrow: a determinant of platelet release and a physiologic version of vascular invasion and metastasis. Trans Assoc Am Physicians. 1977;90:313–23.
47. Junt T, Schulze H, Chen Z, et al. Dynamic visualization of thrombopoiesis within bone marrow. Science. 2007;317:1767–70.
48. Kowata S, Isogai S, Murai K, Ito S, Tohyama K, Ema M, Hitomi J, Ishida Y. Platelet demand modulates the type of intravascular protrusion of megakaryocytes in bone marrow. Thromb Haemost. 2014;112(4):743–56.
49. Nishimura S, Nagasaki M, Kunishima S, Sawaguchi A, Sakata A, Sakaguchi H, Ohmori T, Manabe I, Italiano Jr JE, Ryu T, Takayama N, Komuro I, Kadowaki T, Eto K, Nagai R. IL-1α induces thrombopoiesis through megakaryocyte rupture in response to acute platelet needs. J Cell Biol. 2015;209(3):453–66.
50. Ishida Y, Ito T, Kuriya S. Effects of c-mpl ligand on cytoplasmic maturation of murine megakaryocytes and on platelet production. J Histochem Cytochem. 1998;46(1):49–57.
51. Ito T, Ishida Y, Kashiwagi R, Kuriya S. Recombinant human c-Mpl ligand is not a direct stimulator of proplatelet formation in mature human megakaryocytes. Br J Haematol. 1996;94(2):387–90.
52. Chang Y, Auradé F, Larbret F, Zhang Y, Le Couedic JP, Momeux L, Larghero J, Bertoglio J, Louache F, Cramer E, Vainchenker W, Debili N. Proplatelet formation is regulated by the Rho/ROCK pathway. Blood. 2007;109(10):4229–36.
53. Ishida Y, Yano K, Ito T, Shigematus H, Sasaki K, Kondo S, Kuriya S. Purification of proplatelet formation (PPF) stimulating factor: thrombin/antithrombin III complex stimulates PPF of megakaryocytes in vitro and platelet production in vivo. Thromb Haemost. 2001;85(2):349–55.
54. Tamura S, Suzuki-Inoue K, Tsukiji N, Shirai T, Sasaki T, Osada M, Satoh K, Ozaki Y. Podoplanin-positive periarteriolar stromal cells promote megakaryocyte growth and proplatelet formation in mice by CLEC-2. Blood. 2016;127(13):1701–10.
55. Machlus KR, Johnson KE, Kulenthirarajan R, Forward JA, Tippy MD, Soussou TS, El-Husayni SH, Wu SK, Wang S, Watnick RS, Italiano Jr JE, Battinelli EM. CCL5 derived from platelets increases megakaryocyte proplatelet formation. Blood. 2016;127(7):921–6.
56. Thon JN, Montalvo A, Patel-Hett S, et al. Cytoskeletal mechanics of proplatelet maturation and platelet release. J Cell Biol. 2010;191:861–74.
57. Handagama PJ, Feldman BF, Jain NC, et al. Circulating proplatelets: isolation and quantitation in healthy rats and in rats with induced acute blood loss. Am J Vet Res. 1987;48:962–5.
58. Thon JN, Macleod H, Begonja AJ, et al. Microtubule and cortical forces determine platelet size during vascular platelet production. Nat Commun. 2012;3:852.
59. Zucker-Franklin D, Philipp CS. Platelet production in the pulmonary capillary bed: new ultrastructural evidence for an old concept. Am J Pathol. 2000;157:69–74.

Platelet Membrane Glycoproteins

Hisashi Kato and Yoshiaki Tomiyama

Abstract Platelets are small anucleate blood cells that are produced in the bone marrow from the cytoplasm of megakaryocytes. Circulating platelets are essential for primary hemostasis and also involved in pathological thrombosis. For the platelet hemostatic functions, platelet surface membrane glycoproteins are crucial to form platelet-subendothelial matrix and platelet-platelet interactions. At the site of blood vessel injury, platelets are captured by platelet GPIb-IX-V interaction with von Willebrand factor which bound to exposed collagen followed by direct platelet-collagen interaction by GPIa-IIa (integrin α2β1) and GPVI. Platelet fibrinogen receptor GPIIb-IIIa (integrin αIIbβ3) is the most abundant glycoprotein on platelet surface, and its affinity for fibrinogen is tightly regulated by inside-out signaling. The platelet-platelet interaction mediated by activated GPIIb-IIIa is necessary for platelet accumulation on the layer of adhered platelets at the injured vessel. Both quantitative and qualitative abnormalities in these platelet glycoproteins can be a cause of platelet dysfunctions and bleeding disorders. In addition, platelet glycoproteins are also important in the pathogenesis of idiopathic thrombocytopenic purpura (ITP). In the majority of patients with ITP, antiplatelet autoantibodies in plasma are directed against platelet glycoproteins especially GPIIb-IIIa and GPIb-IX-V.

1 Introduction

Platelet membrane glycoproteins are key receptors for platelet-subendothelial matrix and platelet-platelet interaction during thrombus formation. Among several different receptor families in platelet glycoproteins (integrins, leucine-rich glycoproteins, immunoglobulin cell adhesion molecules, and selectins), three major

---

H. Kato (✉)
Department of Hematology and Oncology, Osaka University Graduate School of Medicine, 2-2 Yamadaoka, Suita, Osaka 565-0871, Japan
e-mail: hisashi@hp-blood.med.osaka-u.ac.jp

Y. Tomiyama
Department of Blood Transfusion, Osaka University Hospital, 2-15 Yamadaoka, Suita, Osaka 565-0871, Japan
e-mail: yoshi@hp-blood.med.osaka-u.ac.jp

Y. Ishida, Y. Tomiyama (eds.), *Autoimmune Thrombocytopenia*,
DOI 10.1007/978-981-10-4142-6_3

Table 1 Platelet membrane receptors

	Ligand	Functions	Copies/platelet
Integrins			
αIIbβ3 (GPIIb-IIIa)	Fibrinogen	Aggregation, adhesion	~80,000
α2β1 (GPIa-IIa)	Collagen	Adhesion	3000–5000
α5β1 (VLA-5)	Fibronectin	Adhesion	1000
α6β1 (VLA-6)	Laminin	Adhesion	1000
αvβ3	Vitronectin	Adhesion	100
Leucine-rich glycoproteins			
GPIb-IX	von Willebrand factor	Adhesion	25,000
GPV			12,500
Immunoglobulin cell adhesion molecules			
GPVI	Collagen	Adhesion, activation	4000–6000
PECAM-1 (CD31)	PECAM-1	Adhesion	8000
Fcg-RII (CD32)		Immune complex binding	~1000
Selectins			
P-selectin (CD62P)	PSGL-1	Platelet-leukocyte adhesion	20,000
Miscellaneous			
GPIV (CD36)	Collagen, thrombospondin, oxidized LDL		20,000
CLEC-2	Podoplanin	Adhesion/activation	

platelet glycoproteins, GPI, II, and III, were identified in the 1970s by electrophoretic procedure. Subsequently, advances in protein separation techniques and its application to the studies on inherited platelet dysfunctional disorders such as Glanzmann thrombasthenia and Bernard-Soulier syndrome made a great contribution for understanding the role of platelet glycoproteins. Several major platelet membrane receptors and their ligands are summarized in Table 1, and some of these glycoproteins are known to be a target of autoantibody which appeared in patients with autoimmune thrombocytopenia (ITP). This chapter will describe the structure and function of glycoproteins expressed in platelet surfaces.

At the site of blood vessel injury, platelet glycoproteins mediate a series of platelet reactions: rolling, tethering, adhesion, and aggregation (Fig. 1). First, circulating platelets form indirect interaction with vessel wall through von Willebrand factor (VWF). Plasma VWF bound to exposed collagen forms a transient bridge between collagen and platelet GPIb. During platelet rolling and tethering on collagen, additional direct collagen-platelet interactions are induced via platelet-collagen receptors GPIa-IIa (integrin α2β1) and GPVI for firm adhesion. Collagen-bound GPVI initiates intracellular signaling leading to cytoskeletal rearrangement, calcium mobilization, and granule release. In addition to ADP and thromboxane A2 (TXA2) released from activated platelets, thrombin generated by the coagulation cascade stimulates platelets as a secondary agonist for further activation. These secondary agonists act through G protein-coupled receptors and induce "inside-out signaling" for fibrinogen receptor GPIIb-IIIa (integrin αIIbβ3) activation which cross-links platelets and leads to platelet aggregation (primary hemostasis).

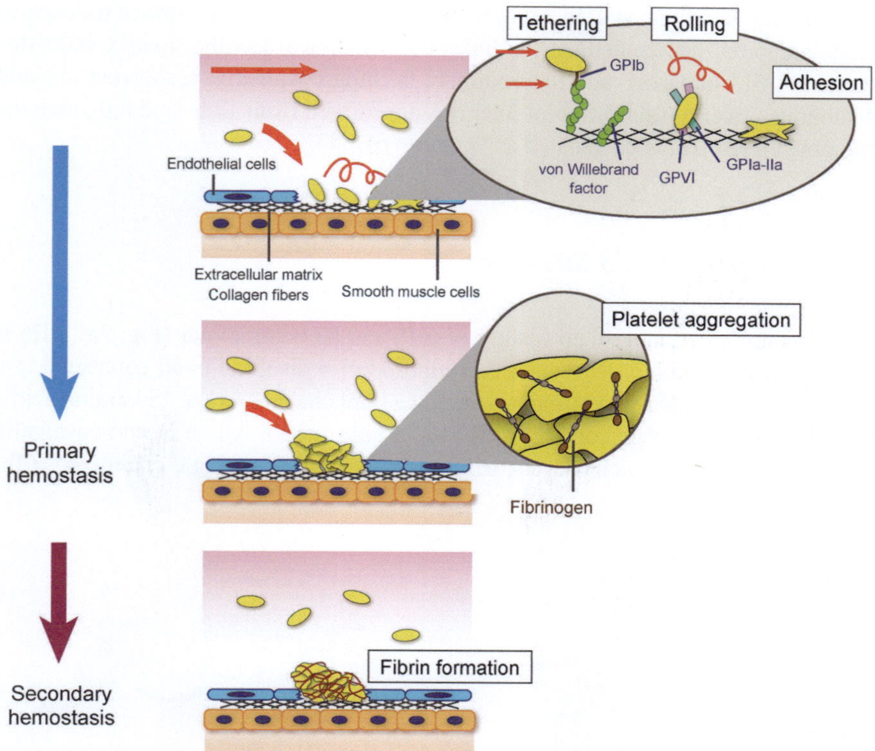

Fig. 1 Primary and secondary hemostasis. At the site of vascular injury, von Willebrand factor mediates transient and indirect interaction of circulating platelets with exposed subendothelial collagen. During platelet rolling on collagen, platelet-collagen receptors, GPVI and GPIa-IIa, form stable direct interaction with collagen followed by firm platelet adhesion. Platelets are activated by thrombin, ADP, and thromboxane A2, and activated GPIIb-IIIa (integrin αIIbβ3) by inside-out signaling forms aggregation via fibrinogen binding (primary hemostasis). In secondary hemostasis, fibrin which is produced by coagulation cascade stabilizes the thrombus formed in primary hemostasis

Following platelet aggregation, insoluble fibrin, which is generated by the coagulation cascade, incorporates into platelet aggregation and stabilizes the platelet aggregation (secondary hemostasis).

2 GPIIb-IIIa (Integrin αIIbβ3)

The fibrinogen receptor GPIIb-IIIa is the major platelet surface glycoprotein which expression is restricted to platelets and megakaryocytes [1]. Each platelet expresses about 80,000 copies of GPIIb-IIIa on their surface [2], and the indispensable role of GPIIb-IIIa for platelet aggregation and hemostasis has been established from the studies of Glanzmann thrombasthenia (GT). GT was first reported in 1918 from a series of patients with an inherited bleeding disorder, and polyacrylamide gel electrophoresis revealed that GPIIb and GPIIIa are deficient in platelets of GT [3, 4].

In 1986, Tamkun et al. started using the word "integrin" for cell surface transmembrane receptors which mediate the linkage between extracellular matrix and cytoskeleton [5]. Integrins are heterodimers of non-covalently associated α- and β-subunits. Twenty-four different integrins are formed from 18 α- and 8 β-subunits, and now GPIIb-IIIa is designated as "integrin αIIbβ3."

2.1 *Integrin αIIbβ3 Structure*

αIIbβ3 is a typical integrin consisting of αIIb and β3 heterodimer (Fig. 2a). αIIb is a 140 kDa glycoprotein [6] which is composed of a disulfide bond connected to a heavy chain (114 kDa, 871 amino acids) and a light chain (23 kDa, 137 amino acids) [7]. β3 is a 116 kDa glycoprotein [8] (762 amino acids), which is non-covalently linked to αIIb. In megakaryocytes, αIIb is synthesized as a single chain (pro-αIIb)

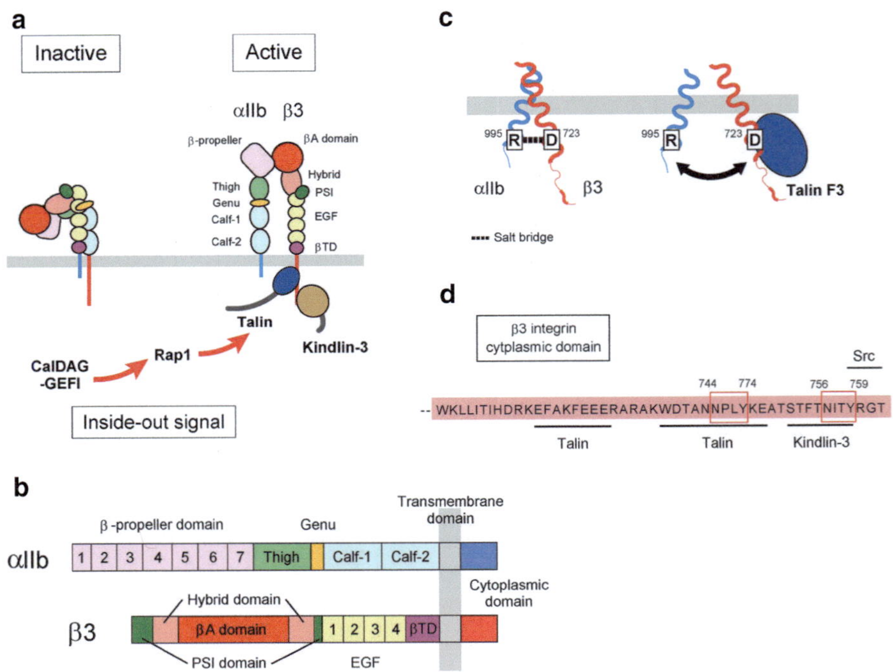

Fig. 2 The structure and inside-out activation of integrin αIIβ3. (**a**, **b**) The domain structure and conformational change of integrin αIIβ3. When αIIbβ3 is in a low-affinity inactive state, αIIbβ3 extracellular domain is in bent conformation. However, once αIIbβ3 is activated by inside-out signaling, talin and kindling-3 interaction with β3 cytoplasmic tail induces conformational change of extracellular domain of αIIbβ3 resulting in extended conformation. (**c**) Disruption of salt bridge in cytoplasmic domain of αIIbβ3 by talin binding. In inactive state αIIbβ3, the salt bridge formed between R995 of αIIb and D723 of β3 is important to keep αIIbβ3 inactive. Inside-out signaling which induced binding of talin head domain to β3 cytoplasmic tail disrupts the salt bridge and induces conformational change of αIIbβ3. (**d**) The binding site of talin, kindlin-3, and Src in β3 cytoplasmic domain

and associates with β3 in the endoplasmic reticulum. The pro-αIIb/β3 complex is transported to the Golgi apparatus, and the proteolytic cleavage of pro-αIIb/β3 yields the mature αIIbβ3. The extracellular domain of αIIb is composed of a seven-bladed β-propeller domain containing ligand-binding sites, thigh domain, calf-1 domain, and calf-2 domain. β3 is composed of βA domain containing ligand-binding sites, plexin/semaphorin/integrin (PSI) domain, hybrid domain, four epidermal growth factor (EGF) repeats, and membrane proximal β-tail domain (βTD) (Fig. 2b). By stable non-covalent association, αIIbβ3 forms an 8 × 12 nm globular head which contains ligand-binding site with 18 nm two rodlike flexible tails [9]. Following the studies of αvβ3 [10, 11], X-ray crystallography revealed the bent conformation of αIIbβ3 [12]. This bent conformation is achieved by the flexibility at the "genu" located between the thigh and calf-1 domain in αIIb and EGF1 and EGF2 in β3. In bent conformation, the ligand-binding face at the globular head is not exposed, and the natural ligands, such as fibrinogen, are not allowed to interact with αIIbβ3. Upon activation, αIIbβ3 can rapidly change its conformation from bent to extended form which is high affinity for fibrinogen (Fig. 2c). Following the short single-spanning transmembrane region, both αIIb- and β3-subunits have short cytoplasmic tail which is important for conformational change of αIIbβ3 (Fig. 2d). In the membrane proximal region, arginine (R) and aspartic acid (D) in the conserved αIIb-GFFKR and β3-HDRKE sequence form a salt bridge. This salt bridge maintains αIIbβ3 in low-affinity inactive state, and αIIbβ3 becomes constitutively active by disruption of the salt bridge [13–16]. Even integrin cytoplasmic domain has no enzymatic or actin-binding activity, and the molecule interactions with cytoplasmic region induce signals for platelet activation [17, 18]. Especially two well-conserved NPXY motifs in β3 tail, NPLY (744–747) and NITY (756–759), are essential for talin and kindling-3 binding, respectively [19]. The last three amino acid residues of β3 is the important binding site for c-Src [20–23].

2.2 *αIIbβ3 Inside-Out Signaling*

The affinity and conformation of αIIbβ3 are tightly regulated by inside-out signaling [24, 25]. Although the precise molecular mechanism of inside-out signaling remains unknown, the direct interaction of talin with β3 cytoplasmic tail is essential at the final step of inside-out αIIbβ3 activation [26–30]. Talin is a 250 kDa actin-binding protein which is composed of a 50 kDa head domain and a 220 kDa rod domain. The N-terminal head domain contains a FERM (band four-point one, ezrin, radixin, and moesin) domain which is further divided into F1, F2, and F3 subdomains [31]. Talin F3 interaction with β3 cytoplasmic first NPXY motif (744–747) [28] disrupts the αIIb-R995/β3-D723 slat bridge followed by the conformational change for αIIbβ3 activation. In genetically modified mice with impaired talin/β3 interaction or talin deficiency, agonist-induced inside-out αIIbβ3 activation is strongly impaired resulting in bleeding diathesis [32–35]. Another FERM domain containing protein kindlin-3 is also essential for αIIbβ3 activation, and deficiency of kindlin-3 is associated with bleeding tendency [36, 37]. In contrast to talin, kindlin-3 F3 domain binds to the membrane-distal second NPXY motif (756–759) [38–40]. Although both talin and kindlin-3 are required for inside-out αIIbβ3 activation, kindlin-3 alone is insufficient for αIIbβ3 activation [41, 42], and probably kindlin-3 cooperates with talin by increasing the avidity of αIIbβ3 [43, 44]. Although no patient with mutation in talin has been reported, mutation in kindling-3 is known to be a cause of leukocyte adhesion deficiency (LAD)-III [45]. In LAD-III, impaired integrin activation in platelets and leukocytes causes bleeding problem and immune defect.

A Ras family member small GTPase Rap1 [46, 47] and calcium- and diacylglycerol-regulated guanine exchange factor-1 (CalDAG-GEFI) [48–51] are the critical molecules at the upstream signaling of talin/β3 interaction. CalDAG-GEFI activates Rap1 by facilitating the release of bound GDP, and activated GTP-bound Rap1 recruits talin to β3 cytoplasmic tail followed by αIIbβ3 activation [52]. Recently, CalDAG-GEFI-deficient patients [53, 54] or a patient expressing CalDAG-GEFI with loss-of-function mutation which causes severe bleeding problems was reported [55].

2.3 *Clinical Importance of αIIbβ3*

GT is an autosomal recessive inherited bleeding disorder due to a quantitative and a qualitative defect in αIIbβ3 [56]. The impaired fibrinogen binding to αIIbβ3 leads to bleeding symptoms such as purpura, petechiae, easy bruising, mucocutaneous bleeding, and excessive bleeding after injury or surgical procedure [57]. In platelet aggregation assay, aggregation response is absent in response to ADP, thrombin, collagen, or arachidonic acid in platelets of patient with typical GT [58]. However, ristocetin-induced aggregation response is induced normally. Flow cytometric analysis of agonist-induced αIIbβ3 activation by binding of activated αIIbβ3-specific monoclonal antibody PAC-1 [59] and molecular genetic analysis [60, 61] of αIIb and β3 is the key to diagnosis. Based on the expression levels of αIIbβ3, GT is classified into three types. The most severe type I platelets express <5%, and type II express 5–20% αIIbβ3 of normal levels. In type III, variant type, platelets express >20% of αIIbβ3. However, expressed αIIbβ3 is functionally impaired and does not support platelet aggregation. Currently, besides platelet transfusion, there is no specific treatment for GT, and the bleeding in GT patients is managed by antifibrinolytic therapy and platelet transfusion, and recombinant activated factor VII is performed [57, 62–64]. In future therapeutic strategy, gene therapy is expected to be a curative treatment for patients with GT [65–67].

3 GPIb-IX-V

Glycoprotein GPIb-IX-V complex is exclusively expressed on platelets and megakaryocytes and an essential receptor for the first step of hemostasis. This essential role of GPIb-IX-V is exemplified by the rare inherited bleeding disorder

Bernard-Soulier syndrome (BSS) which was first reported and described by Jean Bernard and Jean Pierre Soulier in 1948. The acrylamide gel electrophoresis clearly showed the absence of GPIb band in platelets of BSS patient in the 1970s [68]. The clarification that additional two glycoproteins GPV and GPIX are missing in BSS platelets [69] and the cloning of GPIbα [70], GPIbβ [71], GPIX [72], and GPV [11, 12] achieved further develops on the role of GPIb-IX-V.

3.1 GPIb-IX-V Structure

GPIb-IX-V complex (Fig. 3) is the second most abundant platelet glycoprotein (25,000 copies per platelet [73]) next to fibrinogen receptor GPIIb-IIIa. GPIb-IX-V complex consists of four different type I transmembrane subunits, GPIbα (CD42b; 135kDa, 610 amino acids), GPIbβ (CD42c; 26kDa, 181 amino acids), GPIX (20 kDa, 160 amino acids), and GPV (82 kDa, 560 amino acids), with a stoichiometry of 2:2:2:1. Each subunit belongs to the leucine-rich repeat (LRR) protein family which is known to be involved in protein-protein interactions. LRR is the protein structure motif composed of 20–30 amino acid sequences, and the tandem repeat of LRR motifs folds into a horseshoe shape. GPIbα is the largest subunit of the complex, and the N-terminal membrane-distal 282 residues which are composed of seven LRRs are the binding site for VWF. VWF binding region is followed by acidic residue-rich sequence containing sulfated tyrosine, a heavily O-glycosylated macroglycopeptide domain, and stalk region. The extracellular domain is connected to a single transmembrane region and cytoplasmic tail. Both GPIbβ and GPIX are relatively smaller subunits which have a single LRR in the extracellular domain. In contrast to the high sequence similarity of extracellular domain between GPIbβ and GPIX, the short GPIX cytoplasmic tail consisting of five amino acids is different from that of GPIbβ (34 amino acids).

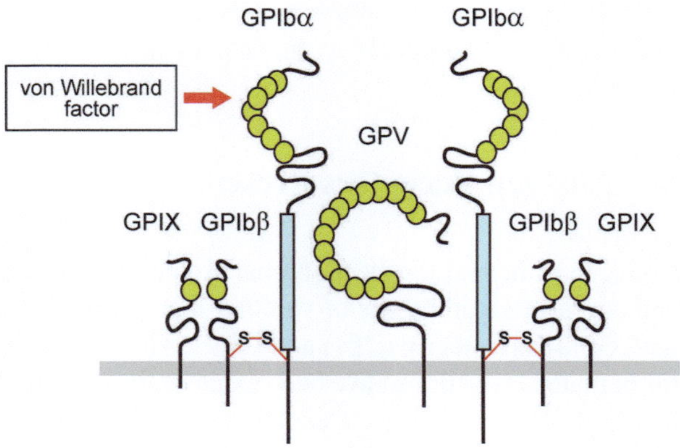

Fig. 3 Schematic representation of the GPIb-IX-V complex. GPIbα, GPIbβ, GPIX, and GPV form GPIb-IX-V complex at a stoichiometry of 2:2:2:1. The N-terminal of GPIbα contains binding sites for von Willebrand factor

3.2 GPIb-IX-V Function

The primary function of GPIb-IX-V is mediating initial platelet attachment to the blood vessel wall by interacting with VWF bound on exposed subendothelial collagen. The synthesized VWF in endothelial cells is stored in Weibel-Palade bodies or secreted into plasma. VWF circulates in plasma as multimer in various sizes ranging from 500 kDa to over 10,000 kDa. The platelet-binding potential of VWF with GPIbα is dependent on the multimer size and conformation of VWF which are regulated by metalloproteinase ADAMTS13 [74] and fluid shear stress [75], respectively. The deficient ADAMTS13 activity results in circulating the unusually large VWF multimers and causes thrombotic thrombocytopenic purpura (TTP) [76, 77]. Although the signaling pathway mediated by GPIb-IX-V for platelet activation remains unclear, VWF/GPIb-IX-V mediated a signaling pathway for platelet activation in which Src family kinase and glycolipid-enriched microdomains (GEMs) are involved [78].

3.3 Clinical Importance of GPIb-IX-V

Bernard-Soulier syndrome (BSS) is a rare autosomal recessive disease due to the genetic defects in *GPIBA*, *GPIBB*, and *GP9* [79, 80] and characterized by bleeding tendency, giant platelets, and low platelet counts (macrothrombocytopenia) [81]. Due to the impaired VWF-mediated initial platelet interaction with exposed collagen, patients show variety of bleeding symptoms from early childhood. Although most mutations in BSS are associated with decreased surface expression or loss of function of GPIb-IX-V, platelet-type von Willebrand disease (VWD), an autosomal dominant disorder, results in gain-of-function phenotype [82–84]. In patients with platelet-type VWD, an excessive spontaneous VWF/GPIb interaction which accelerates the clearance of plasma VWF leads to the bleeding tendency. For the diagnosis of BSS, an isolated defect in ristocetin-induced platelet aggregation is the characteristic abnormality. Flow cytometric analysis of the surface expression levels of GPIb-IX-V, platelet counts, and examination of blood smear to determine large platelets are also important to confirm diagnosis.

4 Collagen Receptors Present on Platelets

Collagen is the major subendothelial protein which is essential for platelet adhesion and aggregation at the site of vascular injury. Platelets express two collagen receptors, GPIa-IIa (integrin α2β1) and GPVI. Although the roles of each collagen receptor in platelet functions have been extensively studied, the respective roles of GPVI and GPIa-IIa are still not clear. However, GPVI is believed as a central platelet-collagen receptor [85, 86], and GPIa-IIa is considered as a secondary collagen receptor to support platelet firm adhesion on collagen.

4.1 Introduction of GPVI

GPVI was first identified as a 62 kDa platelet protein recognized by autoantibody from the patient with idiopathic thrombocytopenic purpura (ITP) suffering from recurrent bleeding problem regardless of normal platelet count with corticosteroid treatment [87]. The patient's platelets exhibited defective aggregation to collagen, and the 62 kDa protein was later identified as GPVI [88]. GPVI expression is restricted to platelets and megakaryocytes [89, 90] with varying GPVI expression levels [91–93].

4.2 GPVI Structure and Signaling Pathway

GPVI was cloned in 2000 and identified as a type I transmembrane glycoprotein which belongs to the immunoglobulin (Ig) superfamily [89] (Fig. 4). GPVI (62 kDa, 319 amino acids) is expressed at 4000–6000 copies per platelets as a complex with

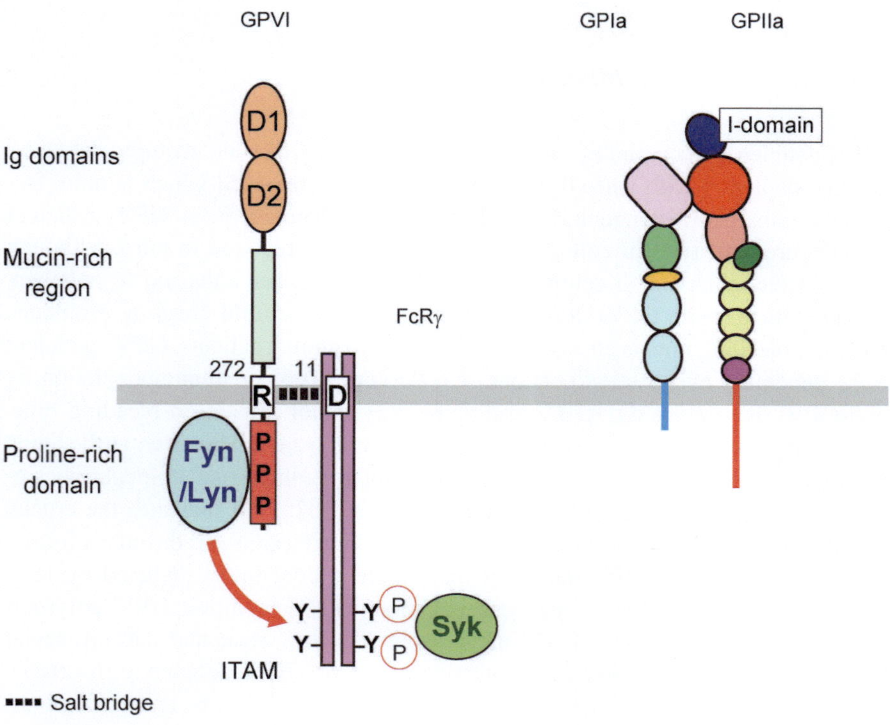

Fig. 4 Collagen receptor GPVI and GPIa-IIa. GPVI consists of two Ig domains followed by mucin-rich region in its extracellular domain. The R272 in transmembrane domain is important to form salt bridge with FcRγ chain. The binding of Src family kinase Fyn and Lyn phosphorylates the tyrosine in ITAM in cytoplasmic domain of FcRγ chain which leads to the Syk interaction and downstream signaling cascade. The extracellular domain of GPIIa has I-domain which is important for ligand binding

FcRγ subunit [94, 95]. GPVI has two Ig-like domains (D1 and D2) and a highly O-glycosylated mucin-rich stalk region in its extracellular domain. A 19-amino acid transmembrane domain is critical for linking to FcRγ subunit by salt bridge between GPVI Arg272 and Asp11 of FcRγ. A 51-amino acid cytoplasmic tail contains a calmodulin-binding basic motif, and constitutive calmodulin binding protects GPVI from shedding in resting platelets [96]. Upon platelet activation, calmodulin dissociation from GPVI leads to the cleavage of GPVI by metalloproteinase which results in decrease of GPVI expression probably to control platelet reactivity. The circulating 55 kDa GPVI ectodomain fragment could be a marker for platelet activation state. Proline-rich domain in cytoplasmic domain provides binding site for Src family kinase, Fyn and Lyn, which are critical for downstream signaling events through FcRγ chain [23]. Following the phosphorylation of immunoreceptor tyrosine-based activation motif (ITAM) in FcRγ by Fyn and Lyn, the recruited tyrosine kinase Syk forms a signaling complex with adaptor proteins (SLP-67 and LAT) and phospholipase Cγ2 (PLCγ2) which leads to calcium mobilization, integrin activation, and granule release for further platelet activation [78, 97, 98].

4.3 *Clinical Importance of GPVI*

GPVI deficiency is caused by congenital mutation [99–102] and acquired defect by immunodepletion with anti-GPVI autoantibody [87, 103–105] which is more frequent compared to congenital GPVI deficiency. Platelets from GPVI-deficient patients are defective for collagen-induced platelet aggregation in vitro. Although GPVI is recognized as a central receptor for firm platelet adhesion to collagen, human patients with GPVI deficiency usually have only mild bleeding problems, and their bleeding time is almost normal. Similar to human patients, GPVI-deficient mice generated by genetic knockout of *GP6* gene [106] or immunodepletion by anti-GPVI antibody JAQ1 [107] also show only minor impact on bleeding time, suggesting that GPVI is not essential for normal hemostasis. However, in the lethal thromboembolism model by intravenous injection of collagen and epinephrine, significantly higher survival of GPVI-deficient mice [107, 108] indicates the crucial role of GPVI in arterial thrombosis. In fact, platelet adhesion and thrombus formation were reduced in GPVI-deficient mice after arterial injury induced by laser [109], $FeCl_3$ [109, 110], wire, and vessel ligation [111]. In addition, GPVI polymorphisms in healthy subjects [112] are associated with stroke and cardiovascular events [113–117], and now the protective effect of GPVI deficiency in arterial thrombosis, not in normal hemostasis, suggests that GPVI may be an attractive target for antithrombotic therapies [118, 119].

4.4 *GPIa-IIa (Integrin α2β1)*

GPIa-IIa, which is now also designated as very late antigen-2 (VLA-2) [120] or integrin α2β1, was first recognized as a platelet-collagen receptor from the patient with bleeding problem in 1985 [121]. Following the cloning of GPIa [122] and GPIIa [123], the studies revealed the supportive role of GPIa-IIa in platelet adhesion on collagen.

GPIa-IIa, integrin α2β1, is a member of integrin family and consists of non-covalently associated α2 and β1 integrin, and platelets express 3000–5000 copies of GPIa-IIa per platelet. The extracellular domain of α2 integrin has 220 amino acid insertions, called I-domain, in the N-terminal β-propeller region. The sequence of I-domain is homologous to the collagen binding region of other proteins such as VWF and critical for α2β1 interaction with collagen types I, II, IV, and XI [124, 125].

4.5 *GPIa-IIa Function and Clinical Importance*

In patients with decreased GPIa, platelets are not responsive to collagen stimulation in aggregation study [121]. The affinity of GPIa-IIa for collagen is regulated by inside-out signaling, and agonist stimulation increases the binding of collagen to GPIa-IIa [126–128]. In contrast to GPIa-IIa, another platelet-collagen receptor GPVI does not need to be pre-activated for collagen interaction, and GPVI-collagen interaction induces intracellular signals for GPIa-IIa activation [86]. The number of GPIa-IIa on platelets is related to platelet response to collagen in normal population [129]. As shown in GPIa polymorphism C807T [130], GPIa polymorphism is associated with the expression levels of GPIa-IIa, and the linkage between GPIa-IIa expression levels [115] and polymorphism with thrombotic event [131, 132] is reported, suggesting the importance of GPIa-IIa in clinical outcomes. In experimental thrombus formation in vivo, the thrombus formed in the carotid artery by laser injury was significantly decreased in GPIa-IIa-deficient mice [133, 134].

5 Conclusions

Platelets are involved in both normal hemostasis and pathological thrombosis such as myocardial infarction and ischemic stroke. Platelet membrane glycoproteins are essential as adhesion molecules for platelet functions to communicate with the blood vessel wall and other cells. Starting from the analysis of patients with bleeding symptoms, the technical development and the application of genetically modified mice revealed the role of membrane glycoproteins in the process of thrombus formation. Further elucidation of the detail of platelet functions is expected from the recent genomic and proteomic techniques.

References

1. Coller BS, Shattil SJ. The GPIIb/IIIa (integrin alphaIIbbeta3) odyssey: a technology-driven saga of a receptor with twists, turns, and even a bend. Blood. 2008;112:3011–25.
2. Wagner CL, et al. Analysis of GPIIb/IIIa receptor number by quantification of 7E3 binding to human platelets. Blood. 1996;88:907–14.
3. Nurden AT, Caen JP. An abnormal platelet glycoprotein pattern in three cases of Glanzmann's thrombasthenia. Br J Haematol. 1974;28:253–60.
4. Phillips DR, Agin PP. Platelet membrane defects in Glanzmann's thrombasthenia. Evidence for decreased amounts of two major glycoproteins. J Clin Invest. 1977;60:535–45.
5. Tamkun JW, et al. Structure of integrin, a glycoprotein involved in the transmembrane linkage between fibronectin and actin. Cell. 1986;46:271–82.
6. Poncz M, et al. Structure of the platelet membrane glycoprotein IIb. Homology to the alpha subunits of the vitronectin and fibronectin membrane receptors. J Biol Chem. 1987;262: 8476–82.
7. Kolodziej MA, Vilaire G, Gonder D, Poncz M, Bennett JS. Study of the endoproteolytic cleavage of platelet glycoprotein IIb using oligonucleotide-mediated mutagenesis. J Biol Chem. 1991;266:23499–504.
8. Fitzgerald LA, Steiner B, Rall Jr SC, Lo SS, Phillips DR. Protein sequence of endothelial glycoprotein IIIa derived from a cDNA clone. Identity with platelet glycoprotein IIIa and similarity to "integrin". J Biol Chem. 1987;262:3936–9.
9. Weisel JW, Nagaswami C, Vilaire G, Bennett JS. Examination of the platelet membrane glycoprotein IIb-IIIa complex and its interaction with fibrinogen and other ligands by electron microscopy. J Biol Chem. 1992;267:16637–43.
10. Xiong JP, et al. Crystal structure of the extracellular segment of integrin alpha Vbeta3. Science. 2001;294:339–45.
11. Xiong JP, et al. Crystal structure of the extracellular segment of integrin alpha Vbeta3 in complex with an Arg-Gly-Asp ligand. Science. 2002;296:151–5.
12. Xiao T, Takagi J, Coller BS, Wang JH, Springer TA. Structural basis for allostery in integrins and binding to fibrinogen-mimetic therapeutics. Nature. 2004;432:59–67.
13. Hughes PE, et al. Breaking the integrin hinge. A defined structural constraint regulates integrin signaling. J Biol Chem. 1996;271:6571–4.
14. Kunishima S, et al. Heterozygous ITGA2B R995W mutation inducing constitutive activation of the alphaIIbbeta3 receptor affects proplatelet formation and causes congenital macrothrombocytopenia. Blood. 2011;117:5479–84.
15. Peyruchaud O, et al. R to Q amino acid substitution in the GFFKR sequence of the cytoplasmic domain of the integrin IIb subunit in a patient with a Glanzmann's thrombasthenia-like syndrome. Blood. 1998;92:4178–87.
16. Weljie AM, Hwang PM, Vogel HJ. Solution structures of the cytoplasmic tail complex from platelet integrin alpha IIb- and beta 3-subunits. Proc Natl Acad Sci U S A. 2002;99:5878–83.
17. Legate KR, Fassler R. Mechanisms that regulate adaptor binding to beta-integrin cytoplasmic tails. J Cell Sci. 2009;122:187–98.

18. Zou ZY, Chen H, Schmaier AA, Hynes RO, Kahn ML. Structure-function analysis reveals discrete beta 3 integrin inside-out and outside-in signaling pathways in platelets. Blood. 2007;109:3284–90.
19. Calderwood DA, Campbell ID, Critchley DR. Talins and kindlins: partners in integrin-mediated adhesion. Nat Rev Mol Cell Biol. 2013;14:503–17.
20. Arias-Salgado EG, et al. Src kinase activation by direct interaction with the integrin beta cytoplasmic domain. Proc Natl Acad Sci U S A. 2003;100:13298–302.
21. Shattil SJ. Integrins and Src: dynamic duo of adhesion signaling. Trends Cell Biol. 2005;15:399–403.
22. Ablooglu AJ, Kang J, Petrich BG, Ginsberg MH, Shattil SJ. Antithrombotic effects of targeting alphaIIbbeta3 signaling in platelets. Blood. 2009;113:3585–92.
23. Senis YA, Mazharian A, Mori J. Src family kinases: at the forefront of platelet activation. Blood. 2014;124:2013–24.
24. Kim C, Ye F, Ginsberg MH. Regulation of integrin activation. Annu Rev Cell Dev Biol. 2011;27:321–45.
25. Luo BH, Springer TA. Integrin structures and conformational signaling. Curr Opin Cell Biol. 2006;18:579–86.
26. Tadokoro S, et al. Talin binding to integrin beta tails: a final common step in integrin activation. Science. 2003;302:103–6.
27. Calderwood DA, et al. The Talin head domain binds to integrin beta subunit cytoplasmic tails and regulates integrin activation. J Biol Chem. 1999;274:28071–4.
28. Wegener KL, et al. Structural basis of integrin activation by talin. Cell. 2007;128:171–82.
29. Anthis NJ, Campbell ID. The tail of integrin activation. Trends Biochem Sci. 2011;36:191–8.
30. Shattil SJ, Kim C, Ginsberg MH. The final steps of integrin activation: the end game. Nature reviews. Mol Cell Biol. 2010;11:288–300.
31. Critchley DR, Gingras AR. Talin at a glance. J Cell Sci. 2008;121:1345–7.
32. Petrich BG, et al. The antithrombotic potential of selective blockade of talin-dependent integrin alpha IIb beta 3 (platelet GPIIb-IIIa) activation. J Clin Invest. 2007;117:2250–9.
33. Stefanini L, et al. A talin mutant that impairs talin-integrin binding in platelets decelerates alphaIIbbeta3 activation without pathological bleeding. Blood. 2014;123:2722–31.
34. Nieswandt B, et al. Loss of talin1 in platelets abrogates integrin activation, platelet aggregation, and thrombus formation in vitro and in vivo. J Exp Med. 2007;204:3113–8.
35. Petrich BG, et al. Talin is required for integrin-mediated platelet function in hemostasis and thrombosis. J Exp Med. 2007;204:3103–11.
36. Malinin NL, et al. A point mutation in KINDLIN3 ablates activation of three integrin subfamilies in humans. Nat Med. 2009;15:313–8.
37. Moser M, Nieswandt B, Ussar S, Pozgajova M, Fassler R. Kindlin-3 is essential for integrin activation and platelet aggregation. Nat Med. 2008;14:325–30.
38. Karakose E, Schiller HB, Fassler R. The kindlins at a glance. J Cell Sci. 2010;123:2353–6.
39. Rognoni E, Ruppert R, Fassler R. The kindlin family: functions, signaling properties and implications for human disease. J Cell Sci. 2016;129:17–27.
40. Moser M, Legate KR, Zent R, Fassler R. The tail of integrins, talin, and kindlins. Science. 2009;324:895–9.
41. Harburger DS, Bouaouina M, Calderwood DA. Kindlin-1 and -2 directly bind the C-terminal region of beta integrin cytoplasmic tails and exert integrin-specific activation effects. J Biol Chem. 2009;284:11485–97.
42. Nakazawa T, et al. Agonist stimulation, talin-1, and kindlin-3 are crucial for alpha(IIb)beta(3) activation in a human megakaryoblastic cell line, CMK. Exp Hematol. 2013;41:79–90.e71.
43. Ye F, et al. The mechanism of kindlin-mediated activation of integrin alphaIIbbeta3. Curr Biol. 2013;23:2288–95.
44. Ye F, Petrich BG. Kindlin: helper, co-activator, or booster of talin in integrin activation? Curr Opin Hematol. 2011;18:356–60.

45. Svensson L, et al. Leukocyte adhesion deficiency-III is caused by mutations in KINDLIN3 affecting integrin activation. Nat Med. 2009;15:306–12.
46. Fischer TH, Gatling MN, Lacal JC, White II GC. rap1B, a cAMP-dependent protein kinase substrate, associates with the platelet cytoskeleton. J Biol Chem. 1990;265:19405–8.
47. Bertoni A, et al. Relationships between Rap1b, affinity modulation of integrin alpha IIbbeta 3, and the actin cytoskeleton. J Biol Chem. 2002;277:25715–21.
48. Stefanini L, Bergmeier W. CalDAG-GEFI and platelet activation. Platelets. 2010;21:239–43.
49. Kawasaki H, et al. A Rap guanine nucleotide exchange factor enriched highly in the basal ganglia. Proc Natl Acad Sci U S A. 1998;95:13278–83.
50. Eto K, et al. Megakaryocytes derived from embryonic stem cells implicate CalDAG-GEFI in integrin signaling. Proc Natl Acad Sci U S A. 2002;99:12819–24.
51. Crittenden JR, et al. CalDAG-GEFI integrates signaling for platelet aggregation and thrombus formation. Nat Med. 2004;10:982–6.
52. Chrzanowska-Wodnicka M, Smyth SS, Schoenwaelder SM, Fischer TH, White II GC. Rap1b is required for normal platelet function and hemostasis in mice. J Clin Invest. 2005;115:680–7.
53. Kato H, et al. Human CalDAG-GEFI deficiency confers severe bleeding tendency and delayed alphaIIbbeta3 activation velocity. Blood. 2016;128:2729–33.
54. Lozano ML, et al. Novel mutations in RASGRP2, which encodes CalDAG-GEFI, abrogate Rap1 activation, causing platelet dysfunction. Blood. 2016;128:1282–9.
55. Canault M, et al. Human CalDAG-GEFI gene (RASGRP2) mutation affects platelet function and causes severe bleeding. J Exp Med. 2014;211:1349–62.
56. Bellucci S, Caen J. Molecular basis of Glanzmann's Thrombasthenia and current strategies in treatment. Blood Rev. 2002;16:193–202.
57. Borhany M, Fatima H, Naz A, Patel H, Shamsi T. Pattern of bleeding and response to therapy in Glanzmann thrombasthenia. Haemophilia. 2012;18:e423–5.
58. Larrieu MJ, et al. Congenital bleeding disorders with long bleeding time and normal platelet count. II. Von Willebrand's disease (report of thirty-seven patients). Am J Med. 1968;45:354–72.
59. Shattil SJ, Hoxie JA, Cunningham M, Brass LF. Changes in the platelet membrane glycoprotein IIb.IIIa complex during platelet activation. J Biol Chem. 1985;260:11107–14.
60. Nurden AT. Glanzmann thrombasthenia. Orphanet J Rare Dis. 2006;1:10.
61. Nurden AT, Fiore M, Nurden P, Pillois X. Glanzmann thrombasthenia: a review of ITGA2B and ITGB3 defects with emphasis on variants, phenotypic variability, and mouse models. Blood. 2011;118:5996–6005.
62. Poon MC, Demers C, Jobin F, Wu JW. Recombinant factor VIIa is effective for bleeding and surgery in patients with Glanzmann thrombasthenia. Blood. 1999;94:3951–3.
63. Poon MC, et al. The international, prospective Glanzmann Thrombasthenia Registry: treatment and outcomes in surgical intervention. Haematologica. 2015;100:1038–44.
64. Di Minno G, et al. The international, prospective Glanzmann Thrombasthenia Registry: treatment modalities and outcomes of non-surgical bleeding episodes in patients with Glanzmann thrombasthenia. Haematologica. 2015;100:1031–7.
65. Nurden AT, Pillois X, Wilcox DA. Glanzmann thrombasthenia: state of the art and future directions. Semin Thromb Hemost. 2013;39:642–55.
66. Sullivan SK, et al. High-level transgene expression in induced pluripotent stem cell-derived megakaryocytes: correction of Glanzmann thrombasthenia. Blood. 2014;123:753–7.
67. Fang J, et al. Platelet gene therapy improves hemostatic function for integrin alphaIIbbeta3-deficient dogs. Proc Natl Acad Sci U S A. 2011;108:9583–8.
68. Nurden AT, Caen JP. Specific roles for platelet surface glycoproteins in platelet function. Nature. 1975;255:720–2.
69. Jenkins CS, et al. Platelet membrane glycoproteins implicated in ristocetin-induced aggregation. Studies of the proteins on platelets from patients with Bernard-Soulier syndrome and von Willebrand's disease. J Clin Invest. 1976;57:112–24.

70. Lopez JA, et al. Cloning of the alpha chain of human platelet glycoprotein Ib: a transmembrane protein with homology to leucine-rich alpha 2-glycoprotein. Proc Natl Acad Sci U S A. 1987;84:5615–9.
71. Lopez JA, et al. The alpha and beta chains of human platelet glycoprotein Ib are both transmembrane proteins containing a leucine-rich amino acid sequence. Proc Natl Acad Sci U S A. 1988;85:2135–9.
72. Hickey MJ, Williams SA, Roth GJ. Human platelet glycoprotein IX: an adhesive prototype of leucine-rich glycoproteins with flank-center-flank structures. Proc Natl Acad Sci U S A. 1989;86:6773–7.
73. Coller BS, Peerschke EI, Scudder LE, Sullivan CA. Studies with a murine monoclonal antibody that abolishes ristocetin-induced binding of von Willebrand factor to platelets: additional evidence in support of GPIb as a platelet receptor for von Willebrand factor. Blood. 1983;61:99–110.
74. Budde U, Schneppenheim R. Interactions of von Willebrand factor and ADAMTS13 in von Willebrand disease and thrombotic thrombocytopenic purpura. Hamostaseologie. 2014;34:215–25.
75. Schneider SW, et al. Shear-induced unfolding triggers adhesion of von Willebrand factor fibers. Proc Natl Acad Sci U S A. 2007;104:7899–903.
76. Sadler JE. Von Willebrand factor, ADAMTS13, and thrombotic thrombocytopenic purpura. Blood. 2008;112:11–8.
77. Zheng XL. ADAMTS13 and von Willebrand factor in thrombotic thrombocytopenic purpura. Annu Rev Med. 2015;66:211–25.
78. Ozaki Y, Suzuki-Inoue K, Inoue O. Platelet receptors activated via mulitmerization: glycoprotein VI, GPIb-IX-V, and CLEC-2. J Thromb Haemost. 2013;11(Suppl 1):330–9.
79. de la Salle C, Lanza F, Cazenave JP. Biochemical and molecular basis of Bernard-Soulier syndrome: a review. Nouv Rev Fr Hematol. 1995;37:215–22.
80. Berndt MC, Andrews RK. Bernard-Soulier syndrome. Haematologica. 2011;96:355–9.
81. Lopez JA, Andrews RK, Afshar-Kharghan V, Berndt MC. Bernard-Soulier syndrome. Blood. 1998;91:4397–418.
82. Woods AI, et al. Identification of p.W246L as a novel mutation in the GP1BA gene responsible for platelet-type von Willebrand disease. Semin Thromb Hemost. 2014;40:151–60.
83. Miller JL, Cunningham D, Lyle VA, Finch CN. Mutation in the gene encoding the alpha chain of platelet glycoprotein Ib in platelet-type von Willebrand disease. Proc Natl Acad Sci U S A. 1991;88:4761–5.
84. Ng C, Motto DG, Di Paola J. Diagnostic approach to von Willebrand disease. Blood. 2015;125:2029–37.
85. Moroi M, Jung SM. Platelet glycoprotein VI: its structure and function. Thromb Res. 2004;114:221–33.
86. Nieswandt B, Watson SP. Platelet-collagen interaction: is GPVI the central receptor? Blood. 2003;102:449–61.
87. Sugiyama T, et al. A novel platelet aggregating factor found in a patient with defective collagen-induced platelet aggregation and autoimmune thrombocytopenia. Blood. 1987;69:1712–20.
88. Moroi M, Jung SM, Okuma M, Shinmyozu K. A patient with platelets deficient in glycoprotein VI that lack both collagen-induced aggregation and adhesion. J Clin Invest. 1989;84:1440–5.
89. Jandrot-Perrus M, et al. Cloning, characterization, and functional studies of human and mouse glycoprotein VI: a platelet-specific collagen receptor from the immunoglobulin superfamily. Blood. 2000;96:1798–807.
90. Berlanga O, et al. Expression of the collagen receptor glycoprotein VI during megakaryocyte differentiation. Blood. 2000;96:2740–5.
91. Furihata K, Clemetson KJ, Deguchi H, Kunicki TJ. Variation in human platelet glycoprotein VI content modulates glycoprotein VI-specific prothrombinase activity. Arterioscler Thromb Vasc Biol. 2001;21:1857–63.

92. Chen H, Locke D, Liu Y, Liu C, Kahn ML. The platelet receptor GPVI mediates both adhesion and signaling responses to collagen in a receptor density-dependent fashion. J Biol Chem. 2002;277:3011–9.
93. Best D, et al. GPVI levels in platelets: relationship to platelet function at high shear. Blood. 2003;102:2811–8.
94. Tsuji M, Ezumi Y, Arai M, Takayama H. A novel association of Fc receptor gamma-chain with glycoprotein VI and their co-expression as a collagen receptor in human platelets. J Biol Chem. 1997;272:23528–31.
95. Schulte V, et al. Targeting of the collagen-binding site on glycoprotein VI is not essential for in vivo depletion of the receptor. Blood. 2003;101:3948–52.
96. Gardiner EE, Arthur JF, Kahn ML, Berndt MC, Andrews RK. Regulation of platelet membrane levels of glycoprotein VI by a platelet-derived metalloproteinase. Blood. 2004;104:3611–7.
97. Schmaier AA, et al. Molecular priming of Lyn by GPVI enables an immune receptor to adopt a hemostatic role. Proc Natl Acad Sci U S A. 2009;106:21167–72.
98. Bergmeier W, Stefanini L. Platelet ITAM signaling. Curr Opin Hematol. 2013;20:445–50.
99. Arthur JF, Dunkley S, Andrews RK. Platelet glycoprotein VI-related clinical defects. Br J Haematol. 2007;139:363–72.
100. Dumont B, et al. Absence of collagen-induced platelet activation caused by compound heterozygous GPVI mutations. Blood. 2009;114:1900–3.
101. Hermans C, et al. A compound heterozygous mutation in glycoprotein VI in a patient with a bleeding disorder. J Thromb Haemost. 2009;7:1356–63.
102. Matus V, et al. An adenine insertion in exon 6 of human GP6 generates a truncated protein associated with a bleeding disorder in four Chilean families. J Thromb Haemost. 2013;11:1751–9.
103. Boylan B, et al. Anti-GPVI-associated ITP: an acquired platelet disorder caused by autoantibody-mediated clearance of the GPVI/FcRgamma-chain complex from the human platelet surface. Blood. 2004;104:1350–5.
104. Akiyama M, et al. Presence of platelet-associated anti-glycoprotein (GP)VI autoantibodies and restoration of GPVI expression in patients with GPVI deficiency. J Thrombo Haemost. 2009;7:1373–83.
105. Gardiner EE, et al. Compromised ITAM-based platelet receptor function in a patient with immune thrombocytopenic purpura. J Thromb Haemost. 2008;6:1175–82.
106. Kato K, et al. The contribution of glycoprotein VI to stable platelet adhesion and thrombus formation illustrated by targeted gene deletion. Blood. 2003;102:1701–7.
107. Nieswandt B, et al. Long-term antithrombotic protection by in vivo depletion of platelet glycoprotein VI in mice. J Exp Med. 2001;193:459–69.
108. Lockyer S, et al. GPVI-deficient mice lack collagen responses and are protected against experimentally induced pulmonary thromboembolism. Thromb Res. 2006;118:371–80.
109. Bender M, Hagedorn I, Nieswandt B. Genetic and antibody-induced glycoprotein VI deficiency equally protects mice from mechanically and FeCl(3) -induced thrombosis. J Thromb Haemost. 2011;9:1423–6.
110. Konstantinides S, et al. Distinct antithrombotic consequences of platelet glycoprotein Ibalpha and VI deficiency in a mouse model of arterial thrombosis. J Thromb Haemost. 2006;4:2014–21.
111. Massberg S, et al. A crucial role of glycoprotein VI for platelet recruitment to the injured arterial wall in vivo. J Exp Med. 2003;197:41–9.
112. Croft SA, et al. Novel platelet membrane glycoprotein VI dimorphism is a risk factor for myocardial infarction. Circulation. 2001;104:1459–63.
113. Bigalke B, et al. Expression of platelet glycoprotein VI is associated with transient ischemic attack and stroke. Eur J Neurol. 2010;17:111–7.
114. Al-Tamimi M, et al. Soluble glycoprotein VI is raised in the plasma of patients with acute ischemic stroke. Stroke. 2011;42:498–500.

115. Samaha FF, et al. Density of platelet collagen receptors glycoprotein VI and alpha-2beta1 and prior myocardial infarction in human subjects, a pilot study. Med Sci Monit. 2005;11:CR224–9.
116. Cabeza N, et al. Surface expression of collagen receptor Fc receptor-gamma/glycoprotein VI is enhanced on platelets in type 2 diabetes and mediates release of CD40 ligand and activation of endothelial cells. Diabetes. 2004;53:2117–21.
117. Takagi S, et al. A GPVI polymorphism is a risk factor for myocardial infarction in Japanese. Atherosclerosis. 2002;165:397–8.
118. Dutting S, Bender M, Nieswandt B. Platelet GPVI: a target for antithrombotic therapy?! Trends Pharmacol Sci. 2012;33:583–90.
119. Induruwa I, Jung SM, Warburton EA. Beyond antiplatelets: the role of glycoprotein VI in ischemic stroke. Int J Stroke. 2016;11:618–25.
120. Kunicki TJ, et al. The human fibroblast class II extracellular matrix receptor mediates platelet adhesion to collagen and is identical to the platelet glycoprotein Ia-IIa complex. J Biol Chem. 1988;263:4516–9.
121. Nieuwenhuis HK, Akkerman JW, Houdijk WP, Sixma JJ. Human blood platelets showing no response to collagen fail to express surface glycoprotein Ia. Nature. 1985;318:470–2.
122. Argraves WS, et al. Amino acid sequence of the human fibronectin receptor. J Cell Biol. 1987;105:1183–90.
123. Takada Y, Hemler ME. The primary structure of the VLA-2/collagen receptor alpha 2 subunit (platelet GPIa): homology to other integrins and the presence of a possible collagen-binding domain. J Cell Biol. 1989;109:397–407.
124. Tuckwell DS, Reid KB, Barnes MJ, Humphries MJ. The A-domain of integrin alpha 2 binds specifically to a range of collagens but is not a general receptor for the collagenous motif. Eur J Biochem. 1996;241:732–9.
125. Tuckwell D, Calderwood DA, Green LJ, Humphries MJ. Integrin alpha 2 I-domain is a binding site for collagens. J Cell Sci. 1995;108(Pt 4):1629–37.
126. Jung SM, Moroi M. Platelets interact with soluble and insoluble collagens through characteristically different reactions. J Biol Chem. 1998;273:14827–37.
127. Jung SM, Moroi M. Activation of the platelet collagen receptor integrin alpha(2)beta(1): its mechanism and participation in the physiological functions of platelets. Trends Cardiovasc Med. 2000;10:285–92.
128. Jung SM, Moroi M. Signal-transducing mechanisms involved in activation of the platelet collagen receptor integrin alpha(2)beta(1). J Biol Chem. 2000;275:8016–26.
129. Kunicki TJ, Orchekowski R, Annis D, Honda Y. Variability of integrin alpha 2 beta 1 activity on human platelets. Blood. 1993;82:2693–703.
130. Corral J, Rivera J, Gonzalez-Conejero R, Vicente V. The number of platelet glycoprotein Ia molecules is associated with the genetically linked 807 C/T and HPA-5 polymorphisms. Transfusion. 1999;39:372–8.
131. Carlsson LE, Santoso S, Spitzer C, Kessler C, Greinacher A. The alpha2 gene coding sequence T807/A873 of the platelet collagen receptor integrin alpha2beta1 might be a genetic risk factor for the development of stroke in younger patients. Blood. 1999;93:3583–6.
132. Moshfegh K, et al. Association of two silent polymorphisms of platelet glycoprotein Ia/IIa receptor with risk of myocardial infarction: a case-control study. Lancet. 1999;353:351–4.
133. He L, et al. The contributions of the alpha 2 beta 1 integrin to vascular thrombosis in vivo. Blood. 2003;102:3652–7.
134. Marjoram RJ, et al. alpha2beta1 integrin, GPVI receptor, and common FcRgamma chain on mouse platelets mediate distinct responses to collagen in models of thrombosis. PLoS One. 2014;9:e114035.

Part III
Epidemiology

Epidemiology

Takaaki Hato and Yoshiyuki Kurata

Abstract ITP is estimated to have incidence between 2.16 and 3.9 per 100,000 person-years. There is a 1.1 to 1.5:1 female to male predominance in the entire ITP patients although ITP was more frequent among males in the age groups less than 5 years and over 75 years old. Intracranial hemorrhage (ICH) is the most devastating bleeding event, and its incidence is 0.37–0.6%. In contrast, recent studies suggest that ITP may have paradoxically an increased risk for thromboembolism. Regarding the treatment of ITP, the rate of splenectomy has been dramatically decreased to only 6% in recent years because patients are increasingly reluctant to undergo splenectomy and new drugs including anti-CD20 monoclonal antibody and thrombopoietin receptor agonists have been developed. Besides the bleeding risk, the infection risk derived from immunosuppressive treatment should be emphasized because bleeding and infection equally contributed to the death of ITP patients.

1 Introduction

Epidemiology is important to identify the cause of disease and health problems. The pathogenesis of ITP remains to be determined although a much greater understanding of immunopathology of ITP has developed. The diagnosis of ITP is still made by excluding other causes of thrombocytopenia, and the disease burden lowers patients' quality of life in spite of a basically benign clinical course. Under these conditions, epidemiological data of ITP would contribute to implementing proper clinical practices and providing effective health care for ITP patients. This chapter will discuss the epidemiology of ITP including the incidence, age distribution, symptoms, treatment, complications, and prognosis. A recent issue regarding thromboembolic events in ITP patients will be also discussed.

T. Hato (✉)
Division of Blood Transfusion and Cell Therapy, Ehime University Hospital, Toon, Ehime 791-0295, Japan
e-mail: takahato@m.ehime-u.ac.jp

Y. Kurata
Shitennoji Hidenin Special Nursing Home for the Aged, 6-1-1 Gakuenmae, Habikino, Osaka 583-0868, Japan
e-mail: kuratayk@gmail.com

Y. Ishida, Y. Tomiyama (eds.), *Autoimmune Thrombocytopenia*,
DOI 10.1007/978-981-10-4142-6_4

2 Incidence and Prevalence

The incidence of ITP has been estimated since several decades ago. The older studies were underpowered to obtain the reliable results because the number of ITP patients surveyed was below 1000 (range, 26–840) [1]. More recent studies surveyed over 1000 patients (range, 1145–7774) from nationwide large database [2–4]. In the United Kingdom, a total of 1145 incident ITP patients were identified from population-based general practice research database (GPRD), and the reported incidence was 3.9 (95% confidence interval [CI], 3.7–4.1) per 100,000 person-years [2]. In France, 3771 incident ITP patients were identified from a nationwide database of the French National Health Insurance System, and the reported incidence was 2.92/100,000 person-years (95% CI, 2.83–3.01) [4]. In Japan, 7774 incident ITP patients were identified from the nationwide ITP registry database of the Ministry of Health, Labour and Welfare of Japan, and the reported incidence was 2.16/100.000 person-years [3]. The variation of incidence among these studies is likely to depend on differences in the diagnostic criteria of ITP, validation of excluding other causes of thrombocytopenia including secondary ITP, characteristics of patients registered to database, and completeness of database. No ethnic disparity among ITP patients is demonstrated. The current evidence indicates that ITP is estimated to have an incidence between 2.16 and 3.9 per 100,000 person-years.

The prevalence of ITP has been also investigated in several studies, and three large studies have been recently reported. In Maryland, USA, 1169 ITP patients were identified from the Medical Care Data Base of the Maryland Health Care Commission, and the age-adjusted prevalence of ITP was 9.5 (95% CI, 8.5–10) per 100,000 persons [5]. This study only included patients under 65 years old. In another study in the United States, 4943 patients with all age groups were identified from the integrated information system database, one of the largest US health-care-managed database, and the reported prevalence was 20.3 (95% CI, 20.1–20.4) per 100,000 persons [6]. In a UK study with GPRD, 3073 patients aged 18 and over were identified, and the reported prevalence was 50.29 (95% CI, 48.51–52.06) per 100,000 persons [7]. From these studies, it is considered that the robust estimates of prevalence of ITP range from 20.3 to 50.29 per 100,000 persons.

3 Age and Gender

Epidemiologic studies in the United Kingdom, France, and Japan have shown that there is a 1.1 to 1.5:1 female to male predominance in the entire ITP patients [2–4]. However, all studies revealed that ITP was more frequent among males in the age groups less than 5 years and over 75 years old. In female patients, the age-specific distribution of ITP patients had a trimodal distribution, with the first peak observed below 4 years, the second among those aged 20–34 years (childbearing age), and the

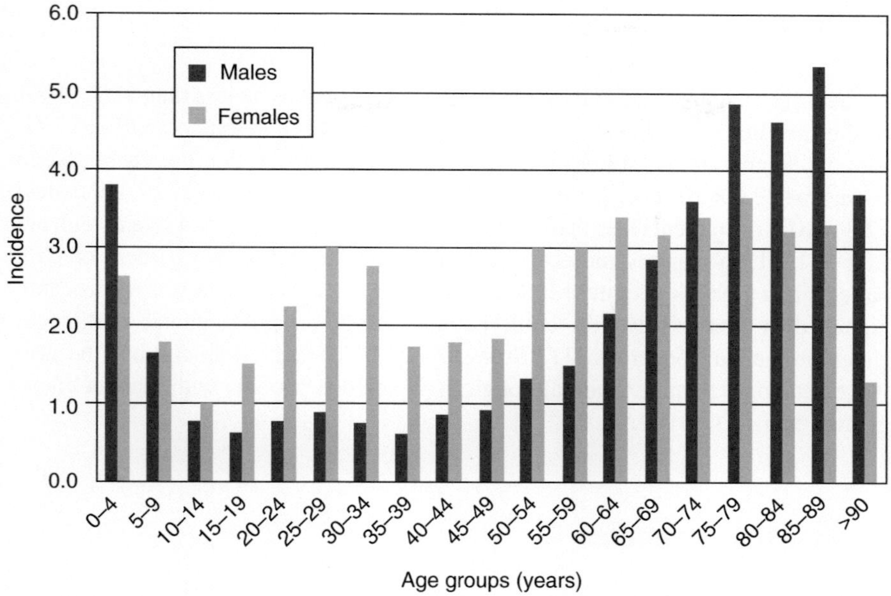

Fig. 1 Age- and gender-specific incidence of ITP per 100,000 population (Adapted from the study by Kurata et al. [3])

third peak among aged over 50 years (Fig. 1). The maximum ratio of female to male was observed in patients aged 20–34 years. The preponderance of females at this childbearing age may include a bias toward an increased opportunity of measurement of platelet count during visits to gynecologists, especially during pregnancy, resulting in fortuitous discovery of thrombocytopenia leading to diagnosis of ITP.

The natural history of ITP is different between children and adult in that childhood ITP takes an acute, self-limited course, whereas the majority of adult ITP progresses to chronic disease [8]. A recent French study showed that 35.7% of childhood ITP became persistent or chronic, whereas 66.7% of adult ITP was persistent or chronic with a mean follow-up of 17.6 ± 6.7 months (range, 6–30 months) [4]. The majority of childhood ITP has been associated with viral infections, suggesting a seasonal variation in incidence. In children, two-thirds of the ITP patients experience flu-like fever during the weeks preceding ITP onset [9]. One study identified an increased incidence of childhood ITP in winter [4], whereas another study found an increased incidence in summer [10]. Additionally, in adult ITP, the peak incidence was reported to be in winter, and infant patients aged 0–1 years, who were most susceptible to viral infections, had a peak incidence in spring [4].

Possible association of ITP with vaccination, especially with MMR immunization, has been debated [11–13]. MMR immunization was associated with an increased risk of ITP; however, a risk-benefit balance of MMR immunization should be considered because immunization-associated ITP is mild, self-limited, and rarer than natural measles or rubella infection-associated ITP [13]. Further studies are necessary to clarify the association of viral infection and immunization with pathogenesis of ITP.

4 Platelet Counts

An international group of ITP defined the platelet count to be less than 100 × 10^9/L as the threshold for diagnosis [14]. A nationwide study in Japan analyzed 7774 patients diagnosed according to this threshold and reported that the mean platelet count was 22.0 × 10^9/L in the total ITP patients (23.7 in females and 19.3 in males), 12.8 × 10^9/L in patients less than 15 years old, 27.2 × 10^9/L at 15–49 years old, and 21.1 × 10^9/L in patients more than 50 years old [3]. Sixty-two percent of child patients had a platelet count of less than 10 × 10^9/L. This percent was significantly higher than that (41.2%) in adult patients. Both an international multicenter (Intercontinental Cooperative ITP Study Group, ICIS) and UK studies had the similar results to a Japanese study although they included patients with platelet counts greater than 100 × 10^9/L [2, 15, 16].

5 Bleeding Symptoms

The most common bleeding symptom of ITP is purpura [3, 16]. Purpura and epistaxis occur more frequently in children than in adults (Table 1). Gastrointestinal bleeding is much less common: 1.11 and 3.9% of entire ITP patients in France and Japan, respectively [3, 4]. There was no significant difference in the frequency of gastrointestinal bleeding between child and adult ITP [3]. However, among adult ITP, there was a linear increasing relation between age and gastrointestinal bleeding [4]. Intracranial hemorrhage (ICH) is the most devastating bleeding event, and its incidence is 0.37–0.6% [3, 4]. Adult patients have more frequent ICH than children, and the older patients, especially over 60 years old, have an exponential increase in ICH. The role of risk factors for adult ICH including hypertension and diabetes mellitus in the onset of ICH remains to be determined. In child ICH, an epidemiologic

Table 1 Hemorrhagic symptoms of child and adult ITP

Bleeding symptoms	Number of cases (%)			p-value (child vs. adult)
	Overall (7774 cases)	Child (929 cases)	Adult (6845 cases)	
Purpura	5160 (66.4)	860 (92.6)	4300 (62.8)	$p < 0.001$
Gingival bleeding	1540 (19.8)	175 (18.8)	1365 (19.9)	ns
Epistaxis	963 (12.4)	276 (29.7)	687 (10.0)	$p < 0.001$
Hematuria	507 (6.5)	54 (5.8)	453 (6.6)	ns
Melena	302 (3.9)	43 (4.6)	259 (3.8)	ns
Hypermenorrhea	275 (3.5)	11 (1.2)	264 (3.9)	$p < 0.001$
Cerebral bleeding	46 (0.6)	1 (0.1)	45 (0.7)	$p < 0.05$
Other bleeding	268 (3.4)	54 (5.8)	214 (3.1)	$p < 0.001$

ns not significant
Adapted from the study by Kurata et al. [3]

study in the United States with a nationwide survey of childhood ITP with ICH showed that the estimated incidence of ICH was 0.19–0.78% and that platelet counts were less than 20×10^9/L in 90% and less than 10×10^9/L in 75% of children with ICH [17]. The ICIS study also reported the similar relationship between platelet counts and ICH in both child and adult patients [16]. However, the US study has revealed that severe thrombocytopenia was not sufficient for child ICH, but head trauma and bleeding symptoms beyond purpura, especially hematuria, were linked to ICH [17]. Such epidemiologic findings may be useful for selection of ITP patients with high risk of ICH.

6 Thrombotic Symptoms

Until recently, thrombosis was not considered as a part of ITP manifestations. Recent several studies suggest that ITP may have paradoxically an increased risk for thromboembolism. A US study with 3131 ITP patients from a database of US health insurance reported that the adjusted incidence rate ratio (IRR) of any vascular, venous, and arterial thromboembolism as compared with the age- and gender-matched reference cohort was 1.70 (95% CI, 1.41–2.05), 2.89 (95% CI, 1.33–6.29), and 1.58 (95% CI, 1.29–1.94), respectively [18]. A Danish population-based study with 391 adult patients from the Danish National Patients Registry showed that the IRR of venous thrombosis as compared with the reference cohort was 2.65 (95% CI, 1.27–5.50) [19]. Another Danish population study with 379 patients showed that the IRR of arterial thrombosis was 1.32 (95% CI, 0.88–1.98), indicating no significant difference [20]. A UK study with 1070 patients from GPRD also reported no significant difference in the IRR of arterial thrombosis, but significantly increased IRR of venous thrombosis [21]. A recent Scandinavian population-based cohort study with 1821 adult patients found that the occurrence of both arterial and venous thromboembolism increased with age and increasing comorbidity burden [22]. Splenectomized ITP patients had the increased risk of both arterial and venous thrombosis compared with non-splenectomized patients with hazard ratios of 3.2 (95% CI, 1.2–8.6) and 4.1 (95% CI, 1.1–15.7), respectively, with an overall hazard ratio of thrombosis in splenectomized of 3.5 (95% CI, 1.6–7.6) [23]. For ages >60 years, more than two classical risk factors for thrombosis at diagnosis and steroid use were independently associated with an increased risk of thrombosis. No independent investigations have explored the thrombotic risk associated with thrombopoietin receptor agonists although several clinical trials showed a certain rate of thrombotic events in ITP patients who received thrombopoietin receptor agonists [24]. This rate did not increase over time. Taken together, there seems to be a slight increase in venous thrombosis in chronic ITP, except for splenectomized and elderly patients [23, 24]. Although such thrombophilia may not be worthy to demand clinical intervention [23], the stratification of a high-risk group would be of value in the establishment of thrombosis-associated subgroup of ITP and choice of treatment.

7 Treatment

The treatment strategy differs between child and adult ITP patients. In child ITP, the most common prescription is intravenous immunoglobulin [3, 16]. This is likely because high-dose immunoglobulin therapy results in a more rapid increase in platelet counts than other therapies when it is administered for management of bleeding symptoms at the acute onset of child ITP. In adult ITP, the most common prescription is corticosteroid that is recommended as a first-line therapy for adult ITP by the international consensus report and the American Society of Hematology guideline [8, 25]. The eradication of *Helicobacter pylori* in adult patients is performed more frequently in Japan than in western countries [3]. The rate of splenectomy was 29% of adult patients in the clinical practice of two decades ago [26], and it has been dramatically decreased to only 6% in recent years [2, 27], because patients are increasingly reluctant to undergo splenectomy and new drugs including anti-CD20 monoclonal antibody and thrombopoietin receptor agonists have been developed [28]. The frequency of each treatment will be altered over time, and an epidemiologic approach to thrombopoietin receptor agonists will have a considerable impact on the management and the burden of this disease.

8 Prognosis

The previous population-based cohort studies have found a significantly increased risk of bleeding, infection, and hematologic malignancies in patients with chronic ITP than in the age- and gender-matched general population [2, 26, 29]. In a Danish population-based study, the adjusted 5-year relative ratio (RR) was 3.2 (95% CI, 1.2–9.0) for ICH and 4.4 (95% CI, 2.3–8.3) for other hospitalized hemorrhage [29]. In a recent French study, 30% of patients hospitalized for ICH and 8% for gastrointestinal bleeding died [27]. Besides the bleeding risk, the infection risk should be emphasized. In a retrospective study of 152 ITP patients with a mean follow-up period of 10.5 years, bleeding and infection equally contributed to the death of the patients [30]. This finding is in accordance with the results of the UK study with GPRD in which death was related to bleeding in 13% and infection in 19% of ITP patients whom the cause of death was specified in the registry record [2]. Immunosuppressive treatment for ITP is likely to be responsible for severe infection, suggesting serious consideration of risk assessment of the treatment strategies for ITP. The increase in hematologic malignancies among ITP patients may be due to misdiagnosis with ITP during the initial stage of hematologic malignancy because ITP is a diagnosis of exclusion. The hazard ratio of all-cause mortality was 1.5 (95% CI, 1.2–1.8) to 2.3 (95% CI, 1.8–3.0) for ITP patients compared with the age- and gender-matched general population [2, 26, 29]. However, the difference in mortality rates between ITP patients and the general population was much less pronounced when ITP patients with comorbidity were compared with general population members with comorbidity, indicating that the major cause of death is more strongly associated with comorbidity than with ITP itself [26].

The prognosis of childhood ITP is much better than that of adult ITP. In the recent ICIS study with 1345 child ITP patients, the majority of patients underwent remissions within 12 months, and 28% of patients have chronic ITP with platelet counts less than 100×10^9/L at 12 months after diagnosis [31]. Severe thrombocytopenia (less than 20×10^9/L) at 12 months was only 7%, and even in such patients, major hemorrhage was infrequent. Neither ICH- nor ITP-related death was observed. In a retrospective survey of 247 child ITP patients in Japan, 67 patients (27%) had persistent or chronic ITP, and the risk factors for transition from newly diagnosed ITP to persistent or chronic ITP were older age, higher initial platelet count, positive medical history or comorbidity, the absence of preceding infection or vaccination, and the absence of an increase in immunoglobulin [32]. Chronic child ITP tends to achieve remission over time, and the overall time required for 50% resolution in chronic child ITP was reported to be 5.6 years [32].

References

1. Terrell DR, Beebe LA, Vesely SK, Neas BR, Segal JB, George JN. The incidence of immune thrombocytopenic purpura in children and adults: a critical review of published reports. Am J Hematol. 2010;85:174–80.
2. Schoonen WM, Kucera G, Coalson J, Li L, Rutstein M, Mowat F, Fryzek J, Kaye JA. Epidemiology of immune thrombocytopenic purpura in the General Practice Research Database. Br J Haematol. 2009;145:235–44.
3. Kurata Y, Fujimura K, Kuwana M, Tomiyama Y, Murata M. Epidemiology of primary immune thrombocytopenia in children and adults in Japan: a population-based study and literature review. Int J Hematol. 2011;93:329–35.
4. Moulis G, Palmaro A, Montastruc JL, Godeau B, Lapeyre-Mestre M, Sailler L. Epidemiology of incident immune thrombocytopenia: a nationwide population-based study in France. Blood. 2014;124:3308–15.
5. Segal JB, Powe NR. Prevalence of immune thrombocytopenia: analyses of administrative data. J Thromb Haemost. 2006;4:2377–83.
6. Feudjo-Tepie MA, Robinson NJ, Bennett D. Prevalence of diagnosed chronic immune thrombocytopenic purpura in the US: analysis of a large US claim database: a rebuttal. J Thromb Haemost. 2008;6:711–712; author reply 713, 2008.
7. Bennett D, Hodgson ME, Shukla A, Logie JW. Prevalence of diagnosed adult immune thrombocytopenia in the United Kingdom. Adv Ther. 2011;28:1096–104.
8. Provan D, Stasi R, Newland AC, Blanchette VS, Bolton-Maggs P, Bussel JB, Chong BH, Cines DB, Gernsheimer TB, Godeau B, Grainger J, Greer I, Hunt BJ, Imbach PA, Lyons G, McMillan R, Rodeghiero F, Sanz MA, Tarantino M, Watson S, Young J, Kuter DJ. International consensus report on the investigation and management of primary immune thrombocytopenia. Blood. 2010;115:168–86.
9. Rand ML, Wright JF. Virus-associated idiopathic thrombocytopenic purpura. Transfus Sci. 1998;19:253–9.
10. Kuhne T, Imbach P, Bolton-Maggs PH, Berchtold W, Blanchette V, Buchanan GR, Intercontinental Childhood ITPSG. Newly diagnosed idiopathic thrombocytopenic purpura in childhood: an observational study. Lancet. 2001;358:2122–5.

11. Cecinati V, Principi N, Brescia L, Giordano P, Esposito S. Vaccine administration and the development of immune thrombocytopenic purpura in children. Hum Vaccin Immunother. 2013;9:1158–62.
12. Rinaldi M, Perricone C, Ortega-Hernandez OD, Perricone R, Shoenfeld Y. Immune thrombocytopaenic purpura: an autoimmune cross-link between infections and vaccines. Lupus. 2014;23:554–67.
13. Mantadakis E, Farmaki E, Buchanan GR. Thrombocytopenic purpura after measles-mumps-rubella vaccination: a systematic review of the literature and guidance for management. J Pediatr. 2010;156:623–8.
14. Rodeghiero F, Stasi R, Gernsheimer T, Michel M, Provan D, Arnold DM, Bussel JB, Cines DB, Chong BH, Cooper N, Godeau B, Lechner K, Mazzucconi MG, McMillan R, Sanz MA, Imbach P, Blanchette V, Kuhne T, Ruggeri M, George JN. Standardization of terminology, definitions and outcome criteria in immune thrombocytopenic purpura of adults and children: report from an international working group. Blood. 2009;113:2386–93.
15. Yong M, Schoonen WM, Li L, Kanas G, Coalson J, Mowat F, Fryzek J, Kaye JA. Epidemiology of paediatric immune thrombocytopenia in the General Practice Research Database. Br J Haematol. 2010;149:855–64.
16. Kuhne T, Berchtold W, Michaels LA, Wu R, Donato H, Espina B, Tamary H, Rodeghiero F, Chitlur M, Rischewski J, Imbrach P. Newly diagnosed immune thrombocytopenia in children and adults: a comparative prospective observational registry of the Intercontinental Cooperative Immune Thrombocytopenia Study Group. Haematologica. 2011;96:1831–7.
17. Psaila B, Petrovic A, Page LK, Menell J, Schonholz M, Bussel JB. Intracranial hemorrhage (ICH) in children with immune thrombocytopenia (ITP): study of 40 cases. Blood. 2009;114:4777–83.
18. Enger C, Bennett D, Forssen U, Fogarty PF, McAfee AT. Comorbidities in patients with persistent or chronic immune thrombocytopenia. Int J Hematol. 2010;92:289–95.
19. Severinsen MT, Engebjerg MC, Farkas DK, Jensen AO, Norgaard M, Zhao S, Sorensen HT. Risk of venous thromboembolism in patients with primary chronic immune thrombocytopenia: a Danish population-based cohort study. Br J Haematol. 2011;152:360–2.
20. Norgaard M, Severinsen MT, Lund Maegbaek M, Jensen AO, Cha S, Sorensen HT. Risk of arterial thrombosis in patients with primary chronic immune thrombocytopenia: a Danish population-based cohort study. Br J Haematol. 2012;159:109–11.
21. Sarpatwari A, Bennett D, Logie JW, Shukla A, Beach KJ, Newland AC, Sanderson S, Provan D. Thromboembolic events among adult patients with primary immune thrombocytopenia in the United Kingdom General Practice Research Database. Haematologica. 2010;95:1167–75.
22. Norgaard M, Cetin K, Maegbaek ML, Kristensen NR, Ghanima W, Bahmanyar S, Stryker S, Christiansen CF. Risk of arterial thrombotic and venous thromboembolic events in patients with primary chronic immune thrombocytopenia: a Scandinavian population-based cohort study. Br J Haematol. 2015;174:639–42.
23. Ruggeri M, Tosetto A, Palandri F, Polverelli N, Mazzucconi MG, Santoro C, Gaidano G, Lunghi M, Zaja F, De Stefano V, Sartori R, Fazi P, Rodeghiero F, Gruppo Italiano Malattie EdAA, Thrombocytopenias Working Party GSITP. Thrombotic risk in patients with primary immune thrombocytopenia is only mildly increased and explained by personal and treatment-related risk factors. J Thromb Haemost. 2014;12:1266–73.
24. Rodeghiero F. Is ITP a thrombophilic disorder? Am J Hematol. 2016;91:39–45.
25. Neunert C, Lim W, Crowther M, Cohen A, Solberg Jr L, Crowther MA, American Society of Hematology. The American Society of Hematology 2011 evidence-based practice guideline for immune thrombocytopenia. Blood. 2011;117:4190–207.
26. Frederiksen H, Maegbaek ML, Norgaard M. Twenty-year mortality of adult patients with primary immune thrombocytopenia: a Danish population-based cohort study. Br J Haematol. 2014;166:260–7.
27. Michel M, Suzan F, Adoue D, Bordessoule D, Marolleau JP, Viallard JF, Godeau B. Management of immune thrombocytopenia in adults: a population-based analysis of the French hospital discharge database from 2009 to 2012. Br J Haematol. 2015;170:218–22.

28. Rodeghiero F, Ruggeri M. Is splenectomy still the gold standard for the treatment of chronic ITP? Am J Hematol. 2008;83:91.
29. Norgaard M, Jensen AO, Engebjerg MC, Farkas DK, Thomsen RW, Cha S, Zhao S, Sorensen HT. Long-term clinical outcomes of patients with primary chronic immune thrombocytopenia: a Danish population-based cohort study. Blood. 2011;117:3514–20.
30. Portielje JEA, Westendorp RGJ, Kluin-Nelemans HC, Brand A. Morbidity and mortality in adults with idiopathic thrombocytopenic purpura. Blood. 2001;97:2549–54.
31. Neunert CE, Buchanan GR, Imbach P, Bolton-Maggs PH, Bennett CM, Neufeld E, Vesely SK, Adix L, Blanchette VS, Kuhne T. Bleeding manifestations and management of children with persistent and chronic immune thrombocytopenia: data from the Intercontinental Cooperative ITP Study Group (ICIS). Blood. 2013;121:4457–62.
32. Kubota M, Adachi S, Usami I, Okada M, Kitoh T, Shiota M, Taniguchi Y, Tanizawa A, Nanbu M, Hamahata K, Fujino H, Matsubara K, Wakazono Y, Nakahata T. Characterization of chronic idiopathic thrombocytopenic purpura in Japanese children: a retrospective multi-center study. Int J Hematol. 2010;91:252–7.

Part IV
Pathophysiology

Autoantigens in ITP

Yoshiaki Tomiyama

Abstract Antiplatelet autoantibodies play a critical role in autoimmune thrombocytopenia (ITP). Thus, characterization of autoantigens recognized by autoantibodies is a prerequisite for elucidating its pathophysiology. Platelet glycoprotein (GP) IIb-IIIa and/or GPIb-IX are the two major autoantigens in ITP. This capture reviews recent advance in the characterization and localization of autoantigens in ITP.

1 Introduction

Autoimmune thrombocytopenia (ITP) is an acquired immune-mediated disorder characterized by early platelet destruction due to antiplatelet autoantibodies. Platelet destruction results from subsequent complement-mediated lysis and/or phagocytosis by the reticuloendothelial system (RES) mainly in the spleen [1–5]. Experiments performed by Harrington et al. in 1951 and following experiments by Schulman et al. in the mid-1960s revealed the immunologic etiology of the disease on the basis of the development of transient thrombocytopenia in healthy recipients after the passive transfer of plasma, including immunoglobulin (Ig) G-rich fractions, from ITP patients [6, 7]. The direct antiglobulin test (DAT) is a reliable method for the diagnosis of autoimmune hemolytic anemia (AIHA). To develop an equivalent assay in ITP to DAT in AIHA, several assays to detect antiplatelet antibodies as platelet-associated IgG (PAIgG) on platelets have been reported in the 1970s [1]. However, elevated levels of PAIgG were not specific for ITP, but were often observed in patients with nonimmune thrombocytopenia [8, 9]. PAIgG should contain "true" antiplatelet IgG autoantibody bound to a platelet antigen (autoantigen) through the Fab terminus of the IgG molecule. In addition to the "true" antibody, PAIgG could contain immune complex bound to the platelet Fcγ receptor (FcγRII) and nonspecific IgG bound to platelets, which resulted in the low specificity (~27%) of PAIgG

Y. Tomiyama, M.D.
Department of Blood Transfusion, Osaka University Hospital, 2-15 Yamadaoka, Suita, Osaka 565-0871, Japan
e-mail: yoshi@hp-blood.med.osaka-u.ac.jp

Y. Ishida, Y. Tomiyama (eds.), *Autoimmune Thrombocytopenia*,
DOI 10.1007/978-981-10-4142-6_5

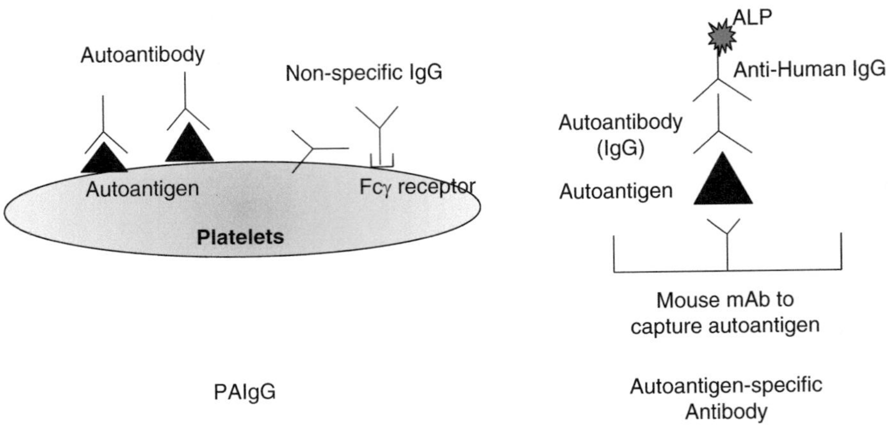

Fig. 1 Comparison between platelet-associated IgG (PAIgG) and autoantigen-specific antibody in ITP. In addition to autoantibody, PAIgG could contain an immune complex bound to the platelet Fcγ receptor (FcγRII) and nonspecific IgG bound to platelets, which results in the low specificity of PAIgG for the diagnosis of ITP

for the diagnosis of ITP [8] (Fig. 1). Thus, the assay to measure IgG associated with platelet is not sufficient for understanding the pathophysiology of ITP or for the diagnostic test for ITP.

To overcome the disadvantage of PAIgG measurement and reveal the pathophysiology of ITP, an autoantigen that binds autoantibody should be identified and then the autoantigen-specific antibody should be evaluated.

2 Platelet-Associated Autoantibodies

van Leeuwen et al. firstly showed that platelet-associated (PA) antibodies eluted from platelets of 42 chronic ITP patients bound to all normal platelets tested, but 32 of these eluates (76%) did not react with platelets obtained from Glanzmann thrombasthenia (GT) [9]. Because GT is a congenital bleeding disorder that is caused by a quantitative defect in platelet membrane glycoprotein (GP)IIb-IIIa [10, 11], the findings of van Leeuwen et al. suggested the importance of GPIIb-IIIa as a major autoantigen in chronic ITP. Varon and Karpatkin showed impaired binding of the monoclonal antibody 3B2, which is specific for GPIIb, to platelets obtained from 15 of 16 chronic ITP patients. Their data also suggested that GPIIb-IIIa may be important as an autoantigen in ITP, and the autoantigen may locate close to the 3B2-binding site because of the possible inhibition of the 3B2 binding by ITP autoantibodies [12]. Subsequently, direct evidence for the presence of anti-GPIIb-IIIa and/or anti-GPIb-IX autoantibodies in ITP has been provided by several different assays including monoclonal antibody-based antigen-specific assays such as the immunobead

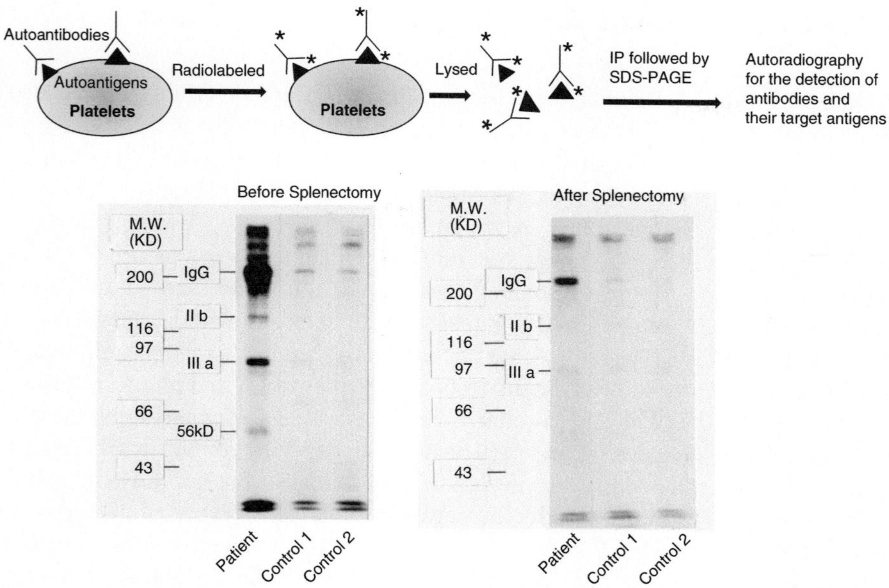

Fig. 2 Demonstration of platelet-associated (PA) antibodies and their target antigens by a direct immunoprecipitation procedure in ITP. *Upper left panel*: Procedure for direct immunoprecipitation assay. *Lower panel*: Direct immunoprecipitation experiments before and after splenectomy are shown. Note that anti-GPIIb-IIIa autoantibodies disappeared after splenectomy. *IP* immunoprecipitation, *IgG* immunoglobulin G; *MW* molecular weight

assay and monoclonal antibody immobilization of platelet antigens (MAIPA) (Fig. 1) [13–15]. Tomiyama et al. developed a direct immunoprecipitation assay: ITP platelets with autoantibodies were directly radiolabeled and solubilized without adding any antibody, and then platelet antigen-antibody complexes were immunoprecipitated by protein A and analyzed by SDS-PAGE. This method allows us to analyze both PA autoantibodies and their target antigens (i.e., autoantigens) simultaneously. Employing this procedure, GPIIb-IIIa and a 56 kd protein were identified as autoantigens for PA autoantibodies in four and three of six ITP patients, respectively, and suggested that the levels of these PA autoantibodies were related to the disease activity (Fig. 2) [16, 17]. Prospective studies revealed that PA autoantibodies were detected in 50–60% ITP patients, and the most frequently detected antibodies were anti-GPIIb-IIIa followed by anti-GPIb-IX antibodies [18, 19]. Although not all but 50–60% ITP possessed PA autoantibodies, the specificity of these autoantibodies for ITP was high (>90%), and the degree of their positivity increased with the severity of ITP [19]. Moreover, corticosteroids and splenectomy resulted in a decrease in PA autoantibody levels associated with an improvement in the platelet count [20]. Taken together, these data indicate that PA autoantibodies play a crucial role in the pathophysiology of ITP.

3 Serum Autoantibodies

Serum (or plasma) antibodies specific for GPIIb-IIIa and/or GPIb-IX have also been demonstrated in ITP by monoclonal antibody-based antigen-specific assays [14]. However, serum autoantibodies were less frequently detected than PA autoantibodies (43.2 vs. 79.7%) [14, 21]. Some serum anti-GPIIb or anti-GPIIIa antibodies could be demonstrated in an immunoblot assay, suggesting that these antibodies might recognize linear structure rather than tertiary structure of GPIIb or GPIIIa [22, 23]. Moreover, some of these serum antibodies showed a different specificity from PA autoantibodies. Fujisawa et al. demonstrated that plasma samples from chronic ITP patients contained antibodies against a cytoplasmic region of GPIIIa and clearly showed the different specificities of PA and plasma autoantibodies to GPIIb-IIIa [24, 25]. Similarly, Kosugi, et al. also demonstrated the different specificity between PA and plasma antibodies specific for GPIIb-IIIa and the presence of anti-αvβ3 antibodies in sera from chronic ITP but not in PA autoantibodies [26, 27]. Moreover, antibodies against vinculin, an intracellular protein, have been detected in ITP sera and control sera. The incidence of antivinculin antibodies in ITP sera (67%; 55 of 82 sera) was significantly higher than that in control sera (40%; 32 of 80 sera), and there is a significant difference between the mean levels of antivinculin antibodies in ITP and control sera [28]. It is possible that antivinculin antibodies may secondarily be induced by platelet destruction in ITP. Taken together, the presence of antibodies against a cytoplasmic region of GPIIIa and/or vinculin in ITP sera as well as the different specificity between PA and serum (plasma) antibodies strongly suggest that sera in chronic ITP may contain antibodies secondarily caused by platelet destruction. Accordingly, in order to reveal the pathophysiology of ITP, we should investigate autoantigens recognized by PA autoantibodies.

4 Characterization of PA Anti-GPIIb-IIIa Autoantibodies

PA anti-GPIIb-IIIa autoantibodies are most frequently detected in ITP [18, 19]. GPIIb and GPIIIa forms a non-covalently associated, divalent cation-dependent heterodimer (αIIbβ3), which is a prototypic integrin and plays a crucial role in normal hemostasis and platelet aggregation as a physiologic receptor for fibrinogen and von Willebrand factor. Dissociation of the GPIIb-IIIa complex into free GPIIb and GPIIIa by EDTA treatment markedly impaired the reactivity of PA anti-GPIIb-IIIa autoantibodies [26, 29]. These findings suggest that most PA autoantibodies recognize cation-dependent conformation(s) of either GPIIb or GPIIIa or conformation(s) formed by both GPIIb and GPIIIa. Bowditch et al. examined the reactivity of PA autoantibodies against five large recombinant GPIIIa peptides. However, they failed to localize the autoantigenic epitopes on GPIIIa [30]. GPIIb-IIIa (αIIbβ3) and αvβ3 share the same β subunit, and GPIIb and αv show strong similarities in primary structure (34% amino acid sequence identity). We took advantage of molecular similarities between these two integrins and investigated whether PA anti-GPIIb-IIIa autoantibodies might also react with αvβ3 expressed on human umbilical vein endothelial cells. We did not detect PA anti-αvβ3 autoantibodies in chronic ITP, and we found that PA anti-GPIIb-IIIa autoantibodies did not recognize αvβ3. Because even topographic epitopes on GPIIIa, such as HPA-1a and HPA-4a, are expressed on both GPIIb-IIIa and αvβ3, these findings suggest that PA autoantibodies are highly GPIIb-IIIa-specific and recognize the tertiary structure of intact GPIIb-IIIa [27].

5 Autoantigenic Epitopes on GPIIb-IIIa

PA anti-GPIIb-IIIa autoantibodies failed to react with αvβ3, suggesting an important role of GPIIb as an autoantigen. Extracellular domain of GPIIb (αIIb) consists of four domains: β-propeller domain, thigh domain, calf-1 domain, and calf-2 domain. The N-terminal globular head of αIIbβ3, which contains a ligand-binding site of this integrin, is formed by a seven-bladed β-propeller domain (W1–W7) from GPIIb and a β I-domain from GPIIIa (β3) (Fig. 3). In addition to the quantitative defect, a qualitative defect in GPIIb-IIIa is responsible for GT phenotype (variant

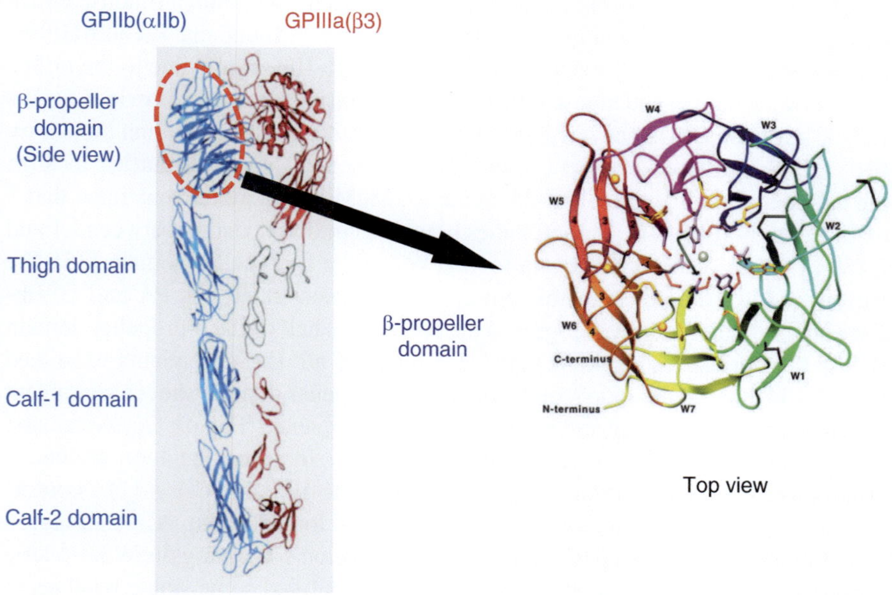

Fig. 3 Structure of extracellular domain of GPIIb-IIIa (integrin αIIbβ3) and β-propeller domain of GPIIb (αIIb). The N-terminal portion of GPIIb, known as the β-propeller domain, contains seven radially arranged β-sheets, termed "W" because of their topology. Each W structure has four antiparallel β-strands and four connecting loops

GT) [10, 11]. Molecular characterization of variant GT is informative in defining functionally important site(s) in GPIIb-IIIa, and ligand-binding sites within the N-terminal globular head have been identified in both GPIIb and GPIIIa [11]. By the characterization of a variant GT, CAM, Loftus et al. first demonstrated Asp residue at 119 in GPIIIa as one of the critical residues for ligand binding [31]. Honda et al. demonstrated that a 2-amino acid insertion (Arg-Thr) between amino acid residues 160 and 161 within the GPIIb W3 4-1 loop is responsible for a ligand-binding defect in a variant GT, KO [32]. Both KO and CAM variants GPIIb-IIIa showed markedly impaired ligand binding without disturbing surface expression or inducing major structural change in the receptor. To localize the autoantigenic epitope(s), we examined the reactivity of platelet eluates (PA autoantibodies) against KO mutant or CAM mutant GPIIb-IIIa-expressing 293T cells. Interestingly, 11 of 34 chronic ITP patients (32%) with PA anti-GPIIb-IIIa autoantibodies showed marked decrease in the reactivity with KO GPIIb-IIIa, but not with CAM GPIIb-IIIa [17, 33]. Thus, in one-third of ITP patients, the W3 4-1 loop and its surrounding regions of β-propeller domain in GPIIb may directly or indirectly participate in the formation of autoantigens.

Autoantigenic epitopes on GPIIb-IIIa were localized on W3 4-1 loop of β-propeller domain in one-third of ITP patients [33]. However, they still remained elusive in the other two-third of ITP patients. In order to further characterize autoantigenic epitopes on GPIIb-IIIa in ITP patients including the remaining two-thirds of ITP patients, Kiyomize et al. systematically examined the reactivity of PA anti-GPIIb-IIIa autoantibodies obtained from 15 ITP patients with human-mouse GPIIb chimeras complexed with human GPIIIa [34]. Firstly, we found that PA anti-GPIIb-IIIa autoantibodies poorly reacted with mouse GPIIb-IIIa mainly due to the difference between human and mouse GPIIb, which is consistent with the previous results [27, 33]. Mouse GPIIb shows higher homology with human GPIIb than human αv (81 vs. 34% amino acid sequence homology), which enabled us to further localize the epitopes. Employing αIIb-αvβ3 chimeras, McMillan et al. demonstrated that 8 of 14 PA anti-GPIIb-IIIa autoantibodies bound to epitopes existing between L1 and Q459 in GPIIb, which correspond to W1–W7 in the β-propeller domain [35]. We narrowed down the autoantigenic epitopes and demonstrated that PA anti-GPIIb-IIIa autoantibodies mainly recognized the N-terminal half of the β-propeller domain (L1-W235 corresponding to W1–W4 4-1 loop) in all 15 ITP patients examined (Fig. 4) [34]. Antigenic loop structures in the β-propeller domain show a significant difference between human and mouse amino acid sequence (Fig. 4). Our systematic examination with human-mouse αIIb chimeras by focusing the loop structures found three main recognition sites for PA anti-GPIIb-IIIa antibodies: (1) a conformational epitope composed of W1:1-2 and W2:3-4 loops (Group A), (2) a region containing the W1:2-3 loop (Group B), and (3) a region containing the W3:4-1 loop (Group C) [34]. It is noteworthy that we further identified some single residues in these loops that were critical for the reactivity of PA autoantibodies obtained from three ITP patients (Pt 17, 23, and 36), suggesting that some PA autoantibodies behaves like monospecific antibodies (Fig. 5) [34]. In addition, we and others demonstrated that many of PA anti-GPIIb-IIIa antibodies showed apparent clonality

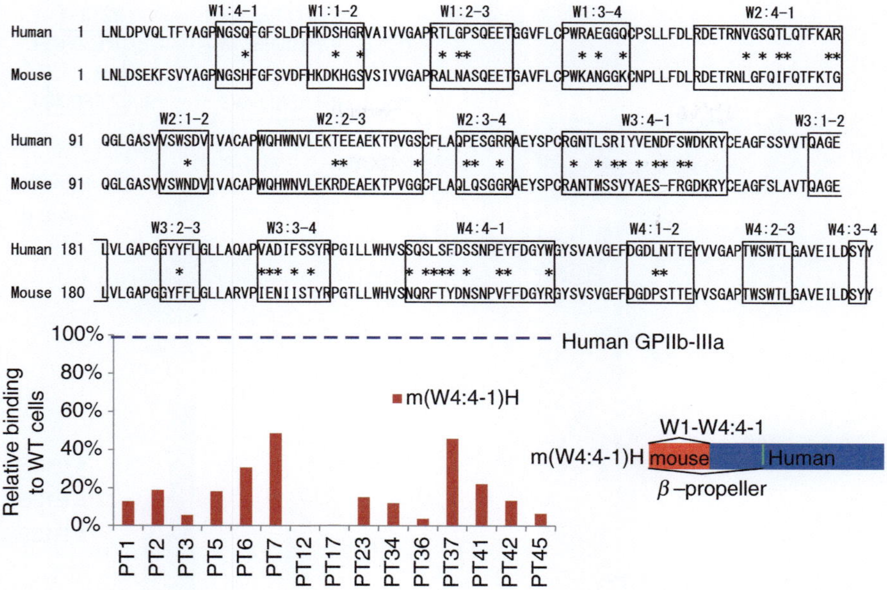

Fig. 4 Autoantigenic epitopes of platelet-associated (PA) anti-GPIIb-IIIa are mainly localized in the N-terminal half of the β-propeller domain (L1-W235 corresponding to W1–W4 4-1 loop). *Upper panel*: Alignment of the β-propeller domain of GPIIb between human and mouse. The boxes indicate the small loop structure of each β-sheet domain, and the asterisks indicate amino acid difference between human and mouse sequence. *Lower panel*: Reactivity of platelet-associated (PA) anti-GPIIb-IIIa autoantibodies with m(W4:4-1)H complexed with human GPIIIa. Their reactivity with human GPIIb-IIIa as 100%. m(W4:4-1)H: human GPIIb carrying mouse sequence from the N-terminus to W4:4-1 loop

because of the restricted κ/λ light chain usage [34, 36, 37], which is consistent of the findings that antigenic epitopes for PA anti-GPIIb-IIIa antibodies are limited [34, 35].

6 Autoantigenic Epitopes on GPIb-IX

He, et al. localized autoantigens on GPIb-IX employing 16 ITP sera containing anti-GPIb-IX and 2 PA autoantibodies in a selected experiment [38]. Reactivity of 16 ITP sera with glycocalicin, which contains most of the extracellular of GPIbα, and with two recombinant fragments (fragment 1, amino acids 1–247; fragment 2, amino acids 240–485), was examined. Six out of sixteen ITP sera reacted with recombinant protein fragment 2. Protein fragment 2 contained four highly antigenic segments (P1–P4), and all six sera as well as two platelet eluates (=PA autoantibodies) reacted with P2 peptide (LHPTQESTKEQTTFPPRWTPN, amino acids 326–346). Furthermore, epitope scanning with a panel of overlapping synthetic 15-mer peptides localized the P2 epitope to the GPIbα sequence, TKEQTTFPP (amino acids 333–341).

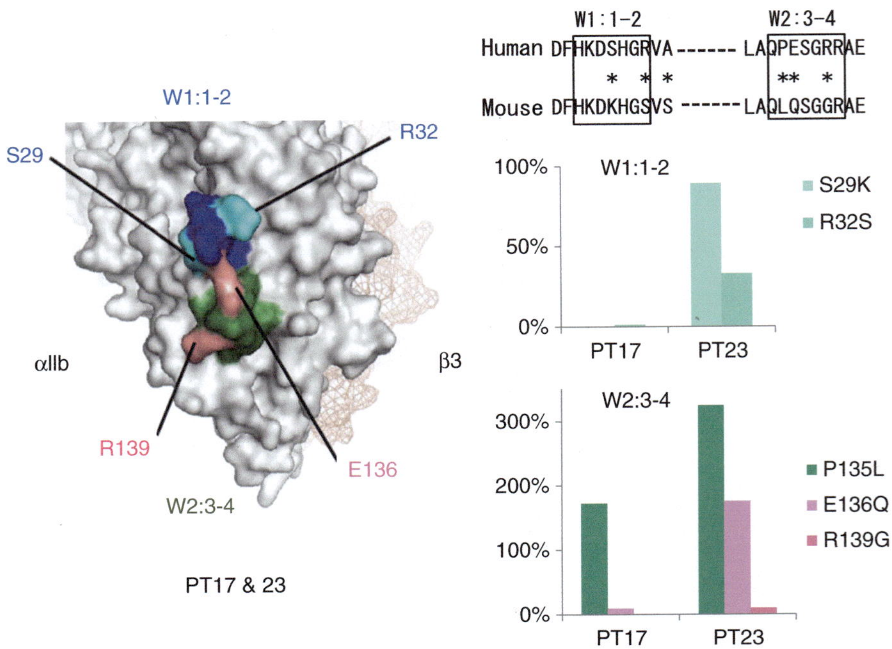

Fig. 5 Structure of the recognition sites for the platelet-associated (PA) antibody obtained from two ITP patients (PT17 and PT23). Note that the single amino acid replacement of human with mouse GPIIb resulted in the marked reduction of the PA antibody binding

7 Summary

The cause of primary ITP remains obscure; however, it has been suggested that molecular mimicry may trigger an immune response against platelet antigens in some secondary forms of ITP [39]. Our understanding regarding autoantigens on GPIIb-IIIa and GPIb-IX is that autoantigenic epitopes for ITP seem limited, and antigenic "hot spots" of GPIIb-IIIa and GPIb-IX may exist on the N-terminal half of the β-propeller domain on GPIIb and amino acids 333–341 of GPIbα, respectively. A recent study reported that many bacterial proteins contained the human integrin-type β-propeller domain [40]; this suggested that conformational mimicry between these bacterial proteins and the β-propeller domain in GPIIb might be involved in the production of PA anti-GPIIb-IIIa Abs. The restricted κ/λ light chain usage further suggests that PA Abs might arise from an antigen-derived clonal expansion rather than from polyclonal B-cell activation triggered by nonspecific stimuli. Further characterization of autoantigenic epitopes would offer insight into the specific treatments as well as the pathophysiology of ITP.

Acknowledgment This work was supported by Grant-in-Aid for Scientific Research from the Ministry of Education, Culture, Sports, Science and Technology in Japan and the Ministry of Health, Labour and Welfare in Japan.

References

1. McMillan R. Chronic idiopathic thrombocytopenic purpura. N Engl J Med. 1981;304: 1135–47.
2. George JN, El-Harase MA, Raskob GE. Chronic idiopathic thrombocytopenic purpura. N Engl J Med. 1994;331:1207–11.
3. Karpatkin S. Autoimmune (idiopathic) thrombocytopenic purpura. Lancet. 1997;349:1531–6.
4. Cines DB, Blanchette VS. Immune thrombocytopenic purpura. N Engl J Med. 2002;346: 995–1008.
5. Kashiwagi H, Tomiyama Y. Pathophysiology and management of primary immune thrombocytopenia. Int J Hematol. 2013;98:24–33.
6. Harrington WJ, Minnich V, Hollingsworth JW, Moore CV. Demonstration of a thrombocytopenic factor in the blood of patients with thrombocytopenic purpura. J Lab Clin Med. 1951;38:1–10.
7. Shulman NR, Marder VJ, Weinrach RS. Similarities between known antiplatelet antibodies and the factor responsible for thrombocytopenia in idiopathic purpura. Physiologic, serologic and isotopic studies. Ann N Y Acad Sci. 1965;124:499–542.
8. Kelton JG, Powers PJ, Carter CJ. A prospective study of the usefulness of the measurement of platelet-associated IgG for the diagnosis of idiopathic thrombocytopenic purpura. Blood. 1982;60:1050–3.
9. Mueller-Eckhardt C, Kayser W, Mersch-Baumert K, Mueller-Eckhardt G, Breidenbach M, Kugel HG, et al. The clinical significance of platelet-associated IgG: a study on 298 patients with various disorders. Br J Haematol. 1980;46:123–31.
10. George JN, Caen JP, Nurden AT. Glanzmann's thrombasthenia: the spectrum of clinical disease. Blood. 1990;75:1383–95.
11. Tomiyama Y. Glanzmann thrombasthenia: integrin αIIbβ3 deficiency. Int J Hematol. 2000;72: 448–54.
12. van Leeuwen EF, van der Ven JTJ, Engelfreit CP, von dem Borne AE. Specificity of autoantibodies in autoimmune thrombocytopenia. Blood. 1982;59:23–6.
13. Woods Jr VL, Oh EH, Mason D, McMillan R. Autoantibodies against the platelet glycoprotein IIb/IIIa complex in patients with chronic ITP. Blood. 1984;63:368–75.
14. McMillan R, Tani P, Millard F, Berchtold P, Renshow L, Woods Jr VL. Platelet-associated and plasma anti-glycoprotein autoantibodies in chronic ITP. Blood. 1987;70:1040–5.
15. Kiefel V, Santoso S, Kaufmann E, Mueller-Eckhardt C. Autoantibodies against platelet glycoprotein Ib/IX: a frequent finding in autoimmune thrombocytopenic purpura. Br J Haematol. 1991;79:256–62.
16. Tomiyama Y, Take H, Honda S, Furubayashi T, Mizutani H, Tsubakio T, et al. Demonstration of platelet antigens that bind platelet-associated autoantibodies in chronic ITP by direct immunoprecipitation procedure. Br J Haematol. 1990;75:92–8.
17. Tomiyama Y, Kosugi S. Autoantigenic epitopes on platelet glycoproteins. Int J Hematol. 2005;81:100–5.
18. Brighton TA, Evans S, Castaldi PA, Chesterman CN, Chong BH. Prospective evaluation of the clinical usefulness of an antigenspecific assay (MAIPA) in idiopathic thrombocytopenic purpura and other immune thrombocytopenias. Blood. 1996;88:194–201.
19. McMillan R, Wang L, Tani P. Prospective evaluation of the immunobead assay for the diagnosis of adult chronic immune thrombocytopenic purpura (ITP). J Thromb Haemost. 2003;1:485–91.
20. Fujisawa K, Tani P, Piro L, McMillan R. The effect of therapy on platelet-associated autoantibody in chronic immune thrombocytopenic purpura. Blood. 1993;81:2872–7.
21. Tani P, Berchtold P, McMillan R. Autoantibodies in chronic ITP. Blut. 1989;59:44–6.
22. Beardsley DS, Spiegel JE, Jacobs MM, Handin RI, Lux SE. Platelet membrane glycoprotein IIIa contains target antigens that bind anti-platelet antibodies in immune thrombocytopenias. J Clin Invest. 1984;74:1701–7.

23. Tomiyama Y, Kurata Y, Mizutani H, et al. Platelet glycoprotein IIb as a target antigen in two patients with chronic idiopathic thrombocytopenic purpura. Br J Haematol. 1987;66:535–8.
24. Fujisawa K, O'Tool TE, Tani P, et al. Autoantibodies to the presumptive cytoplasmic domain of platelet glycoprotein IIIa in patients with chronic immune thrombocytopenic purpura. Blood. 1991;77:2207–13.
25. Fujisawa K, Tani P, O'Toole TE, Ginsberg MH, McMillan R. Different specificities of platelet-associated and plasma autoantibodies to platelet GPIIb-IIIa in patients with chronic immune thrombocytopenic purpura. Blood. 1992;79:1441–6.
26. Kosugi S, Tomiyama Y, Shiraga M, et al. Platelet-associated antiglycoprotein (GP) IIb-IIIa autoantibodies in chronic immune thrombocytopenic purpura mainly recognize cation-dependent conformations: comparison with the epitopes of serum autoantibodies. Thromb Haemost. 1996;75:339–45.
27. Kosugi S, Tomiyama Y, Honda S, et al. Anti-αvβ3 antibodies in chronic immune thrombocytopenic purpura. Thromb Haemost. 2001;85:36–41.
28. Tomiyama Y, Kekomäki R, McFarland J, Kunicki TJ. Antivinculin antibodies in sera of patients with immune thrombocytopenia and in sera of normal subjects. Blood. 1992;79:161–8.
29. Fujisawa K, McMillan R. Platelet-associated antibody to glycoprotein IIb/IIIa from chronic immune thrombocytopenic purpura patients often binds to divalent cation-dependent antigens. Blood. 1993;81:1284–9.
30. Bowditch RD, Tani P, McMillan R. Reactivity of autoantibodies from chronic ITP patients with recombinant glycoprotein IIIa peptides. Br J Haematol. 1995;91:178–84.
31. Loftus JC, O'Tool TE, Plow EF, Glass A, Frelinger III AL, Ginsberg MH. A β3 integrin mutation abolishes ligand binding and alters divalent cation-dependent conformation. Science. 1990;249:915–8.
32. Honda S, Tomiyama Y, Shiraga M, et al. A two amino acid insertion in the Cys46-Cys167 loop of the αIIb subunit is associated with a variant of Glanzmann thrombasthenia. J Clin Invest. 1998;102:1183–92.
33. Kosugi S, Tomiyama Y, Honda S, et al. Platelet-associated anti-GPIIb-IIIa autoantibodies in chronic immune thrombocytopenic purpura recognizing epitopes close to the ligand-binding site of glycoprotein (GP) IIb. Blood. 2001;98:1819–27.
34. Kiyomizu K, Kashiwagi H, Nakazawa T, et al. Recognition of highly restricted regions in the β-propeller domain of αIIb by platelet-associated anti-αIIbβ3 autoantibodies in primary immune thrombocytopenia. Blood. 2012;120:1499–509.
35. McMillan R, Wang L, Lopez-Dee J, Jiu S, Loftus JC. Many αIIbβ3 autoepitopes in chronic immune thrombocytopenic purpura are localized to αIIb between amino acids L1 and Q459. Br J Haematol. 2002;118:1132–6.
36. McMillan R, Lopez-Dee J, Bowditch R. Clonal restriction of platelet-associated anti-GPIIb/IIIa autoantibodies in patients with chronic ITP. Thromb Haemost. 2001;85:821–3.
37. Roark JH, Bussel JB, Cines DB, Siegel DL. Genetic analysis of autoantibodies in idiopathic thrombocytopenic purpura reveals evidence of clonal expansion and somatic mutation. Blood. 2002;100:1388–98.
38. He R, Reid DM, Jones CE, Shulman NR. Extracellular epitopes of platelet glycoprotein Ibα reactive with serum antibodies from patients with chronic idiopathic thrombocytopenic purpura. Blood. 1995;86:3789–96.
39. Nardi MA, Liu LX, Karpatkin S. GPIIIa-(49-66) is a major pathophysiologically relevant antigenic determinant for anti-platelet GPIIIa of HIV-1-related immunologic thrombocytopenia. Proc Natl Acad Sci U S A. 1997;94:7589–94.
40. Chouhan B, Denesyuk A, Heino J. Conservation of the human integrin-type β-propeller domain in bacteria. PLoS One. 2011;6(10):e25069.

T-Cell Abnormalities

Takashi Satoh and Masataka Kuwana

Abstract Immune thrombocytopenia (ITP) is an autoimmune disease characterized by increased platelet destruction and reduced platelet production caused primarily by IgG antiplatelet autoantibodies, which mainly target platelet membrane glycoproteins (GPs), including GPIIb/IIIa and GPIb/IX. GPIIb/IIIa-reactive $CD4^+$ T cells play a central role in the pathogenic process by triggering and maintaining antiplatelet autoantibodies. The mechanism for ongoing antiplatelet antibody production is explained by a "pathogenic loop" model consisting of macrophages in the reticuloendothelial system, GPIIb/IIIa-reactive $CD4^+$ T cells, and B cells producing antiplatelet antibodies. Among T helper (Th) cell subsets, Th1 and Th17 cells as well as newly identified T follicular helper (Tfh) cells, which support B cell maturation and differentiation within the germinal center, are actively involved in antiplatelet antibody production. Finally, platelet-reactive $CD8^+$ cytotoxic T cells directly induce lysis and apoptosis of circulating platelets as well as megakaryocytes. On the other hand, $CD4^+$ regulatory T cells (Tregs), which contribute to maintenance of peripheral immune tolerance, are defective in patients with ITP, through decreased numbers and impaired function of Tregs. In fact, mice lacking Foxp3 Tregs spontaneously develop chronic thrombocytopenia mediated through the production of IgG antiplatelet autoantibodies. Further studies evaluating mechanisms for T-cell dysregulation are useful in elucidating the pathogenesis of ITP and in developing novel treatment strategies.

T. Satoh (✉)
Division of Hematology, Kitasato University School of Allied Health Sciences,
1-15-1, Kitasato, Minami-ku, Sagamihara, Kanagawa 252-0373, Japan

Division of Molecular Hematology, Kitasato University Graduate School of Medical Sciences, 1-15-1, Kitasato, Minami-ku, Sagamihara, Kanagawa 252-0374, Japan
e-mail: takashis@kitasato-u.ac.jp

M. Kuwana
Department of Allergy and Rheumatology, Nippon Medical School Graduate School of Medicine, 1-1-5 Sendagi, Bunkyo-ku, Tokyo 113-8603, Japan
e-mail: kuwanam@nms.ac.jp

Y. Ishida, Y. Tomiyama (eds.), *Autoimmune Thrombocytopenia*,
DOI 10.1007/978-981-10-4142-6_6

1 Introduction

Immune thrombocytopenia (ITP) is an autoimmune disease in association with increased platelet destruction and impaired platelet production, both of which are mediated primarily through IgG antiplatelet autoantibodies reactive with platelet membrane glycoproteins (GPs), such as GPIIb/IIIa and GPIb/IX [1, 2]. There are accumulating lines of evidence demonstrating that cellular immunity in ITP patients is perturbed and shifted toward T helper 1 (Th1) and Th17 pro-inflammatory responses [3]. Moreover, it has been recently found that $CD4^+$ T follicular helper (Tfh) cells are also involved in regulating antiplatelet autoantibody response in ITP patients [4]. However, autoimmune responses observed in patients with ITP, especially those with primary ITP, specifically target platelet GPs. Therefore, the antigen-specific mechanisms should play a central role in the pathogenic process in conjunction with activation of nonspecific immune pathways. Actually, in ITP patients, it has been shown that $CD4^+$ T cells reactive to GPIIb/IIIa are able to stimulate B cells to produce IgG antiplatelet autoantibodies [5]. In addition, platelet-reactive $CD8^+$ cytotoxic T lymphocytes (CTLs) induce the direct destruction of platelets and megakaryocytes [6]. On the other hand, a variety of regulatory T cell (Treg) subsets that contribute to the maintenance of immune tolerance in the periphery, including $CD4^+$ and $CD8^+$ Tregs, are dysfunctional in patients with ITP [7, 8]. Taken together, it is obvious that the dysregulation of a variety of T cell subsets contributes to the complex pathophysiologies of ITP. This review summarizes recent knowledge of aberrant effector and regulatory T cells in the pathogenesis of ITP.

2 Autoreactive Effector $CD4^+$ T Cells

It is now evident that production of high-affinity IgG autoantibodies by B cells requires antigen-specific T cell help. $CD4^+$ T cells that react with autoantigens targeted by IgG autoantibodies have been identified in patients with various systemic or organ-specific autoimmune diseases. These autoantigen-specific $CD4^+$ T cells almost always have an effector phenotype. We have found that GPIIb/IIIa is one of the major target antigens recognized by platelet-reactive $CD4^+$ T cells in an HLA-DR-restricted fashion [5]. In addition, GPIIb/IIIa-reactive T cells obtained from ITP patients are able to stimulate autologous B cells to produce IgG antibodies that bind normal platelet surfaces at least in vitro. In this assay system, a blockade of the CD40/CD154 interaction inhibits in vitro anti-GPIIb/IIIa antibody production, indicating that the engagement of CD40 on B cells with CD154 expressed by activated $CD4^+$ T cells is essential for T-cell helper activity [9]. In addition, CD154 expressed by activated platelets also stimulates B cells to produce antiplatelet autoantibodies in an antigen-independent fashion [10].

Interestingly, GPIIb/IIIa-reactive $CD4^+$ T cells respond to reduced GPIIb/IIIa or tryptic peptides of GPIIb/IIIa, but not to native GPIIb/IIIa, in the presence of antigen-presenting cells, including dendritic cells, macrophages, and B cells [5]. This indicates that the epitopes they recognize are "cryptic" determinants, which are generated at a subthreshold level by the processing of native GPIIb/IIIa under normal circumstances. Therefore, the exposure of "cryptic" peptides of GPIIb/IIIa to the immune system is a critical step for elucidating and maintaining the antiplatelet autoantibody response. In patients with chronic ITP, splenic macrophages are identified as the major antigen-presenting cells for presenting "cryptic" GPIIb/IIIa peptides [11]. In addition, the presentation of the "cryptic" GPIIb/IIIa peptides by macrophages depends on their phagocytosis of a large quantity of opsonized platelets via the Fcγ receptors, leading to an efficient concentration of the small quantities of platelet GP peptides that were previously "cryptic." Therefore, the spleen is the primary site of GPIIb/IIIa-reactive $CD4^+$ T-cell activation and the subsequent antiplatelet antibody production [12]. A recent histologic analysis of ITP spleens indicates that proliferative lymphoid nodules are the primary sites where the T/B--cell interaction for production of antiplatelet autoantibodies occurs [13]. IgG antiplatelet autoantibodies are produced not only by B cells but also by plasma cells; this has been confirmed by partial suppression of antiplatelet antibody production by depletion of $CD20^+$ B cells [14]. Based on accumulating insights of roles of GPIIb/IIIa-reactive $CD4^+$ T cells and B cells in the antiplatelet autoimmune responses, we have proposed a "pathogenic loop" model for the ongoing IgG antiplatelet autoantibody response in ITP patients (Fig. 1) [11]. Namely, macrophages in the reticuloendothelial system capture opsonized platelets via Fcγ receptors and present antigenic platelet GP-derived "cryptic" peptides to T cells in the context of HLA class II molecule. Autoreactive $CD4^+$ T cells to GPIIb/IIIa are then activated by recognition of the antigenic peptides and exert helper activity to stimulate B cells to proliferate, differentiate into plasmoblasts, and produce IgG antiplatelet autoantibodies, which in turn bind to circulating platelets. Theoretically, once this pathogenic loop is established, the production of IgG antiplatelet autoantibodies is endless, irrespective of the triggers that initiated this response.

The majority of current treatment regimens for ITP are aimed to interrupt this pathogenic loop and thereby suppress production of antiplatelet autoantibodies and result in platelet recovery. Specifically, corticosteroids suppress overall immune responses, while splenectomy removes the major site for this pathogenic loop. Cytotoxic immunosuppressants, such as cyclophosphamide and azathioprine, inhibit proliferation of both T and B cells, while cyclosporine and tacrolimus selectively inhibit T-cell activation and rituximab depletes $CD20^+$ B cells. One of the immune regulatory mechanisms involved in the pathogenic process of ITP is an inhibitory Fcγ receptor FcγRIIB expressed on reticuloendothelial macrophages. Interestingly, platelet recovery observed in ITP patients after eradication of *Helicobacter pylori* or treatment of thrombopoietin (TPO) receptor agonists is mediated through a change in Fcγ receptor balance toward the inhibitory FcγRIIB [15, 16].

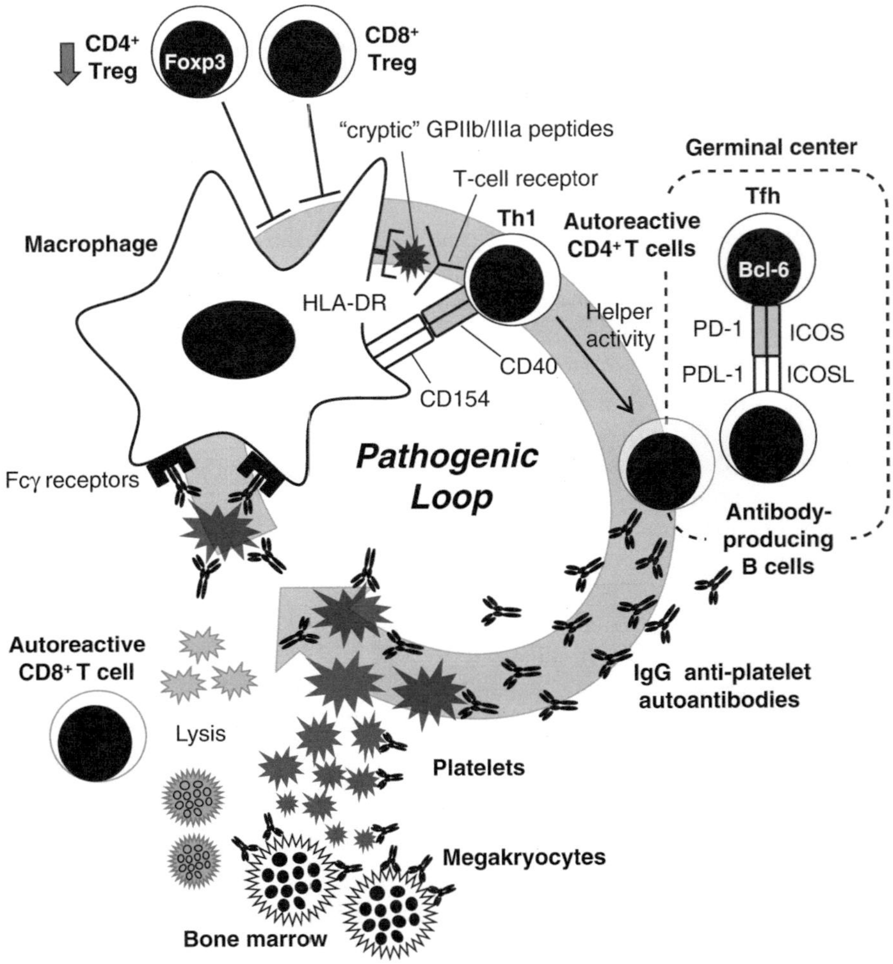

Fig. 1 A schematic model representing the continuous pathogenic loop of ITP, which is carried out by macrophages in the reticuloendothelial system, antibody-producing B cells, and a variety of autoreactive T-cell subsets

3 Dysregulated Treg Function

Tregs are subpopulations of CD4+ T cells specialized in immune suppression and include a variety of subsets, such as Tregs expressing transcription factor forkhead box P3 (Foxp3), T-regulatory 1 (Tr1) cells, and Th3 cells. The negative selection process in the thymus deletes T cells reactive with autoantigenic peptides presented by thymic epithelial cells in high affinity and plays a critical role in the maintenance of central immune tolerance. However, a subset of autoreactive T cells, including those reactive with autoantigenic "cryptic" peptides that are not efficiently expressed in the thymus, escape from the negative selection process and are delivered to periphery. These autoreactive T cells are subsequently suppressed or deleted in periphery through Treg-mediated mechanisms, but Treg deficiency potentially leads to onset of harmful autoimmune conditions [17]. In fact, a reduced frequency of Tregs and defective function of Tregs have been reported in patients with various autoimmune diseases, including type 1 diabetes, multiple sclerosis, and systemic lupus erythematosus [18].

Given a critical role of Tregs in preventing the autoimmune response, dysregulation of Tregs could also be associated with pathophysiology of ITP. Multiple research groups have examined quantity of Foxp3 Tregs in patients with ITP. The majority of studies demonstrated a decreased frequency of Foxp3 Tregs in peripheral blood $CD4^+$ T cells in ITP patients, compared with healthy controls [8]. Some studies failed to represent a significant difference in Treg frequencies between ITP patients and healthy controls, but these inconsistent results might be explained by use of different phenotypes for identification of Foxp3 Tregs, i.e., $CD4^+CD25^{high}$, $CD4^+Foxp3^+$, $CD4^+CD25^{high}Foxp3^+$, and $CD4^+CD25^+CD127^{low}$. The lowest Foxp3 Treg frequency is detected in patients with acute phase of the disease and/or in those with low platelet count, and Foxp3 Treg count is recovered in remission. Foxp3 Treg frequency is also decreased in the bone marrow and spleen from patients with ITP [19–21]. A recent histologic analysis of ITP spleens has found reduced Foxp3 Tregs within the germinal center and proliferative lymphoid nodule, which accommodate B cells proliferating upon antigenic stimulation. In addition, Treg's immunosuppressive function assessed using a principle of allogeneic T-cell response is shown to be inferior in ITP patients than in controls [22–25]. Finally, several studies have evaluated serial changes in frequency and function of Foxp3 Tregs before and after the treatment. High-dose dexamethasone and rituximab increase the proportion of Foxp3 Tregs in responders [24, 26], whereas TPO receptor agonists fail to increase Treg frequency, but improve Treg function [22].

The reduced number and impaired function of Foxp3 Tregs in ITP patients suggest that dysregulation of the peripheral immune tolerance may contribute to development of ITP. This hypothesis has been tested using Foxp3 Treg-deficient mice, which are generated by transferring Foxp3 Treg-depleted $CD4^+CD25^-$ T cells isolated from BALB/c mice into syngeneic nude mice [27]. Three weeks after transfer, approximately one third of Treg-deficient mice spontaneously develop bruises in association with thrombocytopenia, which sustains for at least 12 weeks. IgG antibodies capable of binding to platelets are detected in platelet eluates and in splenocyte culture supernatants from thrombocytopenic Foxp3 Treg-deficient mice. The primary target of antiplatelet autoantibodies produced in these mice was identified as GPIb/IX [28]. These findings indicate that thrombocytopenia observed in Foxp3 Treg-deficient mice is mediated through production of IgG antiplatelet autoantibodies, which is analogous to human ITP. In addition, Foxp3 Tregs can suppress effector T-cell responses through various mechanisms, and we have found that Foxp3 Treg's immunosuppressive property is primarily mediated through engaging cytotoxic T lymphocyte antigen 4 (CTLA4), which suppresses T-cell activation by inhibiting a critical co-stimulatory interaction between CD28 and CD80/CD86. Interestingly, we have happened to find short-term treatment with recombinant TPO could promote the peripheral induction of Foxp3 Tregs and suppress specific T-cell responses to platelet GPs in Foxp3 Treg-deficient mice [29]. This may explain why some patients treated with TPO receptor antagonists maintain their platelet count after cessation of the drug [30]. In another ITP model mouse, in which GPIIIa knockout mice are immunized with wild-type platelets and their splenocytes are transferred into severe combined immunodeficiency mice, severe fatal thrombocytopenia occurs through production of IgG antiplatelet antibodies and induction of platelet-reactive cytotoxic T cells [31]. Interestingly, in this model, Foxp3 Tregs are increased in the thymus, but are decreased in the spleen, in comparison with control mice, proposing an intriguing theory that peripheral Foxp3 Treg deficiency is caused by thymic retention [32]. Therefore, Foxp3 Treg deficiency in secondary lymphoid organs is one of the critical mechanisms that develop and maintain the pathogenic loop of ITP (Fig. 1).

4 Tfh Cells in the Spleen

Tfh cells are a specialized CD4$^+$ T subset that supports B-cell maturation and differentiation within the germinal center [33]. They can be identified by a combination of markers, including high expression of chemokine C-X-C motif receptor 5 (CXCR5), inducible co-stimulator (ICOS), programmed cell death 1 (PD-1), and the transcription repressor B cell lymphoma 6. In the germinal center, Tfh cells interact with antigen-specific B cells through various interactions, such as ICOS-ICOS ligand, PD-1-PD ligand-1, CD40-CD154, and IL-21 receptor-IL-21 in an antigen-dependent and/or -independent manner, resulting in maturation into specialized memory B cells and plasma cells. Increased numbers of Tfh cells and/or dysregulated Tfh function contribute to the development of autoimmune phenotype in mouse models, and expansion of Tfh cells has been reported in peripheral blood from patients with various autoimmune diseases, including systemic lupus erythematosus, Sjögren's syndrome, rheumatoid arthritis, myasthenia gravis, and autoimmune thyroid disease [33–35]. With respect to ITP, some studies have reported an increased proportion of circulating Tfh cells in ITP patients compared to healthy controls and a positive correlation between the percentages of Tfh cells and anti-GPIIb/IIIa or anti-GPIb/IX antibodies [36, 37]. Interestingly, an increased frequency of Tfh cells was also observed in the spleen of ITP patients, and the Tfh proportion was correlated with the expansion of the germinal center structure [4]. In addition, CXCR5 is a B-cell zone homing chemokine receptor and is required for T-cell migration into the follicles for their co-localization with B cells, in response to the specific ligand CXCL13, which is elevated in circulation of ITP patients [38, 39]. Taken together, expansion of Tfh cells in the germinal center of the spleen from ITP patients may promote generation and maintenance of B cells and plasma cells that produce high-affinity IgG antiplatelet autoantibodies, although whether this process is antigen-specific is still controversial.

5 Effector and Regulatory CD8+ T Cells

T-cell-mediated cytotoxicity is an alternative mechanism for platelet destruction in patients with ITP. The involvement of CD8+ CTLs in pathogenic process of ITP was first shown by increased expression of genes involved in cell-mediated cytotoxicity in circulating CD3+ T cells derived from ITP patients [6]. In this landmark study, the authors have successfully demonstrated that CD8+ CTLs from ITP patients are able to induce direct platelet apoptosis or lysis in vitro. In addition, CD8+ T cells in the bone marrow of ITP patients are shown to suppress thrombocytopoiesis by triggering apoptosis and inhibition of maturation in megakaryocytes, leading to a decrease in platelet production, which could be successfully corrected by high-dose dexamethasone [40]. In the ITP mouse model generated by induction of the isoimmune response to GPIIIa followed by transplantation of immune repertoire into severe combined immunodeficiency mice, CD8+ CTLs attack megakaryocytes in the bone marrow and almost completely inhibit platelet production [31]. Using this mouse model, it has been shown that B-cell depletion by treatment with anti-CD20 monoclonal antibody results in suppression of splenic CD8+ CTL proliferation together with normalization of platelet counts [41]. Recently, anti-GPIbα antibodies, but not anti-GPIIb/IIIa antibodies, were shown to induce Fc-independent platelet activation, sialidase neuraminidase-1 translocation, and desialylation, leading to platelet clearance in the liver [42]. This Fc-independent platelet clearance mechanism is fundamentally different from the classical Fc-Fcγ receptor-dependent mechanism, which is mediated through macrophage phagocytosis in the reticuloendothelial system. Moreover, this analogous mechanism is mediated by CD8+ T cells, which induce platelet desialylation and subsequently promote platelet clearance in the liver [43]. Thus, IL-27 may be a promising therapeutic targeting CD8+ T cells in ITP patients because of its ability to inhibit CTL-mediated platelet destruction in vitro [44].

Several lines of recent studies indicate there is a subset of CD8+ cells with regulatory function called CD8+ Tregs [45, 46]. These Tregs exert their immunosuppressive property against effector CD4+ cells and B cells via a cell-cell contact through direct lysis and/or secretion of soluble negative regulates, such as IL-10 and TGF-β. In vitro co-culture studies have revealed that CD8+ Tregs effectively inhibited proliferation of CD4+ T cells and B cells, resulting in suppression of antiplatelet-autoantibody production in the murine model of ITP [7]. In addition, corticosteroid therapy decreased effector CD4+ T cells and B cells, but expanded CD8+ Tregs.

6 Conclusions

A recent accumulating evidence in ITP patients and ITP mouse models has shown that a variety of T cell subsets are involved in pathogenic process of ITP, by promoting IgG antiplatelet autoantibody production and inducing CTLs with capacity to target platelets and megakaryocytes. The elucidation of mechanisms underlying the updated "pathogenic loop" model for the pathophysiology of ITP (Fig. 1) would be useful in developing novel therapeutic strategies.

Acknowledgments We dedicate this chapter to the late Tetsuya Nishimoto, who had contributed to elucidation of autoimmune mechanisms of ITP.

References

1. Cines DB, Blanchette VS. Immune thrombocytopenic purpura. N Engl J Med. 2002;346:995–1008.
2. McMillan R. Autoantibodies and autoantigens in chronic immune thrombocytopenic purpura. Semin Hematol. 2000;37:239–48.
3. Semple JW, Provan D. The immunopathogenesis of immune thrombocytopenia: T cells still take center-stage. Curr Opin Hematol. 2012;19:357–62.
4. Audia S, Rossato M, Santegoets K, et al. Splenic TFH expansion participates in B-cell differentiation and antiplatelet-antibody production during immune thrombocytopenia. Blood. 2014;124:2858–66.
5. Kuwana M, Kaburaki J, Ikeda Y. Autoreactive T cells to platelet GPIIb-IIIa in immune thrombocytopenic purpura. Role in production of anti-platelet autoantibody. J Clin Invest. 1998;102:1393–402.
6. Olsson B, Andersson PO, Jernas M, et al. T-cell-mediated cytotoxicity toward platelets in chronic idiopathic thrombocytopenic purpura. Nat Med. 2003;9:1123–4.
7. Ma L, Simpson E, Li J, et al. $CD8^{+}$ T cells are predominantly protective and required for effective steroid therapy in murine models of immune thrombocytopenia. Blood. 2015;126:247–56.
8. Nishimoto T, Kuwana M. $CD4^{+}CD25^{+}Foxp3^{+}$ regulatory T cells in the pathophysiology of immune thrombocytopenia. Semin Hematol. 2013;1:S43–9.
9. Kuwana M, Kawakami Y, Ikeda Y. Suppression of autoreactive T-cell response to glycoprotein IIb/IIIa by blockade of CD40/CD154 interaction: implications for treatment of immune thrombocytopenic purpura. Blood. 2003;101:621–3.
10. Meabed MH, Taha GM, Mohamed SO, et al. Autoimmune thrombocytopenia: flow cytometric determination of platelet-associated CD154/CD40L and CD40 on peripheral blood T and B lymphocytes. Hematology. 2007;12:301–7.
11. Kuwana M, Okazaki Y, Ikeda Y. Splenic macrophages maintain the anti-platelet autoimmune response via uptake of opsonized platelets in patients with immune thrombocytopenic purpura. J Thromb Haemost. 2009;7:322–9.
12. Kuwana M, Okazaki Y, Kaburaki J, et al. Spleen is a primary site for activation of platelet-reactive T and B cells in patients with immune thrombocytopenic purpura. J Immunol. 2002;168:3675–82.
13. Daridon C, Loddenkemper C, Spieckermann S, et al. Splenic proliferative lymphoid nodules distinct from germinal centers are sites of autoantigen stimulation in immune thrombocytopenia. Blood. 2012;120:5021–31.
14. Mahévas M, Patin P, Huetz F, et al. B cell depletion in immune thrombocytopenia reveals splenic long-lived plasma cell. J Clin Invest. 2013;123:432–42.
15. Asahi A, Nishimoto T, Okazaki Y, et al. *Helicobacter pylori* eradication shifts monocytes Fcγ receptor balance toward inhibitory FcγRIIB in immune thrombocytopenic purpura patients. J Clin Invest. 2008;118:2939–49.
16. Lui XG, Liu S, Feng Q, et al. Thrombopoietin receptor agonists shift the balance of Fcγ receptors toward inhibitory receptor IIb on monocytes in ITP. Blood. 2016;128:852–61.

17. Sakaguchi S, Miyara M, Costantino CM, et al. Foxp3+ regulatory T cells in the human immune system. Nat Rev Immunol. 2010;10:490–500.
18. Buckner JH. Mechanisms of impaired regulation by CD4+CD25+Foxp3+ regulatory T cells in human autoimmune diseases. Nat Rev Immunol. 2010;10:849–59.
19. Audia S, Samson M, Guy J, et al. Immunologic effects of rituximab on the human spleen in immune thrombocytopenia. Blood. 2011;118:4394–400.
20. Olsson B, Ridell B, Carlsson L, et al. Recruitment of T cells into bone marrow of ITP patients possibly due to elevated expression of VLA-4 and CX3CR1. Blood. 2008;112:1078–84.
21. Song Y, Wang YT, Huang XJ, et al. Abnormalities of the bone marrow immune microenvironment in patients with immune thrombocytopenia. Ann Hematol. 2016;95:959–65.
22. Bao W, Bussel JB, Heck S, et al. Improved regulatory T-cell activity in patients with chronic immune thrombocytopenia treated with thrombopoietic agents. Blood. 2010;116:4639–45.
23. Liu B, Zhao H, Poon MC, et al. Abnormality of CD4(+)CD25(+) regulatory T cells in idiopathic thrombocytopenic purpura. Eur J Haematol. 2007;78:139–43.
24. Stasi R, Cooper N, Del Poeta G, et al. Analysis of regulatory T-cell changes in patients with idiopathic thrombocytopenic purpura receiving B cell-depleting therapy with rituximab. Blood. 2008;112:1147–50.
25. Yu J, Heck S, Patel V, et al. Defective circulating CD25 regulatory T cells in patients with chronic immune thrombocytopenic purpura. Blood. 2008;112:1325–8.
26. Ling Y, Cao X, Yu Z, et al. Circulating dendritic cells subsets and CD4+Foxp3+ regulatory T cells in adult patients with chronic ITP before and after treatment with high-dose dexamethasome. Eur J Haematol. 2007;79:310–6.
27. Nishimoto T, Satoh T, Takeuchi T, et al. Critical role of CD4(+)CD25(+) regulatory T cells in preventing murine autoantibody-mediated thrombocytopenia. Exp Hematol. 2012;40:279–89.
28. Nishimoto T, Satoh T, Simpson EK, et al. Predominant autoantibody response to GPIb/IX in a regulatory T-cell-deficient mouse model for immune thrombocytopenia. J Thromb Haemost. 2013;11:369–72.
29. Nishimoto T, Numajiri M, Nakazaki H, et al. Induction of immune tolerance to platelet antigen by short-term thrombopoietin treatment in a mouse model of immune thrombocytopenia. Int J Hematol. 2014;100:341–4.
30. González-López TJ, Pascual C, Álvarez-Román MT, et al. Successful discontinuation of eltrombopag after complete remission in patients with primary immune thrombocytopenia. Am J Hematol. 2015;90:E40–3.
31. Chow L, Aslam R, Speck ER, et al. A murine model of severe immune thrombocytopenia is induced by antibody- and CD8+ T cell-mediated responses that are differentially sensitive to therapy. Blood. 2010;115:1247–53.
32. Aslam R, Hu Y, Gebremeskel S, et al. Thymic retention of CD4+CD25+Foxp3+ T regulatory cells is associated with their peripheral deficiency and thrombocytopenia in a murine model of immune thrombocytopenia. Blood. 2012;120:2127–32.
33. Crotty S. T follicular helper cell differentiation, function, and roles in disease. Immunity. 2014;41:529–42.
34. Craft JE. Follicular helper T cells in immunity and systemic autoimmunity. Nat Rev Rheumatol. 2012;8:337–47.
35. Ma CS, Deenick EK. Human T follicular helper (Tfh) cells and disease. Immunol Cell Biol. 2014;92:64–71.
36. Xie J, Cui D, Liu Y, et al. Changes in follicular helper T cells in idiopathic thrombocytopenic purpura patients. Int J Biol Sci. 2015;11:220–9.
37. Yao X, Li C, Yang J, et al. Differences in frequency and regulation of T follicular helper cells between newly diagnosed and chronic pediatric immune thrombocytopenia. Blood Cells Mol Dis. 2016;61:26–36.
38. Jernas M, Nookaew I, Wadenvik H, et al. MicroRNA regulate immunological pathways in T-cells in immune thrombocytopenia (ITP). Blood. 2013;121:2095–8.
39. Li JQ, Hu SY, Wang ZY, et al. MicroRNA-125-5p targeted CXCL13: a potential biomarker associated with immune thrombocytopenia. Am J Transl Res. 2015b;15:772–80.

40. Li S, Wang L, Zhao C, et al. CD8+ T cells suppress autologous megakaryocyte apoptosis in idiopathic thrombocytopenic purpura. Br J Haematol. 2007;139:605–11.
41. Guo L, Kapur R, Aslam R, et al. CD20+ B-cell depletion therapy suppresses murine CD8+ T-cell-mediated immune thrombocytopenia. Blood. 2016;127:735–8.
42. Li J, van der Wal DE, Zhu G, et al. Desialylation is a mechanism of Fc-independent platelet clearance and a therapeutic target in immune thrombocytopenia. Nat Commun. 2015a;6:7737.
43. Qiu J, Liu X, Li X, et al. CD8(+) T cells induce platelet clearance in the liver via platelet desialylation in immune thrombocytopenia. Sci Rep. 2016;6:27445.
44. Zhou H, Qiu JH, Wang T, et al. Interleukin 27 inhibits cytotoxic T-lymphocyte-mediated platelet destruction in primary immune thrombocytopenia. Blood. 2014;124:3316–9.
45. Lu L, Cantor H. Generation and regulation of CD8(+) regulatory T cells. Cell Mol Immunol. 2008;5:401–6.
46. Tsai YG, Yang KD, Niu DM, et al. TLR2 agonists enhance CD8+Foxp3 regulatory T cells and suppress Th2 immune responses during allergen immunotherapy. J Immunol. 2010;184:7229–37.

Part V
Adult ITP

ITP in Adults

Hirokazu Kashiwagi and Yoshiaki Tomiyama

Abstract Most cases of adult ITP are chronic form, and the onset of the disease is usually insidious. Signs and symptoms vary widely in each case from no hemorrhagic symptom to severe life-threatening bleeding, such as intracranial hemorrhage. In addition to hemorrhagic symptom, treatment-related complications, such as infection and cardiovascular diseases, may lead to poor quality of life of ITP patients. Increase of thrombosis in ITP patients is also demonstrated in epidemiologic studies. Once diagnosed with ITP, screening and eradication of *H. pylori* should be performed in the regions of its high prevalence like Japan. After exclusion of *H. pylori*-associated ITP, treatment of ITP should be initiated to maintain safe platelet counts as a goal. First-line treatment is corticosteroids and second-line is splenectomy. For refractory ITP patients, thrombopoietin receptor agonists are highly recommended. Rituximab may be another option to get sustained response.

1 Clinical Course of Adult ITP

Primary ITP is classified into two categories, acute and chronic ITP, and they differ in incidence, bleeding symptoms, and prognosis (Table 1). Typical ITP in adults is a chronic disease, and the onset of the disease is usually insidious in contrast to children, in which ITP is usually "acute" form preceded by a viral infection, and spontaneous recovery of platelet counts may occur in as many as 90% patients within 6 months [1]. Signs and symptoms vary widely in each case. Severe life-threatening bleeding, such as intracranial hemorrhage (ICH), may be developed; however, hemorrhagic symptoms are often absent or minimal [2, 3], and

H. Kashiwagi, M.D. (✉)
Department of Hematology and Oncology, Graduate School of Medicine, Osaka University, 2-2 Yamadaoka, Suita, Osaka 565-0871, Japan
e-mail: kashi@hp-blood.med.osaka-u.ac.jp

Y. Tomiyama, M.D.
Department of Blood Transfusion, Osaka University Hospital, 2-15 Yamadaoka, Suita, Osaka 565-0871, Japan
e-mail: yoshi@hp-blood.med.osaka-u.ac.jp

Y. Ishida, Y. Tomiyama (eds.), *Autoimmune Thrombocytopenia*, DOI 10.1007/978-981-10-4142-6_7

Table 1 Clinical features of acute and chronic ITP

	Acute ITP	Chronic ITP
Peak age of incidence	Children (2–5 years)	Adults (20–40, 60–80 years)
Sex difference	Female/male = 1:1	Young onset Female/male = 3:1 Old onset Female/male = 1:1
Seasonal predilection	Winter–Spring	None
Antecedent infection	Common (1–3 weeks before) Vaccination	Unusual
Onset of bleeding	Abrupt	Insidious
Bleeding symptoms	Severe (hemorrhagic bullae in mouth is present in severe cases)	Absent in many cases
Prognosis	Spontaneous remissions occur within 6–12 months (an average of 4–6 weeks)	Persist more than 12 months

thrombocytopenia is accidentally identified by routine blood examination in a substantial part of cases. Spontaneous remissions are uncommon, but they do occur in up to 10% in adults with ITP. These usually occur early in the onset of the disease, which are classified as acute ITP; however, spontaneous remissions are possible even after observation periods of 6 months or more [4]. Now, chronicity of ITP is judged on 12 months from diagnosis, and all cases within 3 months from diagnosis are defined as "newly diagnosed" ITP, and cases between 3 and 12 months from diagnosis including patients not reaching spontaneous remission or not maintaining complete response off therapy are defined as "persistent" ITP [5]. Although results of some long-term follow-up studies suggest that ITP is a more benign disease than previously thought [3, 6, 7], a systemic review of prospective clinical studies reported that ICH and non-ICH severe bleeding may occur in 1.4 and 9.6% of patients, respectively [8]. There are also treatment-associated complications, such as infection and cardiovascular diseases, which may affect mortality and quality of life of ITP patients. Studies conducted in Holland, the United Kingdom, and Denmark reported that relative risks (RR) of mortality with adult ITP patients are ranging from 1.3 to 2.2 compared with general population [6, 9–11].

2 Clinical Manifestations

2.1 Hemorrhagic Manifestations

Platelets are essential for primary hemostasis, and thrombocytopenia leads to failure of prevention of blood leakage from small blood vessels. Purpura is the most frequent bleeding symptom in ITP. Purpura includes skin bleeding and mucous membrane bleeding, which are often referred as "dry" and "wet" purpura, respectively [12].

Since wet purpura is usually associated with lower platelet counts and the complication rates higher in those with wet purpura compared with dry purpura [1], wet purpura has been presumed as a sign of serious danger in patients [13]. However, there are no retrospective or prospective data to support the linkage of wet purpura and ICH [14].

Skin and Visual Mucous Membranes

Spontaneous bleeding into the skin is characteristic in ITP. Skin bleeding is classified into petechiae or ecchymosis by size. Petechiae is a red (recent) or purplish (a few days old) discoloration in the epidermis and dermis with a diameter of 0.5–3 mm, and ecchymosis is larger than a petechiae with red, blue, purplish, or yellowish green color [12]. In ITP, subcutaneous hematomas without contusions are rare. Gingival bleeding and epistaxis are common, and hemorrhagic bulla in the oral cavity may be seen in cases of severe thrombocytopenia.

Internal Mucosae of Organs

Bleeding in the genitourinary tract is common in ITP. Menorrhagia may be the only symptom of ITP. Hematuria is also a common symptom, although severe bleeding is rare. Severe bleeding in gastrointestinal tract is possible but rare even in patients with persistent low platelet counts [15].

The Central Nervous System

Although ICH is the most serious complication of ITP, it is fortunately uncommon. A systemic review of all prospective ITP studies that enrolled 20 or more patients showed that the rates of ICH were 1.4% in adults and 0.4% in children [8]. Higher incidence of ICH in cases of more than 60 years with low platelet counts is also reported [15], which may be due to frequent comorbidities or anti-hemostatic medications.

2.2 *Thrombosis*

Although thrombosis has not been considered a part of the spectrum of ITP manifestations, recent epidemiologic studies have revealed unexpected increase of thrombosis in ITP patients [16]. Four epidemiologic studies using large-scale databases from Denmark, the United Kingdom, the United States, and Sweden have been reported [17–21], and a meta-analysis of these observational studies showed that the incidence of arterial thromboembolism per 100 patient-years ranged from

1.0 to 2.8 among ITP patients and from 0.7 to 1.8 among populations without ITP; RR was 1.5 [95% confidence interval (CI): 1.3–1.8] [22]. The incidence of venous thromboembolism was also increased among ITP patients [ITP 0.4–0.7, without ITP 0.1–0.4 per 100 patient-years; RR 1.9 (1.4–2.7)] [22]. Several possible mechanisms of increase of thrombosis in ITP patients have been proposed, which are associated with ITP itself or ITP treatments. Increase of procoagulant microparticles has been reported in ITP [23], and endothelial damages caused by anti-GPIIIa antibodies [24] or antiphospholipid antibodies [25] may also affect the development of thrombosis. More importantly, many of ITP treatments, e.g., corticosteroids, high-dose intravenous immunoglobulin (IVIG), splenectomy, and thrombopoietin receptor agonists (TPO-RAs), may increase risk of thrombosis.

2.3 Treatment-Related Manifestations

A recent Danish population-based cohort study showed increased risk of mortality in ITP patients compared with the general population cohort due to cardiovascular disease (hazard ratio 1.5, 95% CI: 1.1–1.5), infection (2.4, 1.0–5.7), and hematological cancer (5.7, 2.1–15.7) in addition to bleeding (6.2, 2.8–13.25) [9]. These results suggest that ITP treatment-related comorbidities significantly affect prognosis of patients with ITP. Long-term administration of corticosteroids increases the risk of cardiovascular disease, and immunosuppressive therapy, including corticosteroids, increases the risk of infection and malignancy [26–28]. Splenectomy also increases the risk of severe infection [29, 30].

2.4 Quality of Life

Although prognosis of chronic ITP patients is fairly favorable even in the cases with severe thrombocytopenia, ITP itself and its treatments have significant impacts on daily life and physical, psychological, and social functioning. Studies using a health-related quality of life (HRQoL) questionnaire, which is a typical assessment tool of QoL, have been shown that the HRQoL of adult ITP patients was significantly worse than that of control population [31, 32]. In one study, HRQoL was worse than that of patients with hypertension, arthritis, or cancer and similar to that of patients with diabetes mellitus [31]. Fatigue is one of the common and distressful symptoms for patients with a chronic disease. It has been shown that a significant proportion of ITP patients suffer from fatigue, and many feel that they have less energy when the platelet count is low [33]. Despite improvement of thrombocytopenia, bleeding episodes, and QoL, TPO-RAs fail to show a consistent and clinically significant improvement in fatigue [34, 35], suggesting that fatigue in ITP patients is not simply associated with disease severity, and its mechanism is likely to be complex [33].

3 Algorithm of Treatment of Adult Chronic ITP

Before starting treatment of ITP, special attention to thrombocytopenia associated with *H. pylori* infection is needed in the regions of its high prevalence. Since a high prevalence of *H. pylori* and a high platelet response rate to its eradication are well demonstrated in Japan [36], a recent Japanese reference guide for management of adult chronic ITP recommends to screening and eradication of *H. pylori* when ITP is suspected, irrespective of platelet counts (Fig. 1) [37]. However, the value of the screening and eradication of *H. pylori* is uncertain in the regions of its low prevalence and a low platelet response to its eradication, like the United States [36, 38].

After exclusion of *H. pylori*-associated ITP, treatment of ITP should be initiated to maintain safe platelet counts as a goal. Although the safe platelet count may depend on age, comorbidities, and lifestyle of each patient, several observational studies have suggested that bleeding risk is increased with platelets below 20–30 × 10^3/μL [6, 15]. Therefore, many guidelines recommend treating patients with platelets below 20–30 × 10^3/μL and/or severe bleeding ([37, 39–42]). First-line treatment is corticosteroids, usually prednisolone. Seventy to eighty percent of patients will respond to prednisolone initially; however, sustained response would be achieved to a limited portion of patients, and 10-year disease-free survival is estimated as 13–15% [42]. Some studies demonstrated better sustained response of high-dose dexamethasone (HD-DEX) [43, 44]. A recent prospective randomized study performed in China showed that one or two courses of HD-DEX provided better initial response and less toxicity compared with conventional prednisolone therapy with the same sustained response rate [45]. Splenectomy has been recommended for corticosteroid-resistant patients as a second-line treatment. Splenectomy has a

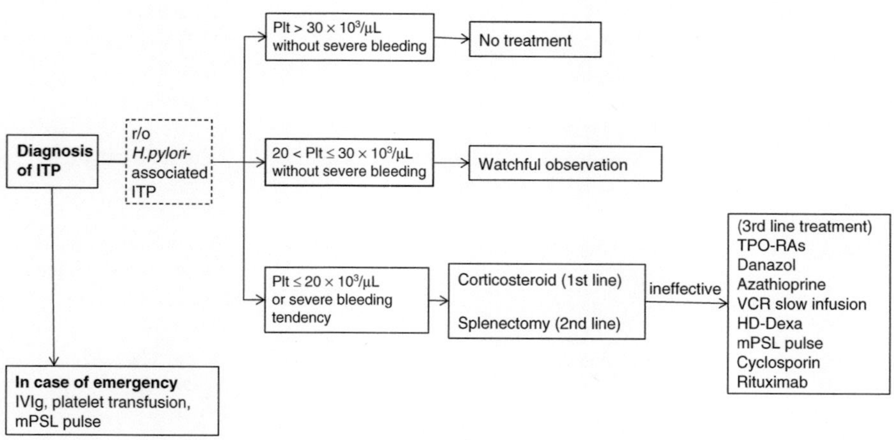

Fig. 1 The 2012 reference guide for management of adult chronic ITP published from the study group of the Specified Disease Treatment Research Program for Intractable Diseases of the Ministry of Health, Labour and Welfare of Japan [37]. *IVIG* intravenous immunoglobulin, *mPSL* methylprednisolone, *TPO-RAs* thrombopoietin receptor agonists, *VCR* vincristine, *HD-Dexa* high-dose dexamethasone

60-year record of success for achieving durable remissions in approximately two-thirds of patients [46]. However, splenectomy increases lifelong risk of severe infection and thrombosis [29]. In elder patients, splenectomy may often be contraindicated because of comorbidity, and a favorable response may be less common in elder patients than in young patients [47]. For refractory ITP patients in whom splenectomy has failed or is avoided by patients' and/or doctors' decision, many drugs have been recommended as third-line treatments, although consistent better outcomes to refractory patients by randomized studies have been shown only in TPO-RAs. Two TPO-RAs, romiplostim and eltrombopag, are currently approved for use in adult ITP in Japan [48]. Randomized studies demonstrate that both drugs are highly effective in both splenectomized and non-splenectomized patients with minimal complications [49, 50]. Extended studies show sustained response and no increase of additional side effects in patients treated with TPO-RAs for up to 5 years [51, 52]. Off-label use of the anti-CD20 antibody rituximab to refractory ITP patients has been widely performed [53], and rituximab provides initial response rates of around 60% and sustained response rates of 20–30% [54]. Other third-line treatments may be also effective in some refractory cases [42, 55] (Table 2); however, the chances of

Table 2 Treatment options for adult ITP [42, 55]

	Dose	Response rate (%)	Time to response	Major toxicities
Azathioprine	1–2 mg/kg/day	40–60	3–6 months	Hepatotoxicity Neutropenia Pancreatitis
Cyclosporine	5–6 mg/kg/day	30–60	3–4 weeks	Neurotoxicity Hypertension Paresthesia Gingival hyperplasia
Cyclophosphamide	0.3–1.0 g/m^2 iv for 1–3 doses or 1–2 mg/kg orally	24–85	1–16 weeks	Neutropenia Nausea
Danazol	50–800 mg/day	10–70	3–6 months	Hepatotoxicity Acne Virilization
Dapsone	75–100 mg	40–75	3 weeks	Hemolysis (in patients with G6PD deficiency) Rash Nausea
Mycophenolate mofetil	250–1000 mg	11–80	4–6 weeks	Headache Diarrhea Nausea Anorexia
Vinca alkaloids	Vincristine: 1–2 mg iv weekly × 3 weeks Vinblastine: 10 mg iv weekly × 3 weeks	10–75	5–7 days	Peripheral neuropathy Fever Neutropenia

Steroids, IVIG, splenectomy, TPO-RAs, and rituximab are described in other chapters administration of these drugs are very limited in these days because of considerable toxicity of these drugs and availability of TPO-RAs in addition to no approval for usage in ITP.

In case of a requirement of rapid platelet increase because of bleeding emergency, surgical procedure, or delivery, IVIG is recommended [37, 39–42]. Administration of 5 days of 0.4 g/kg/day or 1–2 days of 1 g/kg/day IVIG leads to transient increase of platelet with peak on about 1 week after treatment in ~80% patients [42]. High-dose methylprednisolone may also be effective for rapid increase of platelet [56]. Platelet transfusion may be also effective for bleeding emergency, although higher dose of platelet concentrates may be required because of rapid turnover of infused platelets [57]. Platelet transfusion combined with IVIG may work better for rapid restoration of adequate platelet counts [58].

Acknowledgment This work was supported by Grant-in-Aid for Scientific Research from the Ministry of Education, Culture, Sports, Science and Technology and the Ministry of Health, Labour and Welfare in Japan.

References

1. Liel MS, Michae R, Calverley DC. Thrombocytopenia caused by immunologic platelet destruction. In: Greer JP, Arber DA, Glader B, List AF, Means Jr RT, Paraskevas F, Rodgers GM, editors. Wintrobe's clinical hematology. 13th ed. Philadelphia, PA: Lippincott Williams & Wilkins; 2014. p. 1061–76.
2. Frederiksen H, Schmidt K. The incidence of idiopathic thrombocytopenic purpura in adults increases with age. Blood. 1999;94(3):909–13.
3. Neylon AJ, Saunders PW, Howard MR, Proctor SJ, Taylor PR. Clinically significant newly presenting autoimmune thrombocytopenic purpura in adults: a prospective study of a population-based cohort of 245 patients. Br J Haematol. 2003;122(6):966–74.
4. Stasi R, Stipa E, Masi M, Cecconi M, Scimò MT, Oliva F, et al. Long-term observation of 208 adults with chronic idiopathic thrombocytopenic purpura. Am J Med. 1995b;98(5):436–42.
5. Rodeghiero F, Stasi R, Gernsheimer T, Michel M, Provan D, Arnold DM, et al. Standardization of terminology, definitions and outcome criteria in immune thrombocytopenic purpura of adults and children: report from an international working group. Blood. 2009;113(11):2386–93.
6. Portielje JE, Westendorp RG, Kluin-Nelemans HC, Brand A. Morbidity and mortality in adults with idiopathic thrombocytopenic purpura. Blood. 2001;97(9):2549–54.
7. Stasi R, Stipa E, Masi M, Cecconi M, Scimo MT, Oliva F, et al. Long-term observation of 208 adults with chronic idiopathic thrombocytopenic purpura. Am J Med. 1995a;98(5):436–42.
8. Neunert C, Noroozi N, Norman G, Buchanan GR, Goy J, Nazi I, et al. Severe bleeding events in adults and children with primary immune thrombocytopenia: a systematic review. J Thromb Haemost. 2015;13(3):457–64.
9. Frederiksen H, Maegbaek ML, Norgaard M. Twenty-year mortality of adult patients with primary immune thrombocytopenia: a Danish population-based cohort study. Br J Haematol. 2014;166(2):260–7.
10. Norgaard M, Jensen AO, Engebjerg MC, Farkas DK, Thomsen RW, Cha S, et al. Long-term clinical outcomes of patients with primary chronic immune thrombocytopenia: a Danish population-based cohort study. Blood. 2011;117(13):3514–20.
11. Schoonen WM, Kucera G, Coalson J, Li L, Rutstein M, Mowat F, et al. Epidemiology of immune thrombocytopenic purpura in the General Practice Research Database. Br J Haematol. 2009;145(2):235–44.

12. Rodeghiero F, Michel M, Gernsheimer T, Ruggeri M, Blanchette V, Bussel JB, et al. Standardization of bleeding assessment in immune thrombocytopenia: report from the International Working Group. Blood. 2013a;121(14):2596–606.
13. Crosby WH. Editorial: wet purpura, dry purpura. JAMA. 1975;232(7):744–5.
14. Neunert CE. Individualized treatment for immune thrombocytopenia: predicting bleeding risk. Semin Hematol. 2013;50(Suppl 1):S55–7.
15. Cohen YC, Djulbegovic B, Shamai-Lubovitz O, Mozes B. The bleeding risk and natural history of idiopathic thrombocytopenic purpura in patients with persistent low platelet counts. Arch Intern Med. 2000;160(11):1630–8.
16. Rodeghiero F. Is ITP a thrombophilic disorder? Am J Hematol. 2016;91(1):39–45.
17. Enger C, Bennett D, Forssen U, Fogarty PF, McAfee AT. Comorbidities in patients with persistent or chronic immune thrombocytopenia. Int J Hematol. 2010;92(2):289–95.
18. Nørgaard M, Cetin K, Maegbaek ML, Kristensen NR, Ghanima W, Bahmanyar S, et al. Risk of arterial thrombotic and venous thromboembolic events in patients with primary chronic immune thrombocytopenia: a Scandinavian population-based cohort study. Br J Haematol. 2015;174(4):639–42.
19. Nørgaard M, Severinsen MT, Lund Maegbaek M, Jensen A, Cha S, Sørensen HT. Risk of arterial thrombosis in patients with primary chronic immune thrombocytopenia: a Danish population-based cohort study. Br J Haematol. 2012;159(1):109–11.
20. Sarpatwari A, Bennett D, Logie JW, Shukla A, Beach KJ, Newland AC, et al. Thromboembolic events among adult patients with primary immune thrombocytopenia in the United Kingdom General Practice Research Database. Haematologica. 2010;95(7):1167–75.
21. Zoller B, Li X, Sundquist J, Sundquist K. Risk of pulmonary embolism in patients with autoimmune disorders: a nationwide follow-up study from Sweden. Lancet. 2012;379(9812):2 44–9.
22. Langeberg WJ, Schoonen WM, Eisen M, Gamelin L, Stryker S. Thromboembolism in patients with immune thrombocytopenia (ITP): a meta-analysis of observational studies. Int J Hematol. 2016;103(6):655–64.
23. Sewify EM, Sayed D, Abdel Aal RF, Ahmad HM, Abdou MA. Increased circulating red cell microparticles (RMP) and platelet microparticles (PMP) in immune thrombocytopenic purpura. Thromb Res. 2013;131(2):e59–63.
24. Kosugi S, Tomiyama Y, Honda S, Kashiwagi H, Shiraga M, Tadokoro S, et al. Anti-alphavbeta3 antibodies in chronic immune thrombocytopenic purpura. Thromb Haemost. 2001;85(1):36–41.
25. Kim KJ, Baek IW, Yoon CH, Kim WU, Cho CS. Thrombotic risk in patients with immune thrombocytopenia and its association with antiphospholipid antibodies. Br J Haematol. 2013;161(5):706–14.
26. Fardet L, Feve B. Systemic glucocorticoid therapy: a review of its metabolic and cardiovascular adverse events. Drugs. 2014;74(15):1731–45.
27. Marcen R. Immunosuppressive drugs in kidney transplantation: impact on patient survival, and incidence of cardiovascular disease, malignancy and infection. Drugs. 2009;69(16):2227–43.
28. Sorensen HT, Mellemkjaer L, Nielsen GL, Baron JA, Olsen JH, Karagas MR. Skin cancers and non-hodgkin lymphoma among users of systemic glucocorticoids: a population-based cohort study. J Natl Cancer Inst. 2004;96(9):709–11.
29. Boyle S, White RH, Brunson A, Wun T. Splenectomy and the incidence of venous thromboembolism and sepsis in patients with immune thrombocytopenia. Blood. 2013;121(23):4782–90.
30. Thomsen RW, Schoonen WM, Farkas DK, Riis A, Jacobsen J, Fryzek JP, et al. Risk for hospital contact with infection in patients with splenectomy: a population-based cohort study. Ann Intern Med. 2009;151(8):546–55.
31. McMillan R, Bussel JB, George JN, Lalla D, Nichol JL. Self-reported health-related quality of life in adults with chronic immune thrombocytopenic purpura. Am J Hematol. 2008;83(2):150–4.
32. Snyder CF, Mathias SD, Cella D, Isitt JJ, Wu AW, Young J. Health-related quality of life of immune thrombocytopenic purpura patients: results from a web-based survey. Curr Med Res Opin. 2008;24(10):2767–76.

33. Hill QA, Newland AC. Fatigue in immune thrombocytopenia. Br J Haematol. 2015;170(2): 141–9.
34. Cheng G, Saleh MN, Marcher C, Vasey S, Mayer B, Aivado M, et al. Eltrombopag for management of chronic immune thrombocytopenia (RAISE): a 6-month, randomised, phase 3 study. Lancet. 2011;377(9763):393–402.
35. Kuter DJ, Rummel M, Boccia R, Macik BG, Pabinger I, Selleslag D, et al. Romiplostim or standard of care in patients with immune thrombocytopenia. N Engl J Med. 2010;363(20): 1889–99.
36. Kuwana M. Helicobacter pylori-associated immune thrombocytopenia: clinical features and pathogenic mechanisms. World J Gastroenterol. 2014;20(3):714–23.
37. Fujimura K, Miyakawa Y, Kurata Y, Kuwana M, Tomiyama Y, Murata M. Reference guide for management of adult idiopathic thrombocytopenic purpura (ITP) 2012 version. Rinsho Ketsueki. 2012;53(4):433–42.
38. Stasi R, Sarpatwari A, Segal JB, Osborn J, Evangelista ML, Cooper N, et al. Effects of eradication of Helicobacter pylori infection in patients with immune thrombocytopenic purpura: a systematic review. Blood. 2009;113(6):1231–40.
39. British Committee for Standards in Haematology General Haematology Task Force. Guidelines for the investigation and management of idiopathic thrombocytopenic purpura in adults, children and in pregnancy. Br J Haematol. 2003;120(4):574–96.
40. George JN, Woolf SH, Raskob GE, Wasser JS, Aledort LM, Ballem PJ, et al. Idiopathic thrombocytopenic purpura: a practice guideline developed by explicit methods for the American Society of Hematology. Blood. 1996;88(1):3–40.
41. Neunert C, Lim W, Crowther M, Cohen A, Solberg L, Crowther MA, et al. The American Society of Hematology 2011 evidence-based practice guideline for immune thrombocytopenia. Blood. 2011;117(16):4190–207.
42. Provan D, Stasi R, Newland AC, Blanchette VS, Bolton-Maggs P, Bussel JB, et al. International consensus report on the investigation and management of primary immune thrombocytopenia. Blood. 2010;115(2):168–86.
43. Cheng Y, Wong RS, Soo YO, Chui CH, Lau FY, Chan NP, et al. Initial treatment of immune thrombocytopenic purpura with high-dose dexamethasone. N Engl J Med. 2003;349(9): 831–6.
44. Mazzucconi MG, Fazi P, Bernasconi S, De Rossi G, Leone G, Gugliotta L, et al. Therapy with high-dose dexamethasone (HD-DXM) in previously untreated patients affected by idiopathic thrombocytopenic purpura: a GIMEMA experience. Blood. 2007;109(4):1401–7.
45. Wei, Y., Ji, X. B., Wang, Y. W., Wang, J. X., Yang, E. Q., Wang, Z. C., et al. (2016). High-dose dexamethasone vs prednisone for treatment of adult immune thrombocytopenia: a prospective multicenter randomized trial. Blood, 127(3), 296-302; quiz 370.
46. Kojouri K, Vesely SK, Terrell DR, George JN. Splenectomy for adult patients with idiopathic thrombocytopenic purpura: a systematic review to assess long-term platelet count responses, prediction of response, and surgical complications. Blood. 2004;104(9):2623–34.
47. Gonzalez-Porras JR, Escalante F, Pardal E, Sierra M, Garcia-Frade LJ, Redondo S, et al. Safety and efficacy of splenectomy in over 65-yrs-old patients with immune thrombocytopenia. Eur J Haematol. 2013;91(3):236–41.
48. Tomiyama Y. Thrombopoietin receptor agonists. In: Salama A, editor. Current & emerging treatments for immune thrombocytopenia. London: Future Medicine, Ltd.; 2013. p. 89–100.
49. Bussel JB, Provan D, Shamsi T, Cheng G, Psaila B, Kovaleva L, et al. Effect of eltrombopag on platelet counts and bleeding during treatment of chronic idiopathic thrombocytopenic purpura: a randomised, double-blind, placebo-controlled trial. Lancet. 2009;373(9664):641–8.
50. Kuter DJ, Bussel JB, Lyons RM, Pullarkat V, Gernsheimer TB, Senecal FM, et al. Efficacy of romiplostim in patients with chronic immune thrombocytopenic purpura: a double-blind randomised controlled trial. Lancet. 2008;371(9610):395–403.
51. Rodeghiero F, Stasi R, Giagounidis A, Viallard JF, Godeau B, Pabinger I, et al. Long-term safety and tolerability of romiplostim in patients with primary immune thrombocytopenia: a pooled analysis of 13 clinical trials. Eur J Haematol. 2013b;91(5):423–36.

52. Saleh MN, Bussel JB, Cheng G, Meyer O, Bailey CK, Arning M, et al. Safety and efficacy of eltrombopag for treatment of chronic immune thrombocytopenia: results of the long-term, open-label EXTEND study. Blood. 2013;121(3):537–45.
53. Sailler L. Rituximab off label use for difficult-to-treat auto-immune diseases: reappraisal of benefits and risks. Clin Rev Allergy Immunol. 2008;34(1):103–10.
54. Patel VL, Mahevas M, Lee SY, Stasi R, Cunningham-Rundles S, Godeau B, et al. Outcomes 5 years after response to rituximab therapy in children and adults with immune thrombocytopenia. Blood. 2012;119(25):5989–95.
55. Cuker A, Neunert CE. How I treat refractory immune thrombocytopenia. Blood. 2016;128(12):1547–54.
56. Alpdogan O, Budak-Alpdogan T, Ratip S, Firatli-Tuglular T, Tanriverdi S, Karti S, et al. Efficacy of high-dose methylprednisolone as a first-line therapy in adult patients with idiopathic thrombocytopenic purpura. Br J Haematol. 1998;103(4):1061–3.
57. Abrahm J, Ellman L. Platelet transfusion in immune thrombocytopenic purpura. JAMA. 1976;236(16):1847.
58. Spahr JE, Rodgers GM. Treatment of immune-mediated thrombocytopenia purpura with concurrent intravenous immunoglobulin and platelet transfusion: a retrospective review of 40 patients. Am J Hematol. 2008;83(2):122–5.

Part VI
Diagnosis

Diagnosis in General

Hirokazu Kashiwagi and Yoshiaki Tomiyama

Abstract Diagnosis of ITP is carried out by mainly exclusion of thrombocytopenia caused by other etiology and therapeutic responses. Since thrombocytopenia may be associated with a variety of clinical conditions, careful exclusion is necessary. Blood smear examination is especially important to rule out pseudothrombocytopenia and some congenital thrombocytopenia. Bone marrow examination may not be essential to ITP diagnosis, but it should be performed in cases with abnormalities in CBC or blood smear other than thrombocytopenia, atypical clinical course, or refractory to standard treatments. Assessment of reticulated platelets and plasma thrombopoietin concentration may be helpful to distinguish ITP from hypoplastic thrombocytopenia.

1 Principle of ITP Diagnosis

Despite recent advances in understanding of pathophysiology of ITP [1], a definitive test with clinically sufficient sensitivity and specificity for diagnosis of ITP has not been established [2]. Thrombocytopenia may be associated with a variety of clinical conditions (Table 1). Since ITP is mainly diagnosed by exclusion of thrombocytopenia caused by these other etiologies (Fig. 1), reevaluation of diagnosis should be considered when atypical clinical features as ITP, such as progression of anemia/leukopenia or poor response to standard treatments, are emerging.

H. Kashiwagi, M.D. (✉)
Department of Hematology and Oncology, Graduate School of Medicine, Osaka University, 2-2 Yamadaoka, Suita, Osaka 565-0871, Japan
e-mail: kashi@hp-blood.med.osaka-u.ac.jp

Y. Tomiyama, M.D.
Department of Blood Transfusion, Osaka University Hospital, 2-15 Yamadaoka, Suita, Osaka 565-0871, Japan
e-mail: yoshi@hp-blood.med.osaka-u.ac.jp

Y. Ishida, Y. Tomiyama (eds.), *Autoimmune Thrombocytopenia*,
DOI 10.1007/978-981-10-4142-6_8

Table 1 Etiological classification of thrombocytopenia

Artificial thrombocytopenia
Platelet aggregation caused by insufficient anticoagulation
Platelet aggregation caused by EDTA-dependent immunoglobulin (pseudothrombocytopenia)
Giant platelets
Decreased platelet production
Congenital thrombocytopenia
MYH9-related macrothrombocytopenia
Wiskott-Aldrich syndrome
Congenital amegakaryocytic thrombocytopenia (CAMT), etc.
Aplastic anemia
Malignancy with bone marrow infiltration or suppression (e.g., lymphoma, leukemia, solid tumors)
Myelodysplasia
Paroxysmal nocturnal hemoglobinuria
Nutrient deficiencies (e.g., vitamin B12, folate, copper)
Chemotherapy-related suppression
Increased platelet destruction or consumption
Caused by immunologic process
Primary immune thrombocytopenia
Secondary immune thrombocytopenia
Infection associated (e.g., HIV, HCV, *H. pylori*, EBV)
Drug induced (e.g., heparin, quinine, GPIIb/IIIa inhibitors)
Rheumatologic/autoimmune disease associated (e.g., SLE, rheumatoid arthritis)
Alloimmune thrombocytopenia
Neonatal thrombocytopenia
Post-transfusion purpura
Caused by non-immunologic process
Thrombotic microangiopathy (TMA)
Thrombotic thrombocytopenic purpura (TTP)
Hemolytic uremic syndrome (HUS)
HELLP syndrome
Disseminated intravascular coagulation (DIC)
Type 2B or platelet-type von Willebrand disease
Abnormal platelet distribution or pooling
Splenomegaly caused by liver disease, sarcoidosis, granulomatous infections, Gaucher disease, etc.

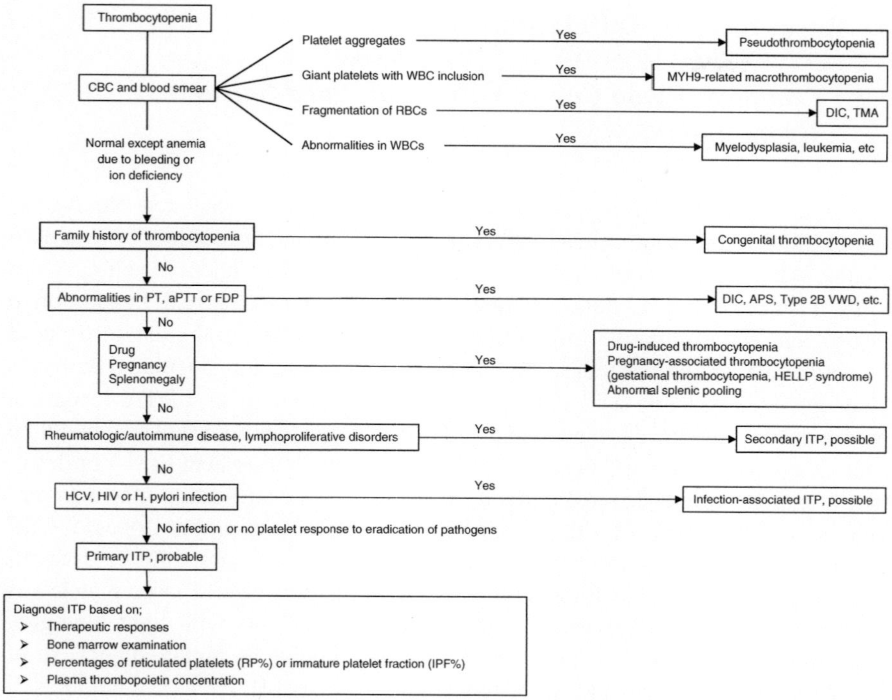

Fig. 1 Algorithm of diagnosis of ITP. ITP is diagnosed by careful exclusion of thrombocytopenia caused by other etiologies. *DIC* disseminated intravascular coagulation, *TMA* thrombotic microangiopathy, *APS* antiphospholipid antibody syndrome

2 Medical History and Physical Examination

Thorough interview of medical history is the first step of ITP diagnosis. Especially, the following information may be helpful: history of thrombocytopenia and bleeding; family history of bleeding diathesis and/or thrombocytopenia; comorbidities and drug exposure; infectious exposures including recent viral, bacterial, or rickettsial infections; vaccination; and chronic HIV or HCV infections.

In physical examination, nature of bleeding should be focused. ITP typically causes skin or mucous membrane bleeding, and bleeding into deep tissues or joints, which is often observed in coagulation abnormalities, is rare. The presence of lymphadenopathy or hepatosplenomegaly may be a sign of an underlying condition responsible for the thrombocytopenia.

3 Basic Tests for Differential Diagnosis

3.1 Complete Blood Count (CBC) and Blood Smear Examination

ITP is characterized by isolated thrombocytopenia with normal red blood cells (RBCs) and white blood cells (WBCs) except anemia due to bleeding or iron deficiency. When a patient presents isolated thrombocytopenia without bleeding symptoms, it is necessary to confirm whether the thrombocytopenia is real. In addition to insufficient anticoagulation in blood collection tubes, platelet aggregation caused by antiplatelet antibodies that react with platelets in blood anticoagulated with ethylenediaminetetraacetic acid (EDTA), which is referred to as EDTA-dependent pseudothrombocytopenia, may lead to false thrombocytopenia [3]. This should be excluded by repeated CBC in blood anticoagulated with other than EDTA or detection of platelet aggregates in blood smear. Blood smear examination may also provide helpful information for the diagnosis in patients with thrombocytopenia. RBC fragmentations suggest the presence of thrombotic microangiopathy or disseminated intravascular coagulation (DIC). Although the presence of large platelets is not uncommon in ITP, excessive number of giant platelets with light blue-gray inclusions in neutrophils, which are called Döhle bodies, is highly suggestive of MYH9-related disorders, such as May-Hegglin anomaly [4]. Excessive numbers of small platelets may suggest Wiskott-Aldrich syndrome or X-linked thrombocytopenia [5]. Details of differential diagnosis of congenital thrombocytopenia are described in chapter "Differential Diagnosis: Congenital Macrothrombocytopenia."

3.2 Coagulation Tests

In ITP, coagulation tests including PT, aPTT, and fibrinogen-degradation product (FDP) are basically normal. However, aPTT may be prolonged due to lupus anticoagulant, which is frequently detected in ITP patients [6, 7]. Abnormalities in aPTT with mild thrombocytopenia and mucosal bleeding may be a sign of type 2B or platelet-type von Willebrand disease [8]. Marked abnormalities in coagulation tests with thrombocytopenia suggest the presence of DIC.

3.3 Helicobacter pylori*, HIV, and HCV Tests*

Persistent thrombocytopenia may be associated with chronic infection of *Helicobacter pylori*, HIV, and HCV [9, 10]. Special attention to *H. pylori* infection is needed in the regions like Japan, in which a high prevalence of *H. pylori* and a high platelet response rate to its eradication have been established [11]. Details of

H. pylori-associated thrombocytopenia are described in chapter "*Helicobacter pylori* (*H. pylori*) Eradication." Chronic HCV infection has been reported to be associated with the development of thrombocytopenia. A variety of pathogenic mechanisms, including hypersplenism and inadequate production of thrombopoietin (TPO) from hepatocytes, may contribute to HCV-associated thrombocytopenia, and this may be present even in the absence of splenomegaly or evident liver dysfunction. Association of chronic HIV infection with thrombocytopenia is also well documented, and multiple mechanisms of HIV-associated thrombocytopenia have been proposed, including the presence of antiplatelet glycoprotein antibodies [12].

3.4 Bone Marrow (BM) Examination

Historically, ITP is defined as isolated thrombocytopenia of undetermined etiology in the presence of normal or increased megakaryocytes in BM [13]; however, the usefulness of BM examination as a diagnostic test for ITP has not been established [14, 15]. In fact, BM examination is no longer recommended as an essential test for ITP diagnosis in recent guidelines [2, 16]. However, BM examination should be considered in patients with abnormalities in CBC or blood smear other than thrombocytopenia, atypical clinical course, or refractory to standard treatments. In cases in which splenectomy is considered, BM examination should be performed to confirm the diagnosis. Before administration of TPO receptor agonists (TPO-RAs), BM examination should also be considered, since TPO-RAs may lead to progression of myelodysplastic syndrome (MDS) to higher-risk MDS or AML [17–19]. Cytogenetic analysis is also important, because MDS may represent with isolated thrombocytopenia [20], and this presentation with minimal morphological dysplasia, which may be easily misdiagnosed as ITP, has been described in patients with an isolated deletion of chromosome 20 [21]. A flow cytometric analysis may be helpful in identifying patients with secondary ITP associated with chronic lymphocytic leukemia (CLL) [22].

3.5 Immunological Tests

Quantitative immunoglobulin levels may be useful to identify underlying immunological abnormalities, such as common variable immunodeficiency (CVID), especially in young patients [2]. Positivity of antinuclear antibody test may be also useful in young patients, because this is a predictor of development of chronic ITP in children [23]. Antiphospholipid syndrome, which is characterized by thrombotic complications with the presence of antiphospholipid antibodies, may be associated with thrombocytopenia, although severe thrombocytopenia and bleeding symptoms are rare [24]. On the other hand, antiphospholipid antibodies, including lupus anticoagulant and anticardiolipin antibodies, are detected in substantial population of

ITP patients, and higher risk of thromboembolism in these patients has been reported [6]. Antithyroid antibodies and thyroid function tests may be useful, since hyper- and hypothyroidism may develop mild thrombocytopenia. Moreover, response to ITP therapy may be improved by resolution of underlying thyroid diseases [2, 25].

4 Specific Tests for ITP

4.1 Antiplatelet Antibody Testing

Although the main pathogenesis of ITP is accelerated destruction of opsonized platelets and impaired thrombopoiesis by antiplatelet antibodies [1], usefulness of assays for antiplatelet antibodies in the diagnosis or management of ITP has not been demonstrated. Elevation of platelet-associated IgG, PAIgG, has been observed in patients with immune as well as nonimmune thrombocytopenia [26, 27]. In contrast, assays for detecting platelet glycoprotein-specific antibodies, e.g., anti-GPIIb/IIIa and anti-GPIb/IX antibodies, may be useful in selected cases for diagnosis of ITP [28–30]. However, sensitivity of the assay is insufficient for routine hematology practice [2]; the positivity of platelet-associated antibodies that recognize GPIIb/IIIa and GPIb/IX in patients with chronic ITP has been reported as 43–57% and 18–50%, respectively [30–32].

4.2 Reticulated Platelets and Plasma Thrombopoietin Concentration

It is sometimes difficult to distinguish ITP from hypoplastic thrombocytopenia, which may progress to aplastic anemia [33]. TPO, a key regulator of thrombopoiesis, is constantly secreted mainly from hepatocytes, and plasma TPO levels are regulated by the total amount of TPO receptor [34], although alternative mechanism of TPO regulation has been recently reported [35]. Plasma TPO levels in ITP patients usually stay in the rage of normal to subnormal, whereas those in patients with hypoplastic thrombocytopenia are highly elevated compared with normal subjects [33, 36]. Reticulated platelets (RP), which is thought to be younger platelets that have been released recently in the circulation, can be measured by staining of RNA with thiazole orange using flow cytometry [37, 38]. In many cases, ITP percentage of RP (RP%), which reflects platelet turnover, is increased, whereas that in patients with aplastic anemia or chemotherapy-induced thrombocytopenia is within normal range [36]. Percentage of immature platelet fraction (IPF%), which can be easily measured by an automated hematology analyzer, may be as useful as RP% detected by flow cytometry [39]. Simultaneous measurement of plasma TPO levels and RP% has high sensitivity and specificity for discrimination of aplastic thrombocytopenia from ITP [29, 36]. Details of differential diagnosis of hypoplastic thrombocytopenia are described in chapter "Differential Diagnosis: Hypoplastic thrombocytopenia."

Acknowledgment This work was supported by Grant-in-Aid for Scientific Research from the Ministry of Education, Culture, Sports, Science and Technology and the Ministry of Health, Labour and Welfare in Japan.

References

1. Kashiwagi H, Tomiyama Y. Pathophysiology and management of primary immune thrombocytopenia. Int J Hematol. 2013;98(1):24–33.
2. Provan D, Stasi R, Newland AC, Blanchette VS, Bolton-Maggs P, Bussel JB, et al. International consensus report on the investigation and management of primary immune thrombocytopenia. Blood. 2010;115(2):168–86.
3. Berkman N, Michaeli Y, Or R, Eldor A. EDTA-dependent pseudothrombocytopenia: a clinical study of 18 patients and a review of the literature. Am J Hematol. 1991;36(3):195–201.
4. Kunishima S, Saito H. Advances in the understanding of MYH9 disorders. Curr Opin Hematol. 2010;17(5):405–10.
5. Bolton-Maggs PH, Chalmers EA, Collins PW, Harrison P, Kitchen S, Liesner RJ, et al. A review of inherited platelet disorders with guidelines for their management on behalf of the UKHCDO. Br J Haematol. 2006;135(5):603–33.
6. Kim KJ, Baek IW, Yoon CH, Kim WU, Cho CS. Thrombotic risk in patients with immune thrombocytopenia and its association with antiphospholipid antibodies. Br J Haematol. 2013;161(5):706–14.
7. Stasi R, Stipa E, Masi M, Oliva F, Sciarra A, Perrotti A, et al. Prevalence and clinical significance of elevated antiphospholipid antibodies in patients with idiopathic thrombocytopenic purpura. Blood. 1994;84(12):4203–8.
8. Nichols WL, Hultin MB, James AH, Manco-Johnson MJ, Montgomery RR, Ortel TL, et al. von Willebrand disease (VWD): evidence-based diagnosis and management guidelines, the National Heart, Lung, and Blood Institute (NHLBI) Expert Panel report (USA). Haemophilia. 2008;14(2):171–232.
9. Liebman HA, Stasi R. Secondary immune thrombocytopenic purpura. Curr Opin Hematol. 2007;14(5):557–73.
10. Stasi R, Willis F, Shannon MS, Gordon-Smith EC. Infectious causes of chronic immune thrombocytopenia. Hematol Oncol Clin North Am. 2009;23(6):1275–97.
11. Kuwana M. *Helicobacter pylori*-associated immune thrombocytopenia: clinical features and pathogenic mechanisms. World J Gastroenterol. 2014;20(3):714–23.
12. Karpatkin S, Nardi MA, Hymes KB. Sequestration of anti-platelet GPIIIa antibody in rheumatoid factor immune complexes of human immunodeficiency virus 1 thrombocytopenic patients. Proc Natl Acad Sci U S A. 1995;92(6):2263–7.
13. Lacey JV, Penner JA. Management of idiopathic thrombocytopenic purpura in the adult. Semin Thromb Hemost. 1977;3(3):160–74.
14. Jubelirer SJ, Harpold R. The role of the bone marrow examination in the diagnosis of immune thrombocytopenic purpura: case series and literature review. Clin Appl Thromb Hemost. 2002;8(1):73–6.
15. Mahabir VK, Ross C, Popovic S, Sur ML, Bourgeois J, Lim W, et al. A blinded study of bone marrow examinations in patients with primary immune thrombocytopenia. Eur J Haematol. 2013;90(2):121–6.

16. Neunert C, Lim W, Crowther M, Cohen A, Solberg L, Crowther MA, et al. The American Society of Hematology 2011 evidence-based practice guideline for immune thrombocytopenia. Blood. 2011;117(16):4190–207.
17. Kantarjian H, Fenaux P, Sekeres MA, Becker PS, Boruchov A, Bowen D, et al. Safety and efficacy of romiplostim in patients with lower-risk myelodysplastic syndrome and thrombocytopenia. J Clin Oncol. 2010;28(3):437–44.
18. Oshima Y, Yuji K, Tanimoto T, Hinomura Y, Tojo A. Association between acute myelogenous leukemia and thrombopoietin receptor agonists in patients with immune thrombocytopenia. Intern Med. 2013;52(19):2193–201.
19. Prica A, Sholzberg M, Buckstein R. Safety and efficacy of thrombopoietin-receptor agonists in myelodysplastic syndromes: a systematic review and meta-analysis of randomized controlled trials. Br J Haematol. 2014;167(5):626–38.
20. Najean Y, Lecompte T. Chronic pure thrombocytopenia in elderly patients. An aspect of the myelodysplastic syndrome. Cancer. 1989;64(12):2506–10.
21. Gupta R, Soupir CP, Johari V, Hasserjian RP. Myelodysplastic syndrome with isolated deletion of chromosome 20q: an indolent disease with minimal morphological dysplasia and frequent thrombocytopenic presentation. Br J Haematol. 2007;139(2):265–8.
22. Mittal S, Blaylock MG, Culligan DJ, Barker RN, Vickers MA. A high rate of CLL phenotype lymphocytes in autoimmune hemolytic anemia and immune thrombocytopenic purpura. Haematologica. 2008;93(1):151–2.
23. Heitink-Polle KM, Nijsten J, Boonacker CW, de Haas M, Bruin MC. Clinical and laboratory predictors of chronic immune thrombocytopenia in children: a systematic review and meta-analysis. Blood. 2014;124(22):3295–307.
24. Artim-Esen B, Diz-Kucukkaya R, Inanc M. The significance and management of thrombocytopenia in antiphospholipid syndrome. Curr Rheumatol Rep. 2015;17(3):14.
25. Meyer O. Symptoms and diagnosis. In: Salama A, editor. Current & emerging treatments for immune thrombocytopenia. London: Future Medicine; 2013. p. 19–29.
26. Kelton JG, Murphy WG, Lucarelli A, Garvey-Williams J, Santos A, Meyer R, et al. A prospective comparison of four techniques for measuring platelet-associated IgG. Br J Haematol. 1989;71(1):97–105.
27. Mueller-Eckhardt C, Kayser W, Mersch-Baumert K, Mueller-Eckhardt G, Breidenbach M, Kugel HG, et al. The clinical significance of platelet-associated IgG: a study on 298 patients with various disorders. Br J Haematol. 1980;46(1):123–31.
28. Kiyomizu K, Kashiwagi H, Nakazawa T, Tadokoro S, Honda S, Kanakura Y, et al. Recognition of highly restricted regions in the β-propeller domain of αIIb by platelet-associated anti-αIIbβ3 autoantibodies in primary immune thrombocytopenia. Blood. 2012;120(7):1499–509.
29. Kuwana M, Kurata Y, Fujimura K, Fujisawa K, Wada H, Nagasawa T, et al. Preliminary laboratory based diagnostic criteria for immune thrombocytopenic purpura: evaluation by multicenter prospective study. J Thromb Haemost. 2006;4(9):1936–43.
30. Warner MN, Moore JC, Warkentin TE, Santos AV, Kelton JG. A prospective study of protein-specific assays used to investigate idiopathic thrombocytopenic purpura. Br J Haematol. 1999;104(3):442–7.
31. Brighton TA, Evans S, Castaldi PA, Chesterman CN, Chong BH. Prospective evaluation of the clinical usefulness of an antigen-specific assay (MAIPA) in idiopathic thrombocytopenic purpura and other immune thrombocytopenias. Blood. 1996;88(1):194–201.
32. McMillan R, Wang L, Tani P. Prospective evaluation of the immunobead assay for the diagnosis of adult chronic immune thrombocytopenic purpura (ITP). J Thromb Haemost. 2003;1(3):485–91.
33. Saito C, Ishiyama K, Yamazaki H, Zaimoku Y, Nakao S. Hypomegakaryocytic thrombocytopenia (HMT): an immune-mediated bone marrow failure characterized by an increased number of PNH-phenotype cells and high plasma thrombopoietin levels. Br J Haematol. 2016;175(2):246–51.

34. Kaushansky K. The molecular mechanisms that control thrombopoiesis. J Clin Invest. 2005;115(12):3339–47.
35. Grozovsky R, Begonja AJ, Liu K, Visner G, Hartwig JH, Falet H, et al. The Ashwell-Morell receptor regulates hepatic thrombopoietin production via JAK2-STAT3 signaling. Nat Med. 2015;21(1):47–54.
36. Kurata Y, Hayashi S, Kiyoi T, Kosugi S, Kashiwagi H, Honda S, et al. Diagnostic value of tests for reticulated platelets, plasma glycocalicin, and thrombopoietin levels for discriminating between hyperdestructive and hypoplastic thrombocytopenia. Am J Clin Pathol. 2001;115(5):656–64.
37. Kienast J, Schmitz G. Flow cytometric analysis of thiazole orange uptake by platelets: a diagnostic aid in the evaluation of thrombocytopenic disorders. Blood. 1990;75(1):116–21.
38. Richards EM, Baglin TP. Quantitation of reticulated platelets: methodology and clinical application. Br J Haematol. 1995;91(2):445–51.
39. Sakuragi M, Hayashi S, Maruyama M, Kabutomori O, Kiyokawa T, Nagamine K, et al. Clinical significance of IPF% or RP% measurement in distinguishing primary immune thrombocytopenia from aplastic thrombocytopenic disorders. Int J Hematol. 2015;101(4):369–75.

Differential Diagnosis: Secondary ITP

Takashi Satoh and Masataka Kuwana

Abstract There is no substantial difference in immunologic pathophysiology between primary and secondary immune thrombocytopenia (ITP): it is characterized by increased platelet destruction in the reticuloendothelial system or reduced platelet production mediated primarily by IgG antiplatelet autoantibodies, resulting in thrombocytopenia. Secondary ITP can occur in the context of a variety of underlying diseases or conditions, including autoimmune diseases, such as systemic lupus erythematosus (SLE) and antiphospholipid syndrome (APS), lymphoproliferative disorders, and chronic infection with certain bacterial or viral microorganisms, including *Helicobacter pylori* (*H. pylori*), hepatitis C virus (HCV), and human immunodeficiency virus (HIV). Therefore, patients diagnosed as having ITP should be further evaluated for symptoms, physical signs, and laboratory tests associated with underlying disorders that potentially cause secondary ITP. It is imperative to consider risk factors in an individual patient basis. For example, elderly in *H. pylori* epidemic countries, such as East Asia and Italy, should be considered for performing *H. pylori* testing, homosexuals and drug abusers for performing HIV and HCV testing, and young women with a rash, fever, or arthralgia for performing a series of autoantibody tests. In clinical practice, identification of underlying diseases or conditions is essential in patients diagnosed as having ITP since treatment strategies are often different between primary and secondary ITP.

T. Satoh (✉)
Division of Hematology, Kitasato University School of Allied Health Sciences, 1-15-1 Kitasato, Minami-ku, Sagamihara, Kanagawa 252-0373, Japan

Division of Molecular Hematology, Kitasato University Graduate School of Medical Sciences, 1-15-1 Kitasato, Minami, Sagamihara, Kanagawa 252-0374, Japan
e-mail: takashis@kitasato-u.ac.jp

M. Kuwana
Department of Allergy and Rheumatology, Nippon Medical School Graduate School of Medicine, 1-1-5 Sendagi, Bunkyo-ku, Tokyo 113-8603, Japan
e-mail: kuwanam@nms.ac.jp

Y. Ishida, Y. Tomiyama (eds.), *Autoimmune Thrombocytopenia*,
DOI 10.1007/978-981-10-4142-6_9

1 Introduction

Based on the proposal by an international working group organized for the standardization of definitions and classifications for immune thrombocytopenia (ITP), ITP can be divided into two forms [1]. ITP can occur in the absence of an apparent predisposing etiology (primary ITP) or as a sequela of an associated condition (secondary ITP). There is no substantial difference in immunologic pathophysiology between primary and secondary ITP: it is characterized by increased platelet destruction in the reticuloendothelial system or reduced platelet production primarily mediated by antiplatelet autoantibodies to platelet surface glycoproteins (GPs), resulting in thrombocytopenia [2]. Nevertheless, distinction of primary and secondary ITP is a major challenge in clinical setting, because they often require different treatment algorithm. Namely, in secondary ITP, the therapeutic approach should be aimed at the underlying disorders. A variety of diseases or conditions can cause secondary ITP, and those include autoimmune diseases such as systemic lupus erythematosus (SLE), lymphoproliferative disorders, and chronic infection [2, 3] (Table 1). According to the current nomenclature for secondary ITP, the name of the associated disease or pathogen is followed by a designation of ITP in parenthesis, i.e., secondary ITP (SLE-associated ITP). This chapter summarizes the clinical manifestations and pathogenesis of individual diseases or conditions that cause secondary ITP and discusses how to proceed with differential diagnosis.

Table 1 Diseases and conditions that cause secondary ITP

Category	Diseases and conditions
Autoimmune diseases	Systemic lupus erythematosus Anti-phospholipid syndrome Systemic sclerosis (scleroderma) Mixed connective tissue disease Sjögren syndrome Hashimoto's thyroiditis
Lymphoproliferative diseases	Chronic lymphocytic leukemia Hodgkin's disease Non-Hodgkin's lymphoma Large granulocytic leukemia
Infection-related conditions	*Helicobacter pylori* Hepatitis C virus Human immunodeficiency virus Cytomegalovirus Varicella-zoster virus Epstein-Barr virus Mumps-measles-rubella (MMR) vaccination
Miscellaneous	Common variable immunodeficiency Autoimmune lymphoproliferative syndrome (ALPS) Evan's syndrome Posttransplantation Drug induced (i.e., penicillin, cephalosporins, sulphonamides, nonsteroidal anti-inflammatory drugs, quinine, and D-penicillamine)

2 Autoimmune Diseases

2.1 Systemic Lupus Erythematosus (SLE)

SLE is a systemic autoimmune disease that causes a variety of clinical manifestations and resultant multi-organ damage. In SLE, genetic factors and environmental triggers, such as ultraviolet exposure, together contribute to induction of autoimmunity against various self-antigens, resulting in the production of high-affinity pathogenic autoantibodies, including anti-double-stranded DNA antibodies. These autoantibodies typically form immune complexes, which accumulate in the kidneys, blood vessel walls, and many other organs, and trigger complement activation and inflammation. Anti-double-stranded DNA antibodies are not only a diagnostic marker but also are involved in disease progression and reflect disease activity [4, 5]. Thrombocytopenia is one of the major complications in patients with SLE, with a prevalence ranging from 10 to 30% [6]. The pathogenic processes of thrombocytopenia in SLE patients are heterogeneous and include ITP, thrombotic microangiopathy (i.e., thrombotic thrombocytopenic purpura and atypical hemolytic uremic syndrome), disseminated intravascular coagulation, and amegakaryocytic thrombocytopenia, while the most common mechanism is ITP, which is mediated through anti-GPIIb/IIIa and anti-GPIb/IX antibodies, as observed in patients with primary ITP [7, 8]. On the other hand, we have identified new autoantibodies reactive with thrombopoietin (TPO) receptor in patients with SLE [9]. Anti-TPO receptor antibodies often coexist with anti-GPIIb/IIIa antibodies and are associated with megakaryocytic hypoplasia and poor treatment response to corticosteroids or intravenous immunoglobulin (IVIG) [7]. SLE patients with anti-TPO receptor antibody often represent an extremely high level of circulating TPO. A rare manifestation of amegakaryocytic thrombocytopenia can occur in the presence of anti-TPO receptor antibodies. In fact, anti-TPO receptor antibodies are capable of inhibiting megakaryogenesis in vitro [9].

2.2 Antiphospholipid Syndrome (APS)

APS is characterized by recurrent arterial and/or venous thrombosis as well as adverse pregnancy outcomes in association with antiphospholipid (aPL) autoantibodies. According to the revised Sapporo criteria, clinically meaningful aPL positivity is defined by moderate levels of IgG/IgA/IgM anti-cardiolipin antibodies, IgG/IgA/IgM anti-β2GPI antibodies, or lupus anticoagulant, which are confirmed to be positive in two occasions apart from >12 weeks [10]. APS is divided into primary and secondary APS, based on the presence or absence of an underlying autoimmune condition; SLE is the commonest. Thrombocytopenia has been reported in ~40% of patients with primary APS and usually presents mildly without apparent bleeding symptoms [11, 12]. Severe thrombocytopenia in primary APS patients is correlated more closely with the presence of antiplatelet autoantibodies to GPIIb/IIIa and

GPIb/IX [13, 14]. However, rare cases of APS patients who develop severe thrombocytopenia concomitant with repeated episodes of thrombosis have been reported. In these cases, thrombocytopenia is mediated by enhanced platelet consumption in association with accelerated coagulation pathways, and platelet count is fully recovered by treatment with warfarin [15]. aPL is occasionally found in patients with primary ITP without any thrombotic episodes. However, the presence of aPL in patients with primary ITP is a risk factor for future development of APS [16].

3 Lymphoproliferative Disorder (LPD)

Among LPDs, chronic lymphocytic leukemia (CLL) is the condition that develops secondary ITP most commonly. Approximately 5% of CLL patients develop clinically significant ITP during the disease course. Large granular lymphocytic leukemia, Hodgkin's lymphoma, and non-Hodgkin's lymphoma are also associated with secondary ITP, although ITP develops in less than 1% of all cases [17]. The identification of secondary ITP in LPDs may be difficult, given the many confounding events, such as the presence of diffuse bone marrow infiltration by monoclonally expanded lymphocytes and/or chemotherapy-induced toxicity, and platelet sequestration associated with splenomegaly can result in thrombocytopenia. Dysregulated immune system associated with LPDs may contribute to emergence of antiplatelet autoantibodies. The treatment of CLL-associated ITP is challenging since immunosuppressive treatment increases the risk of severe infection. Nevertheless, the treatment regimens are primarily same as those used for treating primary ITP [18].

4 Infection-Related Conditions

4.1 Helicobacter pylori *(*H. pylori*) Infection*

Several lines of evidence have indicated that platelet recovery occurs in a subset of ITP patients infected with *H. pylori*, a gram-negative bacterium that establishes chronic infection in the gastric mucosa, after the successful eradication of *H. pylori* [19]. Potential mechanisms for the role of *H. pylori* infection in ITP pathogenesis include molecular mimicry between *H. pylori* components and platelet antigens and modulation of the host's immune system by *H. pylori* infection [20]. Another intriguing mechanism has also been proposed; *H. pylori* infection could modulate the Fcγ receptor balance of monocytes/macrophages toward inhibitory FcγRIIB, thereby enhancing phagocytosis and antigen presentation [21]. This activated monocyte phenotype was suppressed after *H. pylori* was successfully eradicated. It has been now accepted that ITP that recovered after *H. pylori* eradication is categorized as secondary ITP (*H. pylori*-associated ITP) [22]. Interestingly, platelet recovery after *H. pylori* eradication was observed in nearly half of the patients in cohorts from Japan and Italy, but only in <15% of the patients in cohorts from Spain and the

United States [23]. This apparent ethnic difference suggests a potential role for host genetic factors in the development of ITP in *H. pylori*-infected individuals. In addition, single nucleotide polymorphisms within the genes for tumor necrosis factor-β and FcγRIIB were found to be useful for predicting the response to *H. pylori* eradication treatment [24, 25]. In the majority of ITP patients responding to *H. pylori* eradication therapy, antiplatelet autoantibody response is completely resolved with no relapse for more than 7 years, suggesting that the disease is cured. Therefore, in the *H. pylori* epidemic area, adult patients with ITP should be examined for *H. pylori* infection, and eradication therapy is recommended before any immunosuppressive therapy if the infection is present.

H. pylori infection is occasionally found in patients with other forms of secondary ITP, but platelet recovery was rarely observed in patients with SLE-associated or liver cirrhosis-associated ITP [19]. This finding clearly indicates that *H. pylori* eradication fails to improve the pathogenic process of other forms of secondary ITP. Thus, the efficacy of *H. pylori* eradication therapy is likely to be restricted to patients in a subgroup of *H. pylori*-associated ITP.

4.2 Hepatitis C Virus (HCV) Infection

It has been reported that the prevalence of HCV infection in adult patients with ITP ranged from 10 to 36% [26, 27]. Infection with HCV is known to modulate host immune response and prone to elicit autoimmunity. The pathogenesis of HCV-associated ITP is not understood in detail, but it may involve polyclonal activation of B cells and the production of antibodies cross-reactive with HCV components and GPIIIa [28]. A higher frequency of circulating anti-GPIIb/IIIa antibody-producing B cells in HCV-infected patients with liver cirrhosis than in liver cirrhosis patients with other etiologies might be a consequence of enhanced immune activation in association with HCV infection [29]. Other causes of thrombocytopenia in HCV-infected patients may be related to impairment in hepatic function, such as hypersplenism due to portal hypertension and decreased TPO production from the liver [30]. Successful eradication of HCV by antiviral treatment such as type I interferon has resulted in an improved platelet count in some patients with HCV-associated ITP, supporting a direct role for HCV infection in the pathogenic process of ITP [31, 32]. Thus, anti-HCV treatment should be considered before introduction of any immunosuppressive treatment, including corticosteroids. In case of high risk for fatal bleeding, IVIG is reported to be efficacious.

4.3 Human Immunodeficiency Virus (HIV) Infection

Before wide availability of highly active antiretroviral therapy (HAART), HIV-associated ITP was observed in 5–25% of HIV-1-infected individuals [27]. HIV targets $CD4^{+}$ T cells irrespective of their effector or regulatory subsets. Therefore, acquired immune system is dysregulated in HIV-infected individuals, resulting in increased risk for infection and cancer and, paradoxically, in increased risk for autoimmunity [33]. In addition, it has been shown that IgG anti-GPIIb/IIIa antibodies in patients with HIV-related ITP are able to cross-react with HIV-associated gp120 [34]. These potentially cross-reactive antibodies may trigger harmful autoimmune responses to platelets, resulting in the continuous production of IgG antiplatelet autoantibodies. On the other hand, it has been found that megakaryocytes express CD4 and co-receptors necessary for HIV infection [35]. Therefore, HIV infection to megakaryocytes directly leads to ineffective platelet production and may contribute to thrombocytopenia [36, 37]. Since recovery of platelet counts was reported in association with decreased HIV copies by HAART [38], anti-HIV treatment should be the first-line treatment in patients with HIV-associated ITP.

4.4 Diagnostic Evaluations in Clinical Practice

The diagnosis of primary ITP is based principally on the exclusion of the causes of secondary ITP. Table 2 lists the clinical and laboratory characteristics of selected secondary ITP that distinguish them from primary ITP. It is imperative to consider

Table 2 Clinical and laboratory characteristics of secondary ITP

Disorder	Clinical symptoms	Laboratory findings
Systemic lupus erythematosus (SLE)	Systemic manifestation, including fever, join pain/swelling, and rashes	Leukopenia Positive antinuclear antibodies (ANAs), anti-double-stranded DNA, anti-Sm, and anti-phospholipid autoantibodies Hypocomplementemia
Anti-phospholipid syndrome (APS)	History of thrombosis and pregnancy loss	Positive anti-phospholipid autoantibodies Lupus anticoagulant
Lymphoproliferative disease	History of chronic fatigue, fever, weight loss, pallor, and bone pain Lymphadenopathy Splenomegaly Hepatomegaly may be present	Elevated white blood cell count Anemia Blast cells on peripheral blood smear
Helicobacter pylori (*H. pylori*) infection	No specific clinical sign	The presence of *H. pylori* infection, preferably with the urea breath test or the stool antigen test
Hepatitis C virus (HCV) infection	Hepatomegaly Splenomegaly Jaundice (yellowing of eyes and skin) Dark urine and white stool	Elevated transaminases Positive anti-HCV antibody or HCV RNA
Human immunodeficiency virus (HIV) infection	Systemic signs, including fever, malaise, generalized lymphadenopathy, and generalized rash	HIV serologies confirm the diagnosis

the risk factors for developing disorders potentially cause secondary ITP: i.e., SLE for young women; APS for episode of thrombosis and/or repeated fetal losses; *H. pylori* infection for elderly in the epidemic countries, such as in East Asia and Italy; and HIV infection for homosexuals and drug abusers. Clinical evaluations should be aimed at symptoms and physical findings other than bleeding manifestations, which are commonly found in patients with primary and secondary ITP. Constitutional symptoms, such as fever, joint pain, rashes, malaise, Raynaud phenomenon, weight loss, hepatomegaly, and lymphadenopathy, indicate the presence of underlying disorders, such as SLE, LPD, and infection with HCV or HIV. It is necessary to perform serum tests for antinuclear antibody (ANA) and aPL as well as blood tests for infectious agents (HCV and HIV), according to clinical suspicion based on risk factors and clinical signs [39]. In case of high titer of ANA, specific antibody assays should be further conducted to identify anti-double-stranded DNA, anti-Sm, anti-U1RNP, anti-SSA, and anti-SSB antibodies. Increased counts of small lymphocytes or lymphocytes with granular inclusions in peripheral blood smears suggest a diagnosis of CLL, but flow cytometry may be particularly helpful in identifying patients with CLL [40]. *H. pylori* infection can be detected by urea breath test and/or the stool antigen test, although stomach biopsy under endoscopy should be avoided because of the risk for massive mucosal bleeding after invasive procedure. Anti-*H. pylori* antibody testing is less sensitive or specific and does not prove active infection, and a false-positive result can occur after IVIG therapy. *H. pylori* screening is certainly worthwhile in East Asian countries, South and Middle American countries, and Italy, which are areas with a high background prevalence of the infection. In contrast, in the United States and European countries except Italy, testing for *H. pylori* infection remains controversial.

5 Summary

There are a wide variety of diseases and conditions that cause secondary ITP, including autoimmune diseases, LPDs, and chronic infection with bacterial or viral microorganisms. The clinical diagnosis of primary ITP requires the exclusion of secondary ITP, which is made by careful evaluations of demographics, medical history, symptoms, and physical signs as well as appropriate laboratory tests. Differential diagnosis is critical since treatment strategies for secondary ITP are often different from those for primary ITP.

References

1. Rodeghiero F, Stasi R, Gernsheimer T, et al. Standardization of terminology, definitions and outcome criteria in immune thrombocytopenic purpura of adults and children: report from an international working group. Blood. 2009;113:2386–93.
2. Kistangari G, McCrae KR. Immune thrombocytopenia. Hematol Oncol Clin North Am. 2013;27:495–520.

3. Cines DB, Liebman H, Stasi R. Pathobiology of secondary immune thrombocytopenia. Semin Hematol. 2009;46:S2–14.
4. Hanaoka H, Okazaki Y, Satoh T, et al. Circulating anti-double-stranded DNA antibody-secreting cells in patients with systemic lupus erythematosus: a novel biomarker for disease activity. Lupus. 2012;21:1284–93.
5. Yaniv G, Twig G, Shor DB, et al. A volcanic explosion of autoantibodies in systemic lupus erythematosus: a diversity of 180 different antibodies found in SLE patients. Autoimmun Rev. 2015;14:75–9.
6. Boumpas DT, Austin III HA, Fessler BJ, et al. Systemic lupus erythematosus: emerging concepts. Part 1: Renal, neuropsychiatric, cardiovascular, pulmonary, and hematological disease. Ann Intern Med. 1995;122:940–50.
7. Kuwana M, Kaburaki J, Okazaki Y, et al. Two types of autoantibody-mediated thrombocytopenia in patients with systemic lupus erythematosus. Rheumatology. 2006;45:851–4.
8. Michel M, Lee K, Piette JC, et al. Platelet autoantibodies and lupus-associated thrombocytopenia. Br J Haematol. 2002;119:354–8.
9. Kuwana M, Okazaki Y, Kajihara M, et al. Autoantibody to c-Mpl (thrombopoietin receptor) in systemic lupus erythematosus: relationship to thrombocytopenia with megakaryocytic hypoplasia. Arthritis Rheum. 2002;46:2148–59.
10. Miyakis S, Lockshin MD, Atsumi T, et al. International consensus statement on an update of the classification criteria for definite antiphospholipid syndrome (APS). J Thromb Haemost. 2006;4:295–306.
11. Galli M, Finazzi G, Barbui T. Thrombocytopenia in the antiphospholipid syndrome. Br J Haematol. 1996;93:1–5.
12. Atsumi T, Furukawa S, Amengual O, et al. Antiphospholipid antibody associated thrombocytopenia and the paradoxical risk of thrombosis. Lupus. 2005;14:499–504.
13. Godeau B, Piette JC, Fromont P, et al. Specific antiplatelet glycoprotein autoantibodies are associated with the thrombocytopenia of primary antiphospholipid syndrome. Br J Haematol. 1997;98:873–9.
14. Liebman HA, Stasi R. Secondary immune thrombocytopenic purpura. Curr Opin Hematol. 2007;14:557–73.
15. Kuwana M, Kaburaki J, Hirakata M, et al. Thrombocytopenia responsive to warfarin in a patient with systemic sclerosis–systemic lupus erythematosus overlap. Clin Exp Rheumatol. 1995;13:103–6.
16. Diz-Kucukkaya R, Hacihanefioglu A, Yenerel M, et al. Antiphospholipid antibodies and antiphospholipid syndrome in patients presenting with immune thrombocytopenic purpura: a prospective cohort study. Blood. 2001;98:1760–4.
17. Liebman HA. Recognizing and treating secondary immune thrombocytopenic purpura associated with lymphoproliferative disorders. Semin Hematol. 2009;46:S33–6.
18. Zent CS, Kay NE. Autoimmune complications in chronic lymphocytic leukaemia (CLL). Best Pract Res Clin Haematol. 2010;23:47–59.
19. Kuwana M. *Helicobacter pylori*-associated immune thrombocytopenia: clinical features and pathogenic mechanisms. World J Gastroenterol. 2014;20:714–23.
20. Takahashi T, Yujiri T, Shinohara K, et al. Molecular mimicry by *Helicobacter pylori* CagA protein may be involved in the pathogenesis of *H. pylori*-associated chronic idiopathic thrombocytopenic purpura. Br J Haematol. 2004;124:91–6.
21. Asahi A, Nishimoto T, Okazaki Y, et al. Helicobacter pylori eradication shifts monocytes Fcγ receptor balance toward inhibitory FcγRIIB in immune thrombocytopenic purpura patients. J Clin Invest. 2008;118:2939–49.
22. Fujimura K. *Helicobacter pylori* infection and idiopathic thrombocytopenic purpura. Int J Hematol. 2005;81:113–8.
23. Frydman GH, Davis N, Beck PL, et al. *Helicobacter pylori* eradication in patients with immune thrombocytopenic purpura: a review and the role of biogeography. Helicobacter. 2015;20:239–51.

24. Satoh T, Miyazaki K, Shimohira A, et al. Fcγ receptor IIB gene polymorphism in adult Japanese patients with primary immune thrombocytopenia. Blood. 2013;122:1991–2.
25. Suzuki T, Matsushima M, Shirakura K, et al. Association of inflammatory cytokine gene polymorphisms with platelet recovery in idiopathic thrombocytopenic purpura patients after the eradication of *Helicobacter pylori*. Digestion. 2008;77:73–8.
26. McMillan R. Therapy for adults with refractory chronic immune thrombocytopenic purpura. Ann Intern Med. 1997;126:307–14.
27. Liebman H. Other immune thrombocytopenias. Semin Hematol. 2007;44:S24–34.
28. Zhang W, Nardi MA, Borkowsky W, et al. Role of molecular mimicry of hepatitis C virus protein with platelet GPIIIa in hepatitis C-related immunologic thrombocytopenia. Blood. 2009;113:4086–93.
29. Kajihara M, Kato S, Okazaki Y, et al. A role of autoantibody-mediated platelet destruction in thrombocytopenia in patients with cirrhosis. Hepatology. 2003;37:1267–76.
30. Peck-Radosavljevic M. Thrombocytopenia in liver disease. Can J Gastroenterol. 2000;14: 60D–6D.
31. Iga D, Tomimatsu M, Endo H, et al. Improvement of thrombocytopenia with disappearance of HCV RNA in patients treated by interferon-alpha therapy: possible etiology of HCV-associated thrombocytopenia. Eur J Haematol. 2005;75:417–23.
32. Suarez GJ, Burgaleta C, Hernanz N, et al. HCV-associated thrombocytopenia: clinical characteristics and platelet response after recombinant alpha2b-interferon therapy. Br J Haematol. 2000;110:98–103.
33. Stratton R, Slapak G, Mahungu T, et al. Autoimmunity and HIV. Curr Opin Infect Dis. 2009;22: 49–56.
34. Bettaieb A, Oksenhendler E, Duedari N, et al. Cross-reactive antibodies between HIV-gp120 and platelet gpIIIa (CD61) in HIV-related immune thrombocytopenic purpura. Clin Exp Immunol. 1996;103:19–23.
35. Kowalska MA, Ratajczak J, Hoxie J, et al. Megakaryocyte precursors, megakaryocytes and platelets express the HIV co-receptor CXCR4 on their surface: determination of response to stromal-derived factor-1 by megakaryocytes and platelets. Br J Haematol. 1999;104:220–9.
36. Sakaguchi M, Sato T, Groopman JE. Human immunodeficiency virus infection of megakaryocytic cells. Blood. 1991;77:481–5.
37. Sundell IB, Koka PS. Thrombocytopenia in HIV infection: impairment of platelet formation and loss correlates with increased c-Mpl and ligand thrombopoietin expression. Curr HIV Res. 2006;4:107–16.
38. Aboulafia DM, Bundow D, Waide S, et al. Initial observations on the efficacy of highly active antiretroviral therapy in the treatment of HIV-associated autoimmune thrombocytopenia. Am J Med Sci. 2000;320:117–23.
39. Provan D, Stasi R, Newland AC, et al. International consensus report on the investigation and management of primary immune thrombocytopenia. Blood. 2010;115:168–86.
40. Mittal S, Blaylock MG, Culligan DJ, et al. A high rate of CLL phenotype lymphocytes in autoimmune hemolytic anemia and immune thrombocytopenic purpura. Haematologica. 2008;93:151–2.

Differential Diagnosis: Hypoplastic Thrombocytopenia

Yoshiaki Tomiyama

Abstract There is no "gold standard" test that can reliably establish the diagnosis of ITP. Despite recent advancement in the understanding of its pathophysiology, diagnosis of ITP is mainly based on differential diagnosis. Based on its pathophysiology, several biomarkers such as plasma TPO level and percentage of reticulated platelets could be useful to differentiate ITP from hypoplastic thrombocytopenia.

1 Introduction

Autoimmune thrombocytopenia (ITP) is an acquired immune-mediated disorder characterized by isolated thrombocytopenia, defined as a peripheral blood platelet count less than 100×10^9/L, and the absence of any obvious initiating and/or underlying cause of the thrombocytopenia [1, 2]. Although increased platelet destruction mediated by autoantibodies plays a central role in the mechanism of thrombocytopenia in ITP, additional mechanisms in which both impaired platelet production and T cell-mediated effects have been demonstrated [3]. From a clinical point of view, the diagnosis of ITP is based on differential diagnosis despite recent advancement in the understanding of its pathophysiology. Among isolated thrombocytopenic disorders, the differentiation between ITP and hypoplastic disorders such as mild aplastic anemia (AA) and amegakaryocytic thrombocytopenia is often difficult

Y. Tomiyama, M.D.
Department of Blood Transfusion, Osaka University Hospital,
2-15 Yamadaoka, Suita, Osaka 565-0871, Japan
e-mail: yoshi@hp-blood.med.osaka-u.ac.jp

Y. Ishida, Y. Tomiyama (eds.), *Autoimmune Thrombocytopenia*,
DOI 10.1007/978-981-10-4142-6_10

Table 1 Etiological classification of thrombocytopenia

Decreased platelet production (hypoplastic thrombocytopenia)
Aplastic anemia (AA)
Amegakaryocytic thrombocytopenia
Acute leukemia
Chemotherapy-induced thrombocytopenia (CIT)
Myelodysplastic syndrome (MDS)
Malignancy with bone marrow infiltration or suppression (e.g., lymphoma, leukemia, solid tumors)
Increased platelet destruction or consumption
Autoimmune thrombocytopenia (ITP)
Secondary ITP
Systemic lupus erythematosus (SLE)
Drug-induced immune thrombocytopenia
Infection associated (e.g., HIV, HCV, *H. pylori*, EBV)
Thrombotic microangiopathy
Thrombotic thrombocytopenic purpura (TTP)
Hemolytic uremic syndrome (HUS)
Disseminated intravascular coagulation (DIC)
Antiphospholipid syndrome (APS)

(Table 1). There is no "gold standard" test that can reliably establish the diagnosis [4]. This chapter has dealt with possible diagnostic markers to differentiate ITP from hypoplastic thrombocytopenia.

2 Diagnostic Markers for the Differentiation Between ITP and Other Thrombocytopenic Disorders Due to Increased Platelet Destruction or Consumption

Before discussing differential diagnosis between ITP and hypoplastic thrombocytopenia, differentiation between ITP and other thrombocytopenic disorders due to increased platelet destruction or consumption should be discussed. As shown in Table 2, there are several diagnostic markers available to distinguish other thrombotic disorders from ITP. Schistocytes (=RBC fragments) in peripheral blood smear suggest thrombotic microangiopathy such as thrombotic thrombocytopenic purpura (TTP) and hemolytic uremic syndrome (HUS) [5]. Thus, as compared with differential diagnosis with hypoplastic thrombocytopenia, the differentiation between ITP and other thrombocytopenic disorders due to increased platelet destruction or consumption is not so difficult in daily practice.

Table 2 Diagnostic markers for thrombocytopenia due to increased platelet destruction or consumption

Secondary ITP
Systemic lupus erythematosus (SLE): antinuclear antibodies (ANA) (anti-double-stranded DNA [dsDNA] and anti-Sm)
Drug-induced immune thrombocytopenia: history of medication
Infection associated: tests for HIV, HCV, *H. pylori*, EBV, etc.
Thrombotic microangiopathy: microangiopathic hemolytic anemia (MAHA), schistocytes (RBC fragments)
TTP: ADAMTS13 activity, inhibitor for ADAMTS13
HUS: detection of *Shiga toxin-producing Escherichia coli (STEC)*
DIC: screening tests of coagulation (prothrombin time [PT], activated partial thromboplastin time [aPTT], fibrinogen, and D-dimer)
APS: antiphospholipid antibodies (anticardiolipin antibody, anti-β2-glycoprotein I antibody, lupus anticoagulant)

3 Diagnostic Markers for the Differentiation Between ITP and Hypoplastic Thrombocytopenia

3.1 *Bone Marrow Examination*

The need for bone marrow examination is still a matter of debate. The current American Society of Hematology (ASH) ITP guideline 2011 does not recommend a bone marrow examination in patients presenting with typical ITP, although the previous ASH guideline 1996 and international working group (IWG) consensus report recommended bone marrow examination for patients older than 60 years of age, for those with systemic symptoms or abnormal signs, or for some cases in which splenectomy is considered [4, 6, 7]. AA showing pancytopenia is easy for its diagnosis. However, mild AA with thrombocytopenia is often difficult for its diagnosis even by bone marrow examination (bone marrow aspiration and bone marrow biopsy). For considering the limitation of this procedure and to avoid this invasive procedure as initial screening, we need diagnostic markers for the differential diagnosis between ITP and hypoplastic thrombocytopenia.

3.2 *Platelet-Associated IgG (PAIgG)*

Several assays to detect antiplatelet antibodies as platelet-associated IgG (PAIgG) on platelets have been reported in the 1970s [1]. However, elevated levels of PAIgG were not specific for ITP but were often observed in patients with nonimmune thrombocytopenia including AA [8, 9]. IWG classified PAIgG as a test of uncertain benefit for the diagnosis of ITP [4]. More detailed nature of PAIgG is described in the chapter “Autoantigens in ITP.”

3.3 Platelet-Associated Antiplatelet Autoantibodies

Platelet-associated (PA) anti-GPIIb/IIIa and/or anti-GPIb-IX autoantibodies were detected in 50–60% ITP patients but not in patients with aplastic anemia [10, 11] (refer to the chapter "Autoantigens in ITP"). IWG classified PA antiplatelet autoantibodies (=glycoprotein-specific antibody) as a test of potential utility in the management of an ITP patient [4]. Regarding detection of PA autoantibodies, it has been shown that its specificity for the diagnosis of ITP is very high (80–90%) in prospective studies. However, the drawback in this assay is its relatively low sensitivity (50–60%) as well as being time-consuming, laboratory-based assay such as the immunobead assay and monoclonal antibody immobilization of platelet antigens (MAIPA) [11, 12]. Thus, from a clinical view point, it is difficult to perform this specific assay as a screening test for the diagnosis of ITP.

3.4 Plasma Thrombopoietin (TPO) Level and Percentage of Reticulated Platelets (RP%)

IWG consensus report classified plasma TPO level and RP% as tests of unproven or uncertain benefit for the diagnosis of ITP in 2010 [4]. In contrast, Japanese Working Group for ITP suggested that these markers may be useful for the diagnosis prospectively as well as retrospectively [13, 14]. To date, there are a substantial number of papers showing the usefulness of these markers as differential diagnosis of ITP.

Plasma TPO Level

In 1994, three groups independently cloned TPO, as the ligand for orphan cytokine receptor, c-Mpl [15–17]. TPO is a single 95 kDa glycoprotein consisting of 332-amino acid protein that is the primary regulator of normal platelet production. TPO is synthesized primarily in the liver and is secreted into circulation. Although it has long been thought that hepatic transcription and translation of the TPO gene appear constant, recent study reveals that TPO production is stimulated, at least in part, by desialylated, senescent platelets clearance via hepatocyte Ashwell-Morrell receptor. Hepatocyte Ashwell-Morrell receptor regulates TPO production via JAK2-STAT3 signaling [18, 19]. Secreted TPO is removed from circulation by binding of the TPO receptor (c-Mpl) on platelets and bone marrow megakaryocytes. Thus, plasma TPO levels usually increase in response to the decreased in platelet/megakaryocyte mass. Actually, plasma TPO levels are markedly increased in patients with congenital amegakaryocytic thrombocytopenia, aplastic anemia, or chemotherapy-induced thrombocytopenia (CIT). In sharp contrast, in patients with ITP (or thrombocytopenia due to increased platelet destruction or consumption), plasma TPO levels are within normal range or slightly increased [20–23]. Thus, plasma TPO levels may have diagnostic utility in discriminating between patients with ITP and hypoplastic thrombocytopenia [13, 14, 24].

RP%

Reticulated platelets (RPs) are reported to be younger platelets (i.e., immature platelets) that have been released recently into the circulation and are probably analogous to reticulocytes reflecting erythropoiesis. RPs can be distinguished from mature platelets by their RNA contents using flow cytometry with an RNA-binding fluorochrome, such as thiazole orange, and RP% and absolute number of RPs are reflecting platelet production and hence platelet turnover [25–27]. In patients with ITP, RP% was markedly increased compared with healthy controls, whereas RP% in patients with AA or CIT was within normal range [13, 25, 26]. Thus, RP% could also be a good marker to differentiate ITP from hypoplastic thrombocytopenia. However, the method for the measurement of RP% is a time-consuming, laboratory-based assay and has not been standardized yet, because RP% is measured by flow cytometry. To measure RP% in daily practice, percentage of immature platelet fraction (IPF%) could alternatively be measured by automated hematology analyzer such as Sysmex® XN-1000. As compared to XE-2100 (Sysmex Corp., Kobe, Japan), XN-1000 is a newer generation that uses oxazine to detect RNA and PLT-F channel to more accurately detect platelets (Fig. 1). We have compared RP%, IPF% measured by XE-2100, and IPF% measure by XN-1000 (newer generation) in

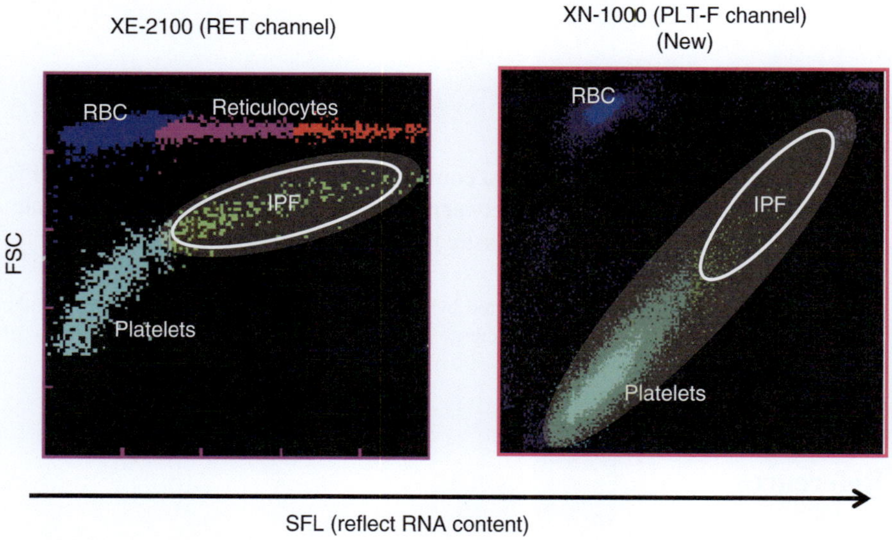

Fig. 1 Comparison between IPF% measured by automated hematology analyzer Sysmex® XE-2100 and XN-1000. In XE-2100, IPF% was measured in RET channel by which reticulocytes and IPF were not well dissociated. *IPF* immature platelet fraction

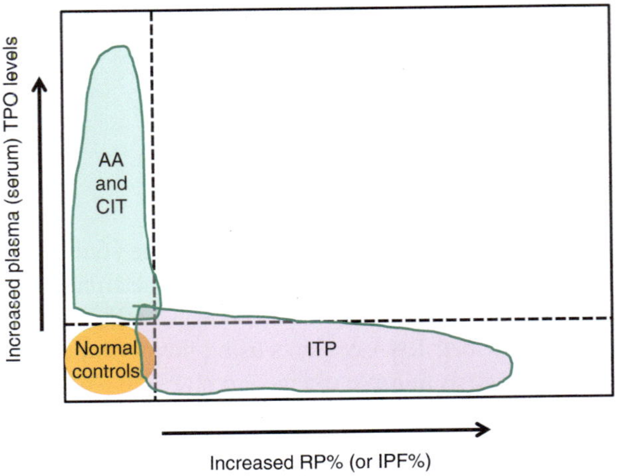

Fig. 2 Discrimination between ITP and hypoplastic thrombocytopenia by the combination of plasma TPO levels and RP% (or IPF%). *Dotted line*: upper limits of normal values

parallel to differentiate patients with ITP from aplastic anemia or CIT who were already well diagnosed. The sensitivity and specificity for the diagnosis of ITP were 83.0 and 75.0% for IPF% (XE), 85.1 and 89.3% for IPF% (XN), and 93.6 and 89.3% for RP%, respectively. Moreover, examination of patients with paroxysmal nocturnal hemoglobinuria (PNH) revealed that hemolysis and/or red blood cell fragments interfered with IPF% (XE) values, but not with RP% or IFP% (XN) values [28]. Thus, IPF% measured by XN-1000 appears comparable to RP% measured by flow cytometry and may have diagnostic utility in discriminating between patients with ITP and hypoplastic thrombocytopenia in daily practice.

4 Summary

Taken together, we have proposed that combination of plasma TPO levels and RP% would more precisely discriminate between thrombocytopenia with increased platelet clearance such as ITP and hypoplastic thrombocytopenia (Fig. 2) [13, 14].

Acknowledgment This work was supported by Grant-in-Aid for Scientific Research from the Ministry of Education, Culture, Sports, Science and Technology in Japan and the Ministry of Health, Labour and Welfare in Japan.

References

1. McMillan R. Chronic idiopathic thrombocytopenic purpura. N Engl J Med. 1981;304:1135–47.
2. Cines DB, Blanchette VS. Immune thrombocytopenic purpura. N Engl J Med. 2002;346: 995–1008.

3. Kashiwagi H, Tomiyama Y. Pathophysiology and management of primary immune thrombocytopenia. Int J Hematol. 2013;98:24–33.
4. Provan D, Stasi R, Newland AC, Blanchette VS, Bolton-Maggs P, Bussel JB, et al. International consensus report on the investigation and management of primary immune thrombocytopenia. Blood. 2010;115:168–86.
5. George JN, Nester CM. Syndrome of thrombotic microangiopathy. N Engl J Med. 2014;371:1847–8.
6. George JN, Woolf SH, Raskob GE, Wasser JS, Aledort LM, Ballem PJ, et al. Idiopathic thrombocytopenic purpura: a practice guideline developed by explicit methods for the American Society of Hematology. Blood. 1996;88:3–40.
7. Neunert C, Lim W, Crowther M, Cohen A, Solberg Jr L, Crowther MA, American Society of Hematology. The American Society of Hematology 2011 evidence-based practice guideline for immune thrombocytopenia. Blood. 2011;117:4190–207.
8. Kelton JG, Powers PJ, Carter CJ. A prospective study of the usefulness of the measurement of platelet-associated IgG for the diagnosis of idiopathic thrombocytopenic purpura. Blood. 1982;60:1050–3.
9. Mueller-Eckhardt C, Kayser W, Mersch-Baumert K, Mueller-Eckhardt G, Breidenbach M, Kugel HG, et al. The clinical significance of platelet-associated IgG: a study on 298 patients with various disorders. Br J Haematol. 1980;46:123–31.
10. Brighton TA, Evans S, Castaldi PA, Chesterman CN, Chong BH. Prospective evaluation of the clinical usefulness of an antigen specific assay (MAIPA) in idiopathic thrombocytopenic purpura and other immune thrombocytopenias. Blood. 1996;88:194–201.
11. McMillan R, Wang L, Tani P. Prospective evaluation of the immunobead assay for the diagnosis of adult chronic immune thrombocytopenic purpura (ITP). J Thromb Haemost. 2003;1:485–91.
12. Kiefel V, Santoso S, Kaufmann E, Mueller-Eckhardt C. Autoantibodies against platelet glycoprotein Ib/IX: a frequent finding in autoimmune thrombocytopenic purpura. Br J Haematol. 1991;79:256–62.
13. Kurata Y, Hayashi S, Kiyoi T, Kosugi S, Kashiwagi H, Honda S, et al. Diagnostic value of tests for reticulated platelets, plasma glycocalicin, and thrombopoietin levels for discriminating between hyperdestructive and hypoplastic thrombocytopenia. Am J Clin Pathol. 2001;115:656–64.
14. Kuwana M, Kurata Y, Fujimura K, Fujisawa K, Wada H, Nagasawa T, et al. Preliminary laboratory based diagnostic criteria for immune thrombocytopenic purpura: evaluation by multicenter prospective study. J Thromb Haemost. 2006;4:1936–43.
15. Bartley TD, Bogenberger J, Hunt P, Li YS, Lu HS, Martin F, et al. Identification and cloning of a megakaryocyte growth and development factor that is a ligand for the cytokine receptor Mpl. Cell. 1994;77:1117–24.
16. Lok S, Kaushansky K, Holly RD, Kuijper JL, Lofton-Day CE, Oort PJ, et al. Cloning and expression of murine thrombopoietin cDNA and stimulation of platelet production in vivo. Nature. 1994;369:565–8.
17. de Sauvage FJ, Hass PE, Spencer SD, Malloy BE, Gurney AL, Spencer SA, et al. Stimulation of megakaryocytopoiesis and thrombopoiesis by the c-Mpl ligand. Nature. 1994;369:533–8.
18. Grozovsky R, Begonja AJ, Liu K, Visner G, Hartwig JH, Falet H, et al. The Ashwell-Morell receptor regulates hepatic thrombopoietin production via JAK2-STAT3 signaling. Nat Med. 2015;21:47–54.
19. Grozovsky R, Giannini S, Falet H, Hoffmeister KM. Regulating billions of blood platelets: glycans and beyond. Blood. 2015;126:1877–84.
20. Kosugi S, Kurata Y, Tomiyama Y, Tahara T, Kato T, Tadokoro S, et al. Circulating thrombopoietin level in chronic immune thrombocytopenic purpura. Br J Haematol. 1996;93:704–6.
21. Emmons RV, Reid DM, Cohen RL, Meng G, Young NS, Dunbar CE, et al. Human thrombopoietin levels are high when thrombocytopenia is due to megakaryocyte deficiency and low when due to increased platelet destruction. Blood. 1996;87:4068–71.

22. Nagata Y, Shozaki Y, Nagahisa H, Nagasawa T, Abe T, Todokoro K. Serum thrombopoietin level is not regulated by transcription but by the total counts of both megakaryocytes and platelets during thrombocytopenia and thrombocytosis. Thromb Hemost. 1997;77:808–14.
23. Schrezenmeier H, Griesshammer M, Hornkohl A, Nichol JL, Hecht T, Heimpel H, et al. Thrombopoietin serum levels in patients with aplastic anaemia: correlation with platelet count and persistent elevation in remission. Br J Haematol. 1998;100:571–6.
24. Makar RS, Zhukov OS, Sahud MA, Kuter DJ. Thrombopoietin levels in patients with disorders of platelet production: diagnostic potential and utility in predicting response to TPO receptor agonists. Am J Hematol. 2013;88:1041–4.
25. Kienast J, Schmitz G. Flow cytometric analysis of thiazole orange uptake by platelets: a diagnostic aid in the evaluation of thrombocytopenic disorders. Blood. 1990;75:116–21.
26. Richards EM, Baglin TP. Quantitation of reticulated platelets: methodology and clinical application. Br J Haematol. 1995;91:445–51.
27. Barsam SJ, Psaila B, Forestier M, Page LK, Sloane PA, Geyer JT, et al. Platelet production and platelet destruction: assessing mechanisms of treatment effect in immune thrombocytopenia. Blood. 2011;117:5723–32.
28. Sakuragi M, Hayashi S, Maruyama M, Kabutomori O, Kiyokawa T, Nagamine K, et al. Clinical significance of IPF% or RP% measurement in distinguishing primary immune thrombocytopenia from aplastic thrombocytopenic disorders. Int J Hematol. 2015;101:369–75.

Differential Diagnosis: Congenital Macrothrombocytopenia

Shinji Kunishima

Abstract Differential diagnosis of congenital thrombocytopenia is important in the diagnosis of autoimmune thrombocytopenia. Congenital macrothrombocytopenia is a heterogeneous group of rare disorders, characterized by abnormally giant platelets and thrombocytopenia since birth. The most common are *MYH9* disorders and heterozygous Bernard-Soulier syndrome. In many of congenital macrothrombocytopenias, defects are associated with platelet cytoskeleton or adhesion molecules and their receptors. Thus, molecular diagnosis targeting subcellular localization or surface expression of defective gene product is available, and thus a definite diagnosis is possible in approximately 60% of cases.

1 Introduction

While congenital thrombocytopenia has been considered extremely rare, it appears that it may not be as rare as previously thought, affecting at least 2.7 in 100,000 [1]. Recent progress in next-generation sequencing (NGS) technologies have enabled identification of 11 causative genes for congenital thrombocytopenia since 2011, and more than 30 genes are presently known [1–5]. This not only improved our understanding of the molecular mechanisms of thrombocytopenia but also allowed the development of specific diagnostic tests [6, 7]. A definite diagnosis can now be achieved in more than half of patients. A series of studies have also shown that there are many patients in which immune thrombocytopenia (ITP) is diagnosed and unnecessarily treated as such. This is mainly because that diagnosis of ITP is basically made by exclusion of other causes of thrombocytopenia. Thus, it is necessary to remind ourselves that the differential diagnosis of congenital thrombocytopenia is necessary in patients with ITP, especially, who do not respond to ITP treatment.

S. Kunishima, Ph.D.
Department of Advanced Diagnosis, Clinical Research Center, National Hospital Organization Nagoya Medical Center, 4-1-1 Sannomaru, Naka-ku, Nagoya 4600001, Japan
e-mail: kunishis@nnh.hosp.go.jp

Y. Ishida, Y. Tomiyama (eds.), *Autoimmune Thrombocytopenia*,
DOI 10.1007/978-981-10-4142-6_11

2 Congenital Thrombocytopenia

The causes of congenital thrombocytopenia vary and can be categorized according to the mode of inheritance and causative genes [2–4]. However, clinically, it is simpler and easier to understand when the condition is categorized according to platelet size, into cases of congenital thrombocytopenia with small platelets (congenital microthrombocytopenia), cases of congenital thrombocytopenia with normal-sized platelets, and congenital thrombocytopenia with giant platelets (congenital macrothrombocytopenia) (Table 1). Mean platelet volume (MPV), which is an indicator of platelet size, can be calculated using automated blood cell counters. However, since the results can be rendered inaccurate by the presence of giant platelets, MPV

Table 1 Congenital thrombocytopenias classified according to platelet size

Platelet size	Disease	OMIM	Inheritance	Gene	Features
Small	Wiskott-Aldrich syndrome	301000	X	*WAS*	Immunodeficiency
	X-linked thrombocytopenia	313900	X	*WAS*	No immunodeficiency
	FYB thrombocytopenia	na	AR	*FYB*	Activated platelets
Normal	*ANKRD26* thrombocytopenia	188000	AD	*ANKRD26*	Predisposition to hematological malignancy
	Platelet disorder, familial, with associated myeloid malignancy	601399	AD	*RUNX1*	Predisposition to myelodysplastic syndrome and leukemia
	Congenital amegakaryocytic thrombocytopenia	604498	AR	*MPL*	Reduced megakaryocytes Development of bone marrow failure
	Thrombocytopenia with absent radii	274000	AR	*RBM8A*	Radial aplasia Platelet count increases with growth
	Congenital thrombocytopenia with radioulnar synostosis	605432	AD	*HOXA11*	Radioulnar synostosis
		616738	AD	*MECOM*	
	CYCS thrombocytopenia	612004	AD	*CYCS*	Platelet apoptosis
	ETV6 thrombocytopenia	na	AD	*ETV6*	Predisposition to hematological malignancy
	SLFN14 thrombocytopenia	616913	AD	*SLFN14*	

Table 1 (continued)

Platelet size	Disease	OMIM	Inheritance	Gene	Features
Large	*MYH9* disorders		AD	*MYH9*	Granulocyte inclusion bodies Alport manifestations
	May-Hegglin anomaly	155100			
	Sebastian syndrome	605249			
	Fechtner syndrome	153640			
	Epstein syndrome	153650			
	Bernard-Soulier syndrome, homozygous	231200	AR	*GP1BA* *GP1BB* *GP9*	Absent ristocetin-induced platelet agglutination
	Bernard-Soulier syndrome, heterozygous	231200	AD	*GP1BA* *GP1BB* *GP9 (?)*	
	DiGeorge syndrome/ velocardiofacial syndrome	188400/ 192430	AD	22q11del *(GP1BB)*	Contiguous gene syndrome
	GPIIb/IIIa macrothrombocytopenia	187800	AD	*ITGA2B* *ITGB3*	Activated GPIIb/ IIIa receptor
	ACTN1 macrothrombocytopenia	615193	AD	*ACTN1*	Platelet anisocytosis
	Type 2B von Willebrand disease	613554	AD	*VWF*	Increased ristocetin-induced platelet agglutination
	Platelet-type von Willebrand disease	177820	AD	*GP1BA*	Increased ristocetin-induced platelet agglutination
	Gray platelet syndrome	139090	AR	*NBEAL2*	Isolated gray platelets Development of myelofibrosis
	GFI1B macrothrombocytopenia	187900	AD	*GFI1B*	Abnormal erythropoiesis
	TUBB1 macrothrombocytopenia	613112	AD	*TUBB1*	Abnormal megakaryocyte/ platelet microtubule assembly
	Paris-Trousseau/ Jacobsen syndrome	188025/ 147791	AD	11q23del *(FLI1)*	Giant platelet α-granules
	X-linked macrothrombocytopenia	300367/ 314040	X	*GATA1*	Abnormal erythropoiesis

(continued)

Table 1 (continued)

Platelet size	Disease	OMIM	Inheritance	Gene	Features
	FLNA macrothrombocytopenia	300049	X	*FLNA*	Periventricular heterotopia
	Sitosterolemia	210250	AR	*ABCG5* *ABCG8*	Stomatocytosis Xanthoma Atherosclerosis
	PRKACG macrothrombocytopenia	616176	AR	*PRKACG*	Filamin A degradation
	CDC42 macrothrombocytopenia	616737	AD	*CDC42*	Lymphedema, developmental delay
	DIAPH1 macrothrombocytopenia	na	AD	*DIAPH1*	Deafness
	TRPM7 macrothrombocytopenia	na	AD	*TRPM7*	Atrial fibrillation
	SRC thrombocytopenia	na	AD	*SRC*	Myelofibrosis, tooth fractures, osteoporosis

AD autosomal dominant, *AR* autosomal recessive, *X* X-linked, *na* not available

values alone must not be used to evaluate platelet size. For this reason, observation of platelet morphology on peripheral blood smears and platelet size determination are particularly important. Large platelets are frequently observed in ITP; however, the majorities are normal in size [8, 9]. In cases of congenital macrothrombocytopenia, on the other hand, the majority of platelets are large. If congenital thrombocytopenia is suspected, then a detailed medical history and family history should be taken, along with information about drugs currently being administered. If the platelet count was normal in the past examinations, the condition is likely to have been acquired. If a history of antecedent infection is not obvious and/or a normal platelet count is not found in the past examinations, it is necessary to consider the differential diagnosis of congenital thrombocytopenia.

3 Congenital Macrothrombocytopenia

The platelet cytoskeleton plays a pivotal role in maintaining and remodeling platelet morphology [10, 11]. It is organized based on actin filaments that are present in a mesh-like lattice throughout the cytoplasm, along with membrane cytoskeleton that lines the platelet membranes. The transmembrane receptors on the platelet membranes not only bind to the cytoskeletal proteins through their intracellular domains but also mediate signal transduction [12–15]. Microtubules contribute to the platelet production through proplatelet formation and regulate maturation and maintaining normal discoid shape of platelets [10, 11].

Congenital macrothrombocytopenia is a heterogeneous group of rare disorders, characterized by abnormally giant platelets and thrombocytopenia since birth [16]. The bleeding tendency varies from very mild in some to severe and life threatening in others. Recently, a significant progress has been made in the identification of new causative genes and the establishment of diagnostic tests for this group [6, 7]. In many of congenital macrothrombocytopenias, defects are associated with platelet cytoskeleton or adhesion receptors and their ligands. Thus, molecular diagnosis targeting subcellular localization or surface expression of defective gene product is available. On the other hand, the diagnosis of congenital thrombocytopenia with normal-sized platelets is more challenging. In many cases, the diagnosis is based solely on genetic analysis with conventional Sanger sequencing of potential candidate genes or recent high-throughput sequencing [17, 18]. This is because in this form of congenital thrombocytopenia, genetic defects are mostly in the transcription factors and thrombopoietin signaling regulating megakaryocyte commitment and growth, and therefore decreased megakaryocytes are the immediate cause for thrombocytopenia.

4 *MYH9* Disorders

MYH9 disorders, the prototype of which is May-Hegglin anomaly (MHA), are autosomal dominant platelet disorders characterized by a triad of giant platelets, thrombocytopenia, and leukocyte inclusion bodies [19, 20]. In addition to MHA, Sebastian, Fechtner, and Epstein syndromes belong to *MYH9* disorders. These disorders are caused by mutations in *MYH9*, the gene encoding for the non-muscle myosin heavy chain-IIA (NMMHC-IIA). From the first description a century ago, the hallmark of the disease is the presence of characteristic Döhle body-like leukocyte cytoplasmic inclusion bodies on conventionally stained peripheral blood smears [21, 22]. They are often faint or even unrecognized. Inclusion bodies are present in granulocytes but not in lymphocytes [23]. Detection of inclusion bodies is a prerequisite for a correct diagnosis, and failure in the detection often leads to misdiagnosis such as ITP. Inclusion bodies are present as a ribonucleoprotein complex consisting of *MYH9* mRNA, clusters of ribosomes, and abnormally accumulated NMMHC-IIA protein [24]. *MYH9* mRNA but not NMMHC-IIA is responsible for the morphological appearance/stainability of inclusion bodies on conventionally stained blood smears [25]. The rapid degradation of *MYH9* mRNA accounts for the time-dependent decrease in the stainability of inclusion bodies.

Immunofluorescence analysis of neutrophil NMMHC-IIA localization has revolutionized the diagnosis of *MYH9* disorders, and this analysis has become a gold standard for diagnosis of the disease [26–28]. The abnormal localization pattern can be classified according to the number, size, and shape of NMMHC-IIA aggregates, into types I, II, and III [26]. Type I comprises one or two large, intensely stained cytoplasmic NMMHC-IIA aggregates. Type II comprises up to 20 small cytoplasmic spots. Type III appears as speckled staining. The pattern of localization correlates with the site of *MYH9* mutation. p.E1841K and frameshift and nonsense mutations in exon 40 are associated with type I localization. Missense mutations such as p.R1165C and p.D1424N are associated with type II localization. Normal NMMHC-IIA localization can exclude the diagnosis of *MYH9* disorders [29]. Although *MYH9* disorders were thought to be very rare, the advent of the immunofluorescence analysis has enabled the detection of even minute abnormal NMMHC-IIA aggregates and more precise diagnosis and classification; thus, *MYH9* disorders are now known to be the most prevalent congenital thrombocytopenia. Patients with *MYH9* disorders often develop non-hematological complications such as glomerulonephritis, sensorineural hearing loss, and cataracts. Because the onset and disease severity of non-hematological complications are related to the site of the *MYH9* mutation, a genetic diagnosis is mandatory [27, 30].

5 Bernard-Soulier Syndrome

Bernard-Soulier syndrome (BSS) is an autosomal recessive bleeding disorder characterized by giant platelets, thrombocytopenia, prolonged bleeding time, and absent ristocetin-induced platelet agglutination [31, 32]. This syndrome is caused by the deficiency of platelet glycoprotein (GP)Ib-IX-V complex, the platelet receptor for von Willebrand factor (VWF), due to compound heterozygous or homozygous mutations in the genes for GPIbα(*GP1BA*), GPIbβ(*GP1BB*), or GPIX(*GP9*). As a result of the absence of GPIb-IX-V complexes on the platelet membrane, platelets are unable to adhere to the vascular subendothelium. Thus, patients manifest a severe bleeding tendency from early childhood, primarily from mucocutaneous tissues; purpura, epistaxis, menorrhagia, and gingival bleeding are common, but hemarthroses and deep visceral hematomas are rare. The cytoplasmic domain of GPIbα, on the other hand, associates with actin via filamin A, and the defective linkage between GPIb-IX-V and cytoskeleton is the primary proposed mechanisms for the large platelet size in BSS [33, 34]. In addition, recent studies indicate that proplatelet formation is defective in megakaryocytes, suggesting defective interactions between GPIb-IX-V and filamin A-actin adversely affect both platelet morphogenesis and megakaryocytopoiesis [35].

Although BSS is a very rare disorder with an estimated prevalence of less than 1 in one million, the calculated frequency of BSS heterozygotes is 1 in 500, indicating that a sizable number of heterozygous carriers are present in the normal population [36, 37]. It is worth to note that although heterozygous BSS carriers are generally asymptomatic with mild or moderate thrombocytopenia, they have large platelets. Individuals with a heterozygous mutation have been often identified as having undifferentiated thrombocytopenia. In Italy, the Bolzano variant (*GP1BA* p. A172V) was found to be responsible for the autosomal dominant macrothrombocytopenia previously known as a Mediterranean macrothrombocytopenia [38, 39]. Likewise, *GP1BB* p. Y113C is prevalent in autosomal dominant macrothrombocytopenia in Japan [40, 41]. In addition, patients with DiGeorge/velocardiofacial syndrome due to a heterozygous chromosome 22q11.2 microdeletion, which includes the *GP1BB* gene, have macrothrombocytopenia [42, 43].

The classical diagnostic features are a prolonged bleeding time, moderate to severe thrombocytopenia, and giant platelets. Especially, giant platelets and the absence of ristocetin-induced platelet agglutination are the laboratory hallmarks of BSS. Flow cytometric determination of platelet GPIb/IX expression is a convenient method for a definite diagnosis. This also allows an evaluation of platelet size, and double labeling of GPIb/IX and GPIIb/IIIa permits determination of comparative expression levels. In a typical case of BSS, the fluorescence intensities of normal mouse IgG and anti-GPIIb/IIIa antibody are increased, which is reflected by giant platelets with a large surface area. In contrast, GPIbα, GPIbβ, and GPIX are all decreased. However, the abnormalities of the GPIb-IX-V complex are heterogeneous; residual amounts of the complex and/or some of the subunits are often present. Evaluating GPIbα, GPIbβ, and GPIX expression highlights selective deficiencies and candidate genes for investigation. Accordingly, the most deficient subunit in the platelets is often found to indicate the genetic basis: patients with residual GPIbβ and GPIX are often associated with a *GP1BA* mutation, and those with residual GPIbα and GPIbβ are often associated with a GP9 mutation [16, 36]. Patients with no substantial expression of each subunit usually have a *GP1BB* mutation, because GPIbβ is the critical subunit linking GPIbα and GPIX [37, 44].

6 *ACTN1* Macrothrombocytopenia

ACTN1 macrothrombocytopenia is recently identified by whole exome sequencing (WES) in families with dominant form of congenital macrothrombocytopenia in which no relevant mutations in the previously reported genes had been identified [45]. Following *MYH9* disorders and heterozygous and homozygous Bernard-Soulier syndrome, *ACTN1* macrothrombocytopenia represents the third most prevalent form of congenital macrothrombocytopenia. It is characterized by mild macrothrombocytopenia, with mild or no bleeding tendency without non-hematologic complications [45, 46]. *ACTN1* gene codes α-actinin-1, of which dimers stabilize the actin filaments and contribute to actin cytoskeletal organization by cross-linking actin filaments [47]. Initially, *ACTN1* mutations were identified within the functional actin-binding and calmodulin-like domains. They cause a disorganized actin-based cytoskeleton in megakaryocytes, resulting in the production of abnormally large proplatelet tips, which were reduced in number [45]. Recently, a p.L395Q mutation within the spacer rod domain, which is composed of spectrin-like repeats, has been found, suggesting that mutations not only affect actin-binding properties but also affect structural organization of actinin can cause *ACTN1* macrothrombocytopenia [48].

Although α-actinin-1 binds to β-integrins and can mediate their signaling, there are no apparent abnormalities in platelet adhesion, aggregation, or clot retraction in *ACTN1* macrothrombocytopenia [45, 46, 49]. Furthermore, there is no apparent abnormal α-actinin-1 localization in resting as well as surface-activated platelets. Accordingly, a molecular genetic analysis was only available for the diagnosis. However, a recent investigation suggested the immunofluorescence analysis to detect NMMHC-IIA in the granulomere zone in surface-activated platelets as a potential diagnostic test for *ACTN1* macrothrombocytopenia [50].

7 GPIIb/IIIa Macrothrombocytopenia

It is well known that congenital deficiency of GPIIb/IIIa (integrin αIIbβ3), platelet receptor for fibrinogen, due to homozygous mutations in the genes for GPIIb (*ITGA2B*) or GPIIIa (*ITGB3*) results in bleeding disorder Glanzmann thrombasthenia [51]. It is also known that homozygous patients and heterozygous carriers have normal platelet count and morphology. However, this is not always the case. Recently, heterozygous, activating mutations in the juxtamembrane region of GPIIb and GPIIIa are found to cause congenital macrothrombocytopenia [52]. Membrane-proximal region of GPIIb/IIIa, especially a salt bridge between GPIIb R995 and GPIIIa D723, maintains the inactive conformation of the receptor [53]. Disruption of the electrostatic interaction produces constitutive, agonist-independent outside-in signaling of GPIIb/IIIa and phosphorylation of signaling proteins such as FAK and leads to perturbation of cytoskeletal reorganization and results in abnormal proplatelet formation [54, 55]. Focal adhesion kinase is known to inhibit Rho and may promote precocious proplatelet formation, which is common among *MYH9* disorders [56, 57].

In GPIIb/IIIa macrothrombocytopenia, GPIIb/IIIa expression is decreased due to accelerated internalization of activated GPIIb/IIIa [58, 59]. While GPIIb/IIIa is constitutively activated, allowing binding of fibrinogen and the ligand-mimetic antibody PAC-1 to resting platelets, no expression of p-selectin is noted, and the platelets themselves are not activated [54, 55]. Thus, flow cytometry is useful for screening GPIIb/IIIa macrothrombocytopenia by detecting decreased GPIIb/IIIa, binding of PAC-1 and fibrinogen, and no expression of p-selectin. Actually, concomitant flow cytometry for GPIb/IX and GPIIb/IIIa can differentiate homozygous and heterozygous Bernard-Soulier syndrome and GPIIb/IIIa macrothrombocytopenia.

8 Type 2B on Willebrand Disease

Von Willebrand disease (VWD) is the most common congenital bleeding disorder of primary hemostasis caused by qualitative or quantitative defects of von Willebrand factor (VWF) [60]. It is classified into three main types: type 1, quantitatively reduced VWF; type 2, qualitatively abnormal VWF; and type 3, absent VWF. Type 2 VWD is categorized into four subtypes: 2A, 2B, 2M, and 2N. Type 2B VWD is a rare autosomal dominant form (5–8% of all VWD) characterized by the increased affinity of mutant VWF to platelet GPIb due to mutations in the A1 domain of VWF that contains the GPIb-binding site. Enhanced VWF-GPIb interactions lead to spontaneous platelet aggregation in vivo and in vitro and result in thrombocytopenia and lack of high molecular weight multimers of VWF. Giant platelets and spontaneous platelet aggregates are often detected on peripheral blood smears [61]. Thrombocytopenia deteriorates during stressors, such as infection, surgery, and pregnancy, and thus patients are often misdiagnosed with ITP. This platelet phenotype was previously described as Montreal platelet syndrome, in which spontaneous platelet is noted, but is now known to be type 2B VWD due to p.V1316M mutation [62].

Platelet aggregates on peripheral blood smears, which are comprised of several to dozens of platelets, are suggestive of type 2B VWD and platelet-type (pseudo) VWD (PT VWD) [61, 63]. While type 2B VWD and PT VWD are characterized by increased ristocetin sensitivity, they can be differentiated by mixing studies of ristocetin-induced platelet agglutination using patient platelets in normal control plasma and normal control platelets in patient plasma. When an unexpected low platelet count and platelet aggregates on a smear are obtained in individuals without bleeding tendency, EDTA-induced pseudothrombocytopenia should be considered [64]. EDTA-induced pseudothrombocytopenia is a common phenomenon caused by in vitro platelet clumping in the presence of EDTA anticoagulant, with a prevalence of as much as 0.1–0.2%. Accurate platelet counts can be usually obtained without anticoagulant or collecting in other anticoagulants such as sodium citrate or heparin.

9 Gray Platelet Syndrome

Gray platelet syndrome (GPS) is an autosomal recessive bleeding disorder that is characterized by macrothrombocytopenia and lack of platelet α-granules [65]. Due to the absence of α-granules and their constituents, platelets appear gray or colorless on May-Grünwald-Giemsa or Wright's stained blood smears. Since α-granules contain fibrinogen and VWF as well as other adhesive molecules and coagulation factors, the condition is closely associated with bleeding tendency. Furthermore, α-granule contents such as platelet-derived growth factor and transforming growth factor-β are synthesized but not properly stored within the granules and released from megakaryocytes into the bone marrow space; myelofibrosis is present in most cases. Although biochemical studies have failed to reveal any genetic alterations, using WES and RNA sequencing, Albers et al., Gunay-Aygun et al., and Kahr et al. simultaneously and independently identified homozygous or compound heterozygous mutations in *NBEAL2* [66–68]. *NBEAL2* contains the Beige and Chediak-Higashi (BEACH) domain, which is critical in vesicle trafficking and also present in *LYST*, a gene responsible for Chediak-Higashi syndrome.

Platelet α-granule deficiencies are also found in ARC syndrome (arthrogryposis-renal dysfunction-cholestasis syndrome) due to homozygous mutation in *VPS33B* and *VIPAS39*, which belong to the Sec1/Munc18 protein family that regulates vesicle formation [69]. Partial deficiency but not complete loss of α-granules can occur in other congenital macrothrombocytopenias due to mutations in *GATA1* and *GFI1B* [70, 71]. GATA-1 is an X-linked megakaryocyte and erythroid-specific transcription factor required for normal growth and differentiation of both lineages [72]. Defective GATA-1 function due to *GATA1* missense mutations causes reduced transcription of its target genes, suggesting that *NBEAL2* may also be dysregulated. Dyserythropoiesis due to diminished or unbalanced synthesis of globin chains is observed in *GATA1* macrothrombocytopenia [73].

10 *GFI1B* Macrothrombocytopenia

Growth factor independence 1b (GFI1B) is a transcriptional repressor containing six zinc finger domains and regulates erythropoiesis and megakaryocytopoiesis [74]. In a family with autosomal dominant macrothrombocytopenia with platelet α-granule deficiencies, genome-wide linkage analysis and candidate gene sequencing led to the identification of a nonsense mutation in *GFI1B* zinc finger 5, which is critical for DNA binding [75]. Functional analyses suggested a dominant negative effect. Subsequently, two other null *GFI1B* mutations that also disrupt zinc finger 5 were identified in patients with autosomal dominant macrothrombocytopenia, a decrease in α-granules, and red blood cell anisopoikilocytosis [70, 76]. Gfl1b mutants dominantly affect the terminal maturation of megakaryocytes and subsequent release of platelets with persistent CD34 expression and decreased CD42b expression.

Although a reduction in platelet α-granules is also observed in *GATA1* macrothrombocytopenia, detecting CD34, which is usually confined to immature hematopoietic progenitors, on platelets by flow cytometry and/or immunofluorescence analysis can differentiate *GFI1B* macrothrombocytopenia [70, 76].

11 *TUBB1* Macrothrombocytopenia

Platelets are released from megakaryocytes through proplatelet formation, which is driven by elongation of microtubules. After being released in the circulation, platelets mature and even divide, where microtubules play a central role [11, 77]. Normal discoid platelet morphology is maintained by marginal band of microtubules. Microtubules are assembled from α- and β-tubulin heterodimers. Among the β-tubulin isoforms, β1-tubulin is the megakaryocyte/platelet specific and the predominant isoform [78]. *TUBB1* mutations interfere with proper microtubule assembly and result in proplatelet-independent platelet release [79, 80]. Platelets from patients with *TUBB1* macrothrombocytopenia as well as from canine and feline *TUBB1* macrothrombocytopenia are large and spherical [81, 82].

12 Paris-Trousseau/Jacobsen Syndrome

Paris-Trousseau thrombocytopenia, a variant of Jacobsen syndrome, is a congenital disorder caused by partial deletions of 11q23 accompanied by developmental abnormalities [83, 84]. The platelet defects include giant platelets with large α-granules, which is due to haploinsufficiency in the transcription factor FLI1, located in the deleted region. FLI1 is a member of the ETS family and cooperates with RUNX1 during megakaryopoiesis [85]. Transient monoallelic expression of *FLI1* is critical for megakaryocyte development; thus, when the deleted or mutated allele is expressed, megakaryocyte development is restricted [86]. Identification of heterozygous point mutations in the ETS DNA-binding domain of FLI1 supports the notion that haploinsufficiency of *FLI1* is responsible for thrombocytopenia in this syndrome [87]. However, the recent identification of a homozygous FLI1 mutation that interferes the autoinhibitory domain regulating DNA binding in two patients with unaffected heterozygous parents has provided evidence that hypofunctional mutations can present with autosomal recessive inheritance [88]. Detecting nonmuscle myosin heavy chain IIB protein remaining in the platelets is an effective diagnosis of the condition [89].

13 Diagnostic Workflow of Congenital Macrothrombocytopenia

We propose a diagnostic flowchart for congenital macrothrombocytopenia, with a definite diagnosis possible in more than 60% of all cases in which congenital macrothrombocytopenia is suspected (Fig. 1). First of all, particularly important is careful morphological examination of peripheral blood smears to examine platelet size and color and the presence of platelet aggregates. Platelet size determination on a peripheral blood smear is useful in the differential diagnosis of congenital macrothrombocytopenia. For example, in *MYH9* disorder and homozygous BSS, many of platelets are giant, larger than 4 μm in diameter. Platelet aggregates are often present in type 2B VWD/PT VWD. Platelets are gray or colorless in GPS and ARC syndrome, and a partial deficiency is found in *GATA1* and *GFI1B* macrothrombocytopenias. In the latter two, abnormal red blood cell morphology is observed, and they can be differentiated by the analysis of platelet CD34 expression. The presence of bleeding tendency is a useful information. If a bleeding tendency is more serious than the thrombocytopenia, ristocetin-induced platelet agglutination can differentiate BSS and type 2B VWD/PT VWD. Absent agglutination suggests BSS. In contrast, agglutination at low concentration suggests type 2B VWD/PT VWD. They can be differentiated by mixing studies of ristocetin-induced platelet agglutination. Then the analysis is proceeded as follows: when the presence of granulocyte inclusion bodies is evident, immunofluorescence analysis of neutrophil NMMHC-IIA followed by *MYH9* gene sequencing corresponding to the localization pattern is performed. When the presence of

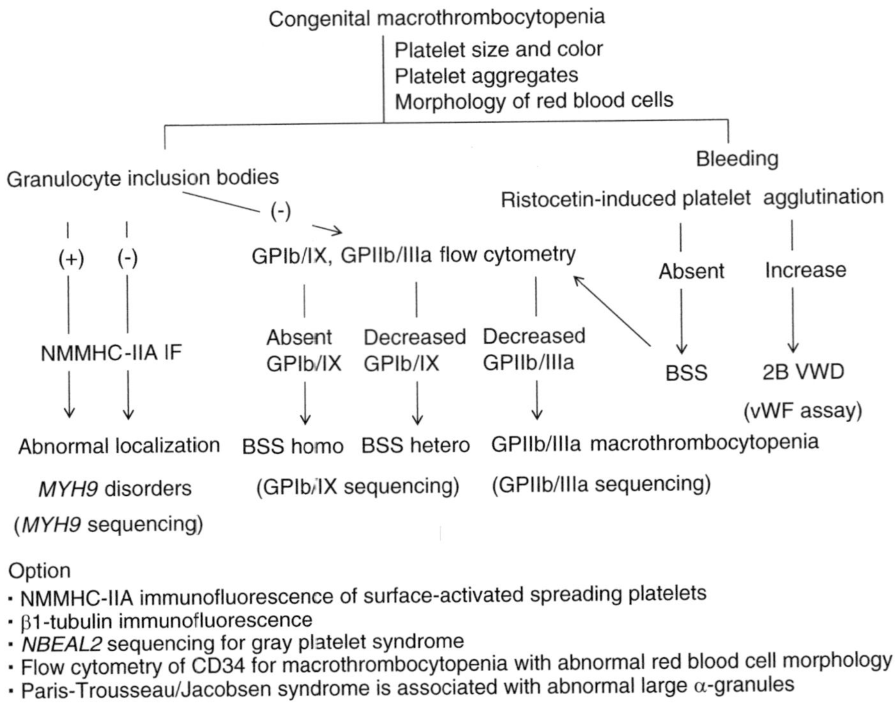

Fig. 1 Diagnostic flowchart for congenital macrothrombocytopenia

granulocyte inclusion bodies is uncertain, then flow cytometry to evaluate the expression levels of GPIb-IX-V and GPIIb/IIIa is simultaneously performed. The optional analyses include NMMHC-IIA localization of surface-activated spreading platelets for *ACTN1* macrothrombocytopenia, platelet β1-tubulin localization for *TUBB1* macrothrombocytopenia, and *NBEAL2* sequencing for gray platelet syndrome.

Despite considerable improvements in the diagnostic armamentarium for ITP, the diagnosis is still one of exclusion and can be challenging. Hematologists and pediatricians should be aware of diagnostic relevance of a careful examination of peripheral blood smears to evaluate platelet morphology.

References

1. Balduini CL, Noris P. Innovation in the field of thrombocytopenias: achievements since the beginning of the century and promises for the future. Haematologica. 2016;101(1):2–4. doi:10.3324/haematol.2015.138149.
2. Balduini CL, Melazzini F, Pecci A. Inherited thrombocytopenias-recent advances in clinical and molecular aspects. Platelets. 2016;28(1):3–13. doi:10.3109/09537104.2016.1171835.
3. Eto K, Kunishima S. Linkage between the mechanisms of thrombocytopenia and thrombopoiesis. Blood. 2016;127(10):1234–41. doi:10.1182/blood-2015-07-607903.

4. Savoia A. Molecular basis of inherited thrombocytopenias. Clin Genet. 2016a;89(2):154–62. doi:10.1111/cge.12607.
5. Savoia A. Molecular basis of inherited thrombocytopenias: an update. Curr Opin Hematol. 2016b;23(5):486–92. doi:10.1097/MOH.0000000000000269.
6. Favier R, Raslova H. Progress in understanding the diagnosis and molecular genetics of macrothrombocytopenias. Br J Haematol. 2015;170(5):626–39. doi:10.1111/bjh.13478.
7. Pecci A. Diagnosis and treatment of inherited thrombocytopenias. Clin Genet. 2016;89(2):141–53. doi:10.1111/cge.12603.
8. Noris P, Biino G, Pecci A, Civaschi E, Savoia A, Seri M, Melazzini F, Loffredo G, Russo G, Bozzi V, Notarangelo LD, Gresele P, Heller PG, Pujol-Moix N, Kunishima S, Cattaneo M, Bussel J, De Candia E, Cagioni C, Ramenghi U, Barozzi S, Fabris F, Balduini CL. Platelet diameters in inherited thrombocytopenias: analysis of 376 patients with all known disorders. Blood. 2014;124(6):e4–10. doi:10.1182/blood-2014-03-564328.
9. Noris P, Klersy C, Gresele P, Giona F, Giordano P, Minuz P, Loffredo G, Pecci A, Melazzini F, Civaschi E, Mezzasoma A, Piedimonte M, Semeraro F, Veneri D, Menna F, Ciardelli L, Balduini CL, Italian Gruppo di Studio delle Piastrine. Platelet size for distinguishing between inherited thrombocytopenias and immune thrombocytopenia: a multicentric, real life study. Br J Haematol. 2013;162(1):112–9. doi:10.1111/bjh.12349.
10. Thon JN, Italiano Jr JE. Does size matter in platelet production? Blood. 2012;120(8):1552–61. doi:10.1182/blood-2012-04-408724.
11. Thon JN, Macleod H, Begonja AJ, Zhu J, Lee KC, Mogilner A, Hartwig JH, Italiano Jr JE. Microtubule and cortical forces determine platelet size during vascular platelet production. Nat Commun. 2012;3:852. doi:10.1038/ncomms1838.
12. Bennett JS. Regulation of integrins in platelets. Biopolymers. 2015;104(4):323–33. doi:10.1002/bip.22679.
13. Coller BS. αIIbβ3: structure and function. J Thromb Haemost. 2015;13(Suppl 1):S17–25. doi:10.1111/jth.12915.
14. Gardiner EE, Andrews RK. Structure and function of platelet receptors initiating blood clotting. Adv Exp Med Biol. 2014;844:263–75. doi:10.1007/978-1-4939-2095-2_13.
15. Ozaki Y, Suzuki-Inoue K, Inoue O. Platelet receptors activated via mulitmerization: glycoprotein VI, GPIb-IX-V, and CLEC-2. J Thromb Haemost. 2013;11(Suppl 1):330–9. doi:10.1111/jth.12235.
16. Kunishima S, Saito H. Congenital macrothrombocytopenias. Blood Rev. 2006;20(2):111–21. doi:10.1016/j.blre.2005.08.001.
17. Lentaigne C, Freson K, Laffan MA, Turro E, Ouwehand WH, BRIDGE-BPD Consortium and the ThromboGenomics Consortium. Inherited platelet disorders: toward DNA-based diagnosis. Blood. 2016;127(23):2814–23. doi:10.1182/blood-2016-03-378588.
18. Simeoni I, Stephens JC, Hu F, Deevi SV, Megy K, Bariana TK, Lentaigne C, Schulman S, Sivapalaratnam S, Vries MJ, Westbury SK, Greene D, Papadia S, Alessi MC, Attwood AP, Ballmaier M, Baynam G, Bermejo E, Bertoli M, Bray PF, Bury L, Cattaneo M, Collins P, Daugherty LC, Favier R, French DL, Furie B, Gattens M, Germeshausen M, Ghevaert C, Goodeve AC, Guerrero JA, Hampshire DJ, Hart DP, Heemskerk JW, Henskens YM, Hill M, Hogg N, Jolley JD, Kahr WH, Kelly AM, Kerr R, Kostadima M, Kunishima S, Lambert MP, Liesner R, Lopez JA, Mapeta RP, Mathias M, Millar CM, Nathwani A, Neerman-Arbez M, Nurden AT, Nurden P, Othman M, Peerlinck K, Perry DJ, Poudel P, Reitsma P, Rondina MT, Smethurst PA, Stevenson W, Szkotak A, Tuna S, van Geet C, Whitehorn D, Wilcox DA, Zhang B, Revel-Vilk S, Gresele P, Bellissimo DB, Penkett CJ, Laffan MA, Mumford AD, Rendon A, Gomez K, Freson K, Ouwehand WH, Turro E. A high-throughput sequencing test for diagnosing inherited bleeding, thrombotic, and platelet disorders. Blood. 2016;127(23):2791–803. doi:10.1182/blood-2015-12-688267.
19. Balduini CL, Pecci A, Savoia A. Recent advances in the understanding and management of MYH9-related inherited thrombocytopenias. Br J Haematol. 2011;154(2):161–74. doi:10.1111/j.1365-2141.2011.08716.x.
20. Kunishima S, Saito H. Advances in the understanding of MYH9 disorders. Curr Opin Hematol. 2010;17(5):405–10. doi:10.1097/MOH.0b013e32833c069c.

21. Hegglin R. Gleichzeitige konstitutionelle Veranderungen an Neutrophilen und Thrombocyten. Helv Med Acta. 1945;12:439–40.
22. May R. Leukozyteneinschlusse. Dtsch Arch Klin Med. 1909;96:1–6.
23. Kunishima S, Hamaguchi M, Saito H. Differential expression of wild-type and mutant NMMHC-IIA polypeptides in blood cells suggests cell-specific regulation mechanisms in MYH9 disorders. Blood. 2008a;111(6):3015–23. doi:10.1182/blood-2007-10-116194.
24. Kunishima S, Hirano K, Hamaguchi M, Saito H. Accumulation of MYH9 mRNA at leukocyte inclusion bodies in MYH9 disorders. Eur J Haematol. 2008b;81(4):325–6. doi:10.1111/j.1600-0609.2008.01119.x.
25. Kunishima S, Yoshinari M, Nishio H, Ida K, Miura T, Matsushita T, Hamaguchi M, Saito H. Haematological characteristics of MYH9 disorders due to MYH9 R702 mutations. Eur J Haematol. 2007;78(3):220–6. doi:10.1111/j.1600-0609.2006.00806.x.
26. Kunishima S, Matsushita T, Kojima T, Sako M, Kimura F, Jo EK, Inoue C, Kamiya T, Saito H. Immunofluorescence analysis of neutrophil nonmuscle myosin heavy chain-A in MYH9 disorders: association of subcellular localization with MYH9 mutations. Lab Investig. 2003;83(1):115–22.
27. Saposnik B, Binard S, Fenneteau O, Nurden A, Nurden P, Hurtaud-Roux MF, Schlegel N, French MYH. Mutation spectrum and genotype-phenotype correlations in a large French cohort of MYH9-related disorders. Mol Genet Genomic Med. 2014;2(4):297–312. doi:10.1002/mgg3.68.
28. Savoia A, De Rocco D, Panza E, Bozzi V, Scandellari R, Loffredo G, Mumford A, Heller PG, Noris P, De Groot MR, Giani M, Freddi P, Scognamiglio F, Riondino S, Pujol-Moix N, Fabris F, Seri M, Balduini CL, Pecci A. Heavy chain myosin 9-related disease (MYH9-RD): neutrophil inclusions of myosin-9 as a pathognomonic sign of the disorder. Thromb Haemost. 2010;103(4):826–32. doi:10.1160/TH09-08-0593.
29. Kitamura K, Yoshida K, Shiraishi Y, Chiba K, Tanaka H, Furukawa K, Miyano S, Ogawa S, Kunishima S. Normal neutrophil myosin IIA localization in an immunofluorescence analysis can rule out MYH9 disorders. J Thromb Haemost. 2013;11(11):2071–3. doi:10.1111/jth.12406.
30. Pecci A, Klersy C, Gresele P, Lee KJ, De Rocco D, Bozzi V, Russo G, Heller PG, Loffredo G, Ballmaier M, Fabris F, Beggiato E, Kahr WH, Pujol-Moix N, Platokouki H, Van Geet C, Noris P, Yerram P, Hermans C, Gerber B, Economou M, De Groot M, Zieger B, De Candia E, Fraticelli V, Kersseboom R, Piccoli GB, Zimmermann S, Fierro T, Glembotsky AC, Vianello F, Zaninetti C, Nicchia E, Guthner C, Baronci C, Seri M, Knight PJ, Balduini CL, Savoia A. MYH9-related disease: a novel prognostic model to predict the clinical evolution of the disease based on genotype-phenotype correlations. Hum Mutat. 2014;35(2):236–47. doi:10.1002/humu.22476.
31. Andrews RK, Berndt MC. Bernard-Soulier syndrome: an update. Semin Thromb Hemost. 2013;39(6):656–62. doi:10.1055/s-0033-1353390.
32. Savoia A, Kunishima S, De Rocco D, Zieger B, Rand ML, Pujol-Moix N, Caliskan U, Tokgoz H, Pecci A, Noris P, Srivastava A, Ward C, Morel-Kopp MC, Alessi MC, Bellucci S, Beurrier P, de Maistre E, Favier R, Hezard N, Hurtaud-Roux MF, Latger-Cannard V, Lavenu-Bombled C, Proulle V, Meunier S, Negrier C, Nurden A, Randrianaivo H, Fabris F, Platokouki H, Rosenberg N, HadjKacem B, Heller PG, Karimi M, Balduini CL, Pastore A, Lanza F. Spectrum of the mutations in Bernard-Soulier syndrome. Hum Mutat. 2014;35(9):1033–45. doi:10.1002/humu.22607.
33. Kanaji T, Ware J, Okamura T, Newman PJ. GPIbα regulates platelet size by controlling the subcellular localization of filamin. Blood. 2012;119(12):2906–13. doi:10.1182/blood-2011-08-376566.
34. Ware J, Russell S, Ruggeri ZM. Generation and rescue of a murine model of platelet dysfunction: the Bernard-Soulier syndrome. Proc Natl Acad Sci U S A. 2000;97(6):2803–8. doi:10.1073/pnas.050582097.
35. Balduini A, Malara A, Balduini CL, Noris P. Megakaryocytes derived from patients with the classical form of Bernard-Soulier syndrome show no ability to extend proplatelets in vitro. Platelets. 2011;22(4):308–11. doi:10.3109/09537104.2010.547960.

36. Kunishima S, Kamiya T, Saito H. Genetic abnormalities of Bernard-Soulier syndrome. Int J Hematol. 2002;76(4):319–27.
37. Lopez JA, Andrews RK, Afshar-Kharghan V, Berndt MC. Bernard-Soulier syndrome. Blood. 1998;91(12):4397–418.
38. Noris P, Perrotta S, Bottega R, Pecci A, Melazzini F, Civaschi E, Russo S, Magrin S, Loffredo G, Di Salvo V, Russo G, Casale M, De Rocco D, Grignani C, Cattaneo M, Baronci C, Dragani A, Albano V, Jankovic M, Scianguetta S, Savoia A, Balduini CL. Clinical and laboratory features of 103 patients from 42 Italian families with inherited thrombocytopenia derived from the monoallelic Ala156Val mutation of GPIbα (Bolzano mutation). Haematologica. 2012;97(1):82–8. doi:10.3324/haematol.2011.050682.
39. Savoia A, Balduini CL, Savino M, Noris P, Del Vecchio M, Perrotta S, Belletti S, Poggi V, Iolascon A. Autosomal dominant macrothrombocytopenia in Italy is most frequently a type of heterozygous Bernard-Soulier syndrome. Blood. 2001;97(5):1330–5.
40. Kunishima S, Lopez JA, Kobayashi S, Imai N, Kamiya T, Saito H, Naoe T. Missense mutations of the glycoprotein (GP) Ibβ gene impairing the GPIbα/β disulfide linkage in a family with giant platelet disorder. Blood. 1997;89(7):2404–12.
41. Kurokawa Y, Ishida F, Kamijo T, Kunishima S, Kenny D, Kitano K, Koike K. A missense mutation (Tyr88 to Cys) in the platelet membrane glycoprotein Ibβ gene affects GPIb/IX complex expression—Bernard-Soulier syndrome in the homozygous form and giant platelets in the heterozygous form. Thromb Haemost. 2001;86(5):1249–56.
42. Trevisan P, Barbosa S, Sperotto G, Costi C, de Omena Filho RL, Silva AP, Varella-Garcia M, Fiegenbaum M, Rosa RF, Zen PR. Macrothrombocytopenia as diagnosis predictor of 22q11 deletion syndrome among patients with congenital heart defects. Am J Med Genet A. 2015;167(6):1406–8. doi:10.1002/ajmg.a.36531.
43. Van Geet C, Devriendt K, Eyskens B, Vermylen J, Hoylaerts MF. Velocardiofacial syndrome patients with a heterozygous chromosome 22q11 deletion have giant platelets. Pediatr Res. 1998;44(4):607–11. doi:10.1203/00006450-199810000-00023.
44. Luo SZ, Mo X, Afshar-Kharghan V, Srinivasan S, Lopez JA, Li R. Glycoprotein Ibα forms disulfide bonds with 2 glycoprotein Ibβ subunits in the resting platelet. Blood. 2007;109(2):603–9. doi:10.1182/blood-2006-05-024091.
45. Kunishima S, Okuno Y, Yoshida K, Shiraishi Y, Sanada M, Muramatsu H, Chiba K, Tanaka H, Miyazaki K, Sakai M, Ohtake M, Kobayashi R, Iguchi A, Niimi G, Otsu M, Takahashi Y, Miyano S, Saito H, Kojima S, Ogawa S. ACTN1 mutations cause congenital macrothrombocytopenia. Am J Hum Genet. 2013;92(3):431–8. doi:10.1016/j.ajhg.2013.01.015.
46. Bottega R, Marconi C, Faleschini M, Baj G, Cagioni C, Pecci A, Pippucci T, Ramenghi U, Pardini S, Ngu L, Baronci C, Kunishima S, Balduini CL, Seri M, Savoia A, Noris P. ACTN1-related thrombocytopenia: identification of novel families for phenotypic characterization. Blood. 2015;125(5):869–72. doi:10.1182/blood-2014-08-594531.
47. Sjoblom B, Salmazo A, Djinovic-Carugo K. α-actinin structure and regulation. Cell Mol Life Sci. 2008;65(17):2688–701. doi:10.1007/s00018-008-8080-8.
48. Yasutomi M, Kunishima S, Okazaki S, Tanizawa A, Tsuchida S, Ohshima Y. ACTN1 rod domain mutation associated with congenital macrothrombocytopenia. Ann Hematol. 2016;95(1):141–4. doi:10.1007/s00277-015-2517-6.
49. Tadokoro S, Nakazawa T, Kamae T, Kiyomizu K, Kashiwagi H, Honda S, Kanakura Y, Tomiyama Y. A potential role for α-actinin in inside-out αIIbβ3 signaling. Blood. 2011;117(1):250–8. doi:10.1182/blood-2009-10-246751.
50. Kunishima S, Kitamura K, Yasutomi M, Kobayashi R. Diagnostic biomarker for ACTN1 macrothrombocytopenia. Blood. 2015;126(22):2525–6. doi:10.1182/blood-2015-08-666180.
51. Nurden AT, Pillois X, Wilcox DA. Glanzmann thrombasthenia: state of the art and future directions. Semin Thromb Hemost. 2013;39(6):642–55. doi:10.1055/s-0033-1353393. Epub 1352013 Aug 1353398
52. Nurden AT, Fiore M, Nurden P, Pillois X. Glanzmann thrombasthenia: a review of ITGA2B and ITGB3 defects with emphasis on variants, phenotypic variability, and mouse models. Blood. 2011;118(23):5996–6005. doi:10.1182/blood-2011-5907-365635. Epub 362011 Sep 365613

53. Lau TL, Kim C, Ginsberg MH, Ulmer TS. The structure of the integrin αIIbβ3 transmembrane complex explains integrin transmembrane signalling. EMBO J. 2009;28(9):1351–61. doi:10.1038/emboj.2009.63.
54. Ghevaert C, Salsmann A, Watkins NA, Schaffner-Reckinger E, Rankin A, Garner SF, Stephens J, Smith GA, Debili N, Vainchenker W, de Groot PG, Huntington JA, Laffan M, Kieffer N, Ouwehand WH. A nonsynonymous SNP in the ITGB3 gene disrupts the conserved membrane-proximal cytoplasmic salt bridge in the αIIbβ3 integrin and cosegregates dominantly with abnormal proplatelet formation and macrothrombocytopenia. Blood. 2008;111(7):3407–14. doi:10.1182/blood-2007-09-112615.
55. Kunishima S, Kashiwagi H, Otsu M, Takayama N, Eto K, Onodera M, Miyajima Y, Takamatsu Y, Suzumiya J, Matsubara K, Tomiyama Y, Saito H. Heterozygous ITGA2B R995W mutation inducing constitutive activation of the αIIbβ3 receptor affects proplatelet formation and causes congenital macrothrombocytopenia. Blood. 2011;117(20):5479–84. doi:10.1182/blood-2010-12-323691.
56. Chang Y, Aurade F, Larbret F, Zhang Y, Le Couedic JP, Momeux L, Larghero J, Bertoglio J, Louache F, Cramer E, Vainchenker W, Debili N. Proplatelet formation is regulated by the Rho/ROCK pathway. Blood. 2007;109(10):4229–36. doi:10.1182/blood-2006-04-020024.
57. Chen Z, Naveiras O, Balduini A, Mammoto A, Conti MA, Adelstein RS, Ingber D, Daley GQ, Shivdasani RA. The May-Hegglin anomaly gene MYH9 is a negative regulator of platelet biogenesis modulated by the Rho-ROCK pathway. Blood. 2007;110(1):171–9. doi:10.1182/blood-2007-02-071589.
58. Bury L, Falcinelli E, Chiasserini D, Springer TA, Italiano Jr JE, Gresele P. Cytoskeletal perturbation leads to platelet dysfunction and thrombocytopenia in variant forms of Glanzmann thrombasthenia. Haematologica. 2016;101(1):46–56. doi:10.3324/haematol.2015.130849.
59. Bury L, Malara A, Gresele P, Balduini A. Outside-in signalling generated by a constitutively activated integrin αIIbβ3 impairs proplatelet formation in human megakaryocytes. PLoS One. 2012;7(4):e34449. doi:10.1371/journal.pone.0034449.
60. Lillicrap D. von Willebrand disease: advances in pathogenetic understanding, diagnosis, and therapy. Blood. 2013;122(23):3735–40. doi:10.1182/blood-2013-06-498303.
61. Federici AB, Mannucci PM, Castaman G, Baronciani L, Bucciarelli P, Canciani MT, Pecci A, Lenting PJ, De Groot PG. Clinical and molecular predictors of thrombocytopenia and risk of bleeding in patients with von Willebrand disease type 2B: a cohort study of 67 patients. Blood. 2009;113(3):526–34. doi:10.1182/blood-2008-04-152280.
62. Jackson SC, Sinclair GD, Cloutier S, Duan Z, Rand ML, Poon MC. The Montreal platelet syndrome kindred has type 2B von Willebrand disease with the VWF V1316M mutation. Blood. 2009;113(14):3348–51. doi:10.1182/blood-2008-06-165233.
63. Othman M, Emsley J. Platelet-type von Willebrand disease: toward an improved understanding of the "sticky situation". Semin Thromb Hemost. 2014;40(2):146–50. doi:10.1055/s-0033-1364182.
64. Barracchia A, Lari R. EDTA induced pseudothrombocytopenia: a misleading artifact causing potentially dangerous clinical errors. Haematologica. 1989;74(3):332–3.
65. Nurden AT, Nurden P. The gray platelet syndrome: clinical spectrum of the disease. Blood Rev. 2007;21(1):21–36. doi:10.1016/j.blre.2005.12.003.
66. Albers CA, Cvejic A, Favier R, Bouwmans EE, Alessi MC, Bertone P, Jordan G, Kettleborough RN, Kiddle G, Kostadima M, Read RJ, Sipos B, Sivapalaratnam S, Smethurst PA, Stephens J, Voss K, Nurden A, Rendon A, Nurden P, Ouwehand WH. Exome sequencing identifies NBEAL2 as the causative gene for gray platelet syndrome. Nat Genet. 2011;43(8):735–7. doi:10.1038/ng.885.
67. Gunay-Aygun M, Falik-Zaccai TC, Vilboux T, Zivony-Elboum Y, Gumruk F, Cetin M, Khayat M, Boerkoel CF, Kfir N, Huang Y, Maynard D, Dorward H, Berger K, Kleta R, Anikster Y, Arat M, Freiberg AS, Kehrel BE, Jurk K, Cruz P, Mullikin JC, White JG, Huizing M, Gahl WA. NBEAL2 is mutated in gray platelet syndrome and is required for biogenesis of platelet α-granules. Nat Genet. 2011;43(8):732–4. doi:10.1038/ng.883.

68. Kahr WH, Hinckley J, Li L, Schwertz H, Christensen H, Rowley JW, Pluthero FG, Urban D, Fabbro S, Nixon B, Gadzinski R, Storck M, Wang K, Ryu GY, Jobe SM, Schutte BC, Moseley J, Loughran NB, Parkinson J, Weyrich AS, Di Paola J. Mutations in NBEAL2, encoding a BEACH protein, cause gray platelet syndrome. Nat Genet. 2011;43(8):738–40. doi:10.1038/ng.884.
69. Urban D, Li L, Christensen H, Pluthero FG, Chen SZ, Puhacz M, Garg PM, Lanka KK, Cummings JJ, Kramer H, Wasmuth JD, Parkinson J, Kahr WH. The VPS33B-binding protein VPS16B is required in megakaryocyte and platelet α-granule biogenesis. Blood. 2012;120(25):5032–40. doi:10.1182/blood-2012-05-431205.
70. Monteferrario D, Bolar NA, Marneth AE, Hebeda KM, Bergevoet SM, Veenstra H, Laros-van Gorkom BA, MacKenzie MA, Khandanpour C, Botezatu L, Fransen E, Van Camp G, Duijnhouwer AL, Salemink S, Willemsen B, Huls G, Preijers F, Van Heerde W, Jansen JH, Kempers MJ, Loeys BL, Van Laer L, Van der Reijden BA. A dominant-negative GFI1B mutation in the gray platelet syndrome. N Engl J Med. 2014;370(3):245–53. doi:10.1056/NEJMoa1308130.
71. Tubman VN, Levine JE, Campagna DR, Monahan-Earley R, Dvorak AM, Neufeld EJ, Fleming MD. X-linked gray platelet syndrome due to a GATA1 Arg216Gln mutation. Blood. 2007;109(8):3297–9. doi:10.1182/blood-2006-02-004101.
72. Ferreira R, Ohneda K, Yamamoto M, Philipsen S. GATA1 function, a paradigm for transcription factors in hematopoiesis. Mol Cell Biol. 2005;25(4):1215–27. doi:10.1128/MCB.25.4.1215-1227.2005.
73. Millikan PD, Balamohan SM, Raskind WH, Kacena MA. Inherited thrombocytopenia due to GATA-1 mutations. Semin Thromb Hemost. 2011;37(6):682–9. doi:10.1055/s-0031-1291378.
74. van der Meer LT, Jansen JH, van der Reijden BA. Gfi1 and Gfi1b: key regulators of hematopoiesis. Leukemia. 2010;24(11):1834–43. doi:10.1038/leu.2010.195.
75. Stevenson WS, Morel-Kopp MC, Chen Q, Liang HP, Bromhead CJ, Wright S, Turakulov R, Ng AP, Roberts AW, Bahlo M, Ward CM. GFI1B mutation causes a bleeding disorder with abnormal platelet function. J Thromb Haemost. 2013;11(11):2039–47. doi:10.1111/jth.12368.
76. Kitamura K, Okuno Y, Yoshida K, Sanada M, Shiraishi Y, Muramatsu H, Kobayashi R, Furukawa K, Miyano S, Kojima S, Ogawa S, Kunishima S. Functional characterization of a novel GFI1B mutation causing congenital macrothrombocytopenia. J Thromb Haemost. 2016;14(7):1462–9. doi:10.1111/jth.13350.
77. Schwertz H, Koster S, Kahr WH, Michetti N, Kraemer BF, Weitz DA, Blaylock RC, Kraiss LW, Greinacher A, Zimmerman GA, Weyrich AS. Anucleate platelets generate progeny. Blood. 2010;115(18):3801–9. doi:10.1182/blood-2009-08-239558.
78. Lecine P, Italiano Jr JE, Kim SW, Villeval JL, Shivdasani RA. Hematopoietic-specific β1 tubulin participates in a pathway of platelet biogenesis dependent on the transcription factor NF-E2. Blood. 2000;96(4):1366–73.
79. Kunishima S, Kobayashi R, Itoh TJ, Hamaguchi M, Saito H. Mutation of the β1-tubulin gene associated with congenital macrothrombocytopenia affecting microtubule assembly. Blood. 2009;113(2):458–61. doi:10.1182/blood-2008-06-162610.
80. Kunishima S, Nishimura S, Suzuki H, Imaizumi M, Saito H. TUBB1 mutation disrupting microtubule assembly impairs proplatelet formation and results in congenital macrothrombocytopenia. Eur J Haematol. 2014;92(4):276–82. doi:10.1111/ejh.12252.
81. Boudreaux MK, Osborne CD, Herre AC, Rivera ER, Spangler EA. Unique structure of the M loop region of β1-tubulin may contribute to size variability of platelets in the family Felidae. Vet Clin Pathol. 2010;39(4):417–23. doi:10.1111/j.1939-165X.2010.00256.x.
82. Davis B, Toivio-Kinnucan M, Schuller S, Boudreaux MK. Mutation in β1-tubulin correlates with macrothrombocytopenia in Cavalier King Charles Spaniels. J Vet Intern Med. 2008;22(3):540–5. doi:10.1111/j.1939-1676.2008.0085.x.
83. Favier R, Jondeau K, Boutard P, Grossfeld P, Reinert P, Jones C, Bertoni F, Cramer EM. Paris-Trousseau syndrome: clinical, hematological, molecular data of ten new cases. Thromb Haemost. 2003;90(5):893–7. doi:10.1267/THRO03050893.

84. Mattina T, Perrotta CS, Grossfeld P. Jacobsen syndrome. Orphanet J Rare Dis. 2009;4:9. doi:10.1186/1750-1172-4-9.
85. Li Y, Luo H, Liu T, Zacksenhaus E, Ben-David Y. The ets transcription factor Fli-1 in development, cancer and disease. Oncogene. 2015;34(16):2022–31. doi:10.1038/onc.2014.162.
86. Raslova H, Komura E, Le Couedic JP, Larbret F, Debili N, Feunteun J, Danos O, Albagli O, Vainchenker W, Favier R. FLI1 monoallelic expression combined with its hemizygous loss underlies Paris-Trousseau/Jacobsen thrombopenia. J Clin Invest. 2004;114(1):77–84. doi:10.1172/JCI21197.
87. Stockley J, Morgan NV, Bem D, Lowe GC, Lordkipanidze M, Dawood B, Simpson MA, Macfarlane K, Horner K, Leo VC, Talks K, Motwani J, Wilde JT, Collins PW, Makris M, Watson SP, Daly ME, Genotyping UK, Phenotyping of Platelets Study Group. Enrichment of FLI1 and RUNX1 mutations in families with excessive bleeding and platelet dense granule secretion defects. Blood. 2013;122(25):4090–3. doi:10.1182/blood-2013-06-506873.
88. Stevenson WS, Rabbolini DJ, Beutler L, Chen Q, Gabrielli S, Mackay JP, Brighton TA, Ward CM, Morel-Kopp MC. Paris-Trousseau thrombocytopenia is phenocopied by the autosomal recessive inheritance of a DNA-binding domain mutation in FLI1. Blood. 2015;126(17):2027–30. doi:10.1182/blood-2015-06-650887.
89. Antony-Debre I, Bluteau D, Itzykson R, Baccini V, Renneville A, Boehlen F, Morabito M, Droin N, Deswarte C, Chang Y, Leverger G, Solary E, Vainchenker W, Favier R, Raslova H. MYH10 protein expression in platelets as a biomarker of RUNX1 and FLI1 alterations. Blood. 2012;120(13):2719–22. doi:10.1182/blood-2012-04-422352.

Part VII
Treatment of Adult ITP

Helicobacter pylori (*H. pylori*) Eradication

Toshiro Takafuta and Kingo Fujimura

Abstract In 1998, Gasbarrini et al. reported that eradication therapy for *Helicobacter pylori* (*H. pylori*) increased platelet counts in most *H. pylori*-positive immune thrombocytopenia (ITP) patients. A large number of retrospective and prospective studies have since been performed in order to evaluate the efficacy of eradication therapy. A positive relationship was reported between ITP and *H. pylori* infection, and the eradication of *H. pylori* resulted in a significant increase in platelet counts in more than 50% of eradication-successful ITP cases. These results suggest that *H. pylori* infection is involved in the mechanisms underlying thrombocytopenia.

1 Introduction

Immune thrombocytopenia (ITP) is an autoimmune disease mediated by antiplatelet autoantibodies that bind to circulating platelets and megakaryocytes, resulting in platelet destruction by the reticuloendothelial system as well as suppressed platelet production [1, 2]. T-cell-mediated destruction also participates in reducing the numbers of platelets and megakaryocytes [3].

Corticosteroids, intravenous immunoglobulin, and splenectomy have been employed in order to suppress platelet destruction mechanisms. In 1998, Gasbarrini et al. reported that the eradication of *Helicobacter pylori* in ITP patients increased platelet counts [4]. The eradication of *H. pylori* in ITP patients has since been attracting attention because the eradication treatment is basically a single course therapy that is cost effective and tolerable. Previous studies that reported the efficacy of *H. pylori* eradication therapy in ITP patients are reviewed herein, and the mechanisms of ITP related to *H. pylori* infection are discussed.

T. Takafuta, M.D., Ph.D. (✉)
Department of Clinical Research, Hiroshima-Nishi Medical Center, Hiroshima, Japan
e-mail: takafuta-th@umin.ac.jp

K. Fujimura, M.D., Ph.D.
Department of Nursing, Yasuda Women's University, Hiroshima, Japan
e-mail: k-fujimu@yasuda-u.ac.jp

Y. Ishida, Y. Tomiyama (eds.), *Autoimmune Thrombocytopenia*,
DOI 10.1007/978-981-10-4142-6_12

2 *H. pylori* Infection and Diseases

H. pylori is a gram-negative bacillus that colonizes the mucous layer of the human stomach. The persistent presence of *H. pylori* in the gastric mucosa induces gastrointestinal disorders including atrophic gastritis, peptic ulcers, and gastric cancer [5]. *H. pylori* has also been shown to activate the host immune system with cytokine signaling and the stimulation of various immune cells including macrophages and lymphocytes. The continuous stimulation of the immune system may induce mucosa-associated lymphoid tissue (MALT) lymphoma and various autoimmune disorders such as chronic thyroiditis, Sjögren disease, systemic sclerosis, rheumatoid arthritis, and ITP [6–8].

Various mechanisms have been proposed in order to explain extra-gastrointestinal disorders related to *H. pylori* infection. However, since these mechanisms have not been elucidated in detail, it is important to analyze the underlying pathophysiologies in order to improve their management.

3 Eradication Regimens for *H. pylori* Therapy

Triple therapy with a proton pump inhibitor (PPI), clarithromycin, and either amoxicillin or metronidazole for 1 or 2 weeks has been used as the standard eradication regimen for *H. pylori* therapy in the most countries worldwide [9]. However, *H. pylori* infection is becoming more difficult to treat because of the increasing failure of therapy. New first-line strategies including non-bismuth quadruple therapy (PPI + amoxicillin + metronidazole + clarithromycin) and bismuth quadruple therapy (PPI + bismuth + metronidazole + tetracycline) are now being recommended as the Toronto Consensus [10]. Another new regimen using a novel potassium-competitive acid blocker (PCAB) in combination with antibiotics has been tested in Japan [11] and may represent an effective option.

4 Effects of Eradication Treatments on Platelet Counts in *H. pylori*-Positive ITP Patients

In 1998, Gasbarrini et al. reported increases in platelet counts after eradication therapy in most *H. pylori*-positive ITP patients [4]. Many studies have since been published on the effects of eradication therapy on platelet responses in *H. pylori*-positive ITP cases. In Italy and Japan, platelet counts were found to increase after *H. pylori* eradication in most (50–80%) *H. pylori*-positive ITP patients [12–23]. However, the effectiveness of eradication was very limited in Spain, France, and the United States [24–27]. Studies performed in Serbia, Turkey, and Iran also reported relatively low response rates [28–30]. The reasons for this discrepancy have not yet been established, but may be attributed to the high proportion of patients with severe and persistent ITP in these countries, differences in immunological backgrounds between populations, or differences in antigenicity [25, 26].

In Japan, a nationwide retrospective study was performed in order to assess the prevalence of *H. pylori* infection, the effects of the eradication of *H. pylori* on platelet counts, and the characteristic clinical features of chronic ITP with *H. pylori* infection [21]. A total of 435 ITP patients were enrolled in this study and *H. pylori* infection was detected in 300 patients. *H. pylori*-positive patients were significantly older, and hyperplastic megakaryocytes in bone marrow were also more frequently detected than in patients without *H. pylori* infection. A total of 207 *H. pylori*-positive ITP patients received *H. pylori* eradication therapy, and platelet counts increased in 63% of eradication-successful patients. Among most responders, the platelet count response started 1 month after eradication therapy, and increases in platelet counts continued without the ITP treatment for more than 12 months. Although most early studies excluded patients with severe thrombocytopenia, this study also reported the efficacy of eradicating *H. pylori* in severe patients with refractory ITP, even after splenectomy. In this study, increases in platelet counts were maintained without additional treatments for more than 12 months. Long-term follow-up studies confirmed that the platelet response after eradication therapy lasted 7 years or longer with very few cases of relapse [31, 32].

The first systematic review with a meta-analysis by Francini et al. reviewed 788 ITP patients including 494 *H. pylori*-positive patients [33]. Platelet counts were significantly higher in *H. pylori*-infected patients after successful *H. pylori* eradication than in the following groups: untreated *H. pylori*-infected patients, *H. pylori*-infected patients who failed eradication, and *H. pylori*-uninfected patients. Stasi et al. performed another systematic review involving 1555 patients and reported similar findings [34]. Therefore, *H. pylori* eradication is strongly related to platelet recovery in ITP patients. In another systematic review, Arnold et al. evaluated the efficacy of eradication therapy in ITP patients by comparing platelet responses in patients with or without *H. pylori* infection [35]. A total of 205 *H. pylori*-positive and 77 *H. pylori*-negative patients received eradication therapy. The odds of platelet counts increasing with eradication therapy were 14.5-fold higher in *H. pylori*-positive patients than in *H. pylori*-negative patients. This finding indicated a clear relationship between increased platelet counts and the successful eradication of *H. pylori* and also strongly suggested that *H. pylori* infection plays a direct role in the pathogenesis of ITP.

Although *H. pylori* eradication therapy is still only one of the treatment options available for patients with refractory ITP or those with ITP and less severe thrombocytopenia in the United States and European countries (other than Italy) [36–39], in a reference guide for managing adult ITP in Japan, *H. pylori* eradication is recommended as an initial strategy for managing ITP in adult patients [40].

5 *H. pylori* Infection in the Pathogenesis of ITP

In ITP, a pathogenic loop has generally been suggested to be established, and platelets and megakaryocytes are continuously impaired by macrophages and lymphocytes [2, 41]. The establishment of this loop may be initiated through the capture of opsonized platelets by the Fcγ receptors of macrophages in the reticuloendothelial system. Macrophages present antigenic peptides derived from platelet-specific glycoproteins including GPIb-IX-V and GPIIb/IIIa, and CD4+ T cells are activated by these autoantigens. These autoreactive T cells activate B cells to produce antiplatelet autoantibodies, which then bind to and destroy platelets and megakaryocytes.

As described, clinical observations suggest the involvement of *H. pylori* infection in the pathogenesis of ITP, and a large number of hypotheses have been proposed to explain the mechanisms responsible.

5.1 Fcγ Receptor Balance of Monocytes/Macrophages

The expression level of FcγRIIB, which exerts inhibitory functions on macrophages and monocytes, was previously reported to be low in the circulating monocytes of *H. pylori*-infected patients, but not in those from uninfected patients [23, 42]. An enhanced phagocytic capacity was also noted in monocytes. When the eradication of *H. pylori* was successful, this activated phenotype of monocytes was suppressed shortly after eradication therapy and platelet counts increased [23]. Alterations in the Fcγ receptor balance of monocytes by *H. pylori* infection may be strongly associated with the pathophysiology of ITP.

*5.2 Platelet Activation by an Anti-*H. pylori *Antibody and von Willebrand Factor*

A previous study reported that a direct association between some *H. pylori* strains and von Willebrand factor (VWF) induced platelet aggregation in the presence of the anti-*H. pylori* antibody IgG [43]. The VWF-*H. pylori*-IgG complex may interact with platelets through the VWF receptor (GPIb-IX-V) and Fcγ receptor IIA (FcγRIIA). These interactions may activate platelets and induce thrombocytopenia through the consumption of platelets. Moreover, macrophages or monocytes may capture *H. pylori* platelet aggregates, present platelet-specific antigens, and induce antiplatelet antibody production.

5.3 The CagA (Cytotoxin-Associated Gene A) Protein

In *H. pylori*, the cag pathogenicity island (cag-PAI) encodes the CagA protein (CagA). After translocating into host cells, the CagA protein is phosphorylated, binds to SHP-2 in host cells, and induces cellular responses and immune reactions [5]. Molecular mimicry is one of the important mechanisms needed to induce autoimmune disorders.

Previous studies reported that platelet-associated IgG from *H. pylori*-positive ITP patients interacted with the CagA protein [17], and anti-Cag A antibodies cross-reacted with a peptide specifically expressed by platelets [44]. In *H. pylori* infection, molecular mimicry between the CagA protein and platelet antigens may be one of the candidates for pathological immune reactions.

A Japanese group found that most Japanese *H. pylori* strains are positive for CagA [45], while an Italian group showed that the prevalence of the *H. pylori* CagA gene was significantly higher in patients with ITP than in a control group [22]. In contrast, the proportion of CagA-positive strains was lower in Western countries [46, 47].

Differences in clinical responses to eradication therapy may occur among ITP patients because of differences in the CagA status of the bacterium.

5.4 Lewis Antibody

Lewis antibody titers were previously reported to be high in some *H. pylori*-infected patients, and Lewis antigens, which are also expressed by some *H. pylori* strains, may be targets for molecular mimicry [48].

These Lewis antibodies have been hypothesized to nonspecifically bind to platelets and induce thrombocytopenia [38, 49].

5.5 Evolution of Antiplatelet Antibodies after H. pylori Infection

Platelet activation and/or molecular mimicry have been suggested to initiate the development of ITP following alterations in the Fcγ receptor balance by *H. pylori* infection [17, 23, 43, 48]. After its initiation, continuous platelet destruction and the presentation of platelet-specific antigens may activate the immune system and produce antiplatelet autoantibodies not related to *H. pylori* antigens. This mechanism may lead to the development of refractory ITP, resulting in the eradication of *H. pylori* [50].

6 Definition of "Secondary ITP (*H. pylori* Associated)"

In 2009, an international working group standardized terminologies and definitions for ITP [51]. The acronym ITP was proposed to stand for immune thrombocytopenia, and ITP was classified into "primary" and "secondary" ITP. The term "primary" indicates the absence of any obvious cause. The term "secondary" indicates that there is an underlying disease or drug exposure, and "secondary ITP" may broadly include all forms of immune thrombocytopenia, except for primary ITP. The panel proposed the diagnosis of improvements in thrombocytopenia after the successful eradication of *H. pylori* as "secondary ITP (H. pylori associated)." There are some refractory ITP patients who do not respond to eradication therapy. These refractory cases may be regarded as primary ITP and a coincidental *H. pylori* infection [41].

7 Conclusion

Although the efficacy of *H. pylori* eradication for the treatment of ITP appears to correlate with geographical locations, eradication therapy is very effective in Japan and Italy. In these countries, *H. pylori* infection has to be tested at the diagnosis of ITP and eradication considered as the initial treatment.

A better understanding of the mechanisms by which *H. pylori* causes ITP may provide important information for elucidating the pathophysiology of "primary" ITP.

References

1. Karpatkin S. Autoimmune (idiopathic) thrombocytopenic purpura. Lancet. 1997;349(9064):1531–6. doi:10.1016/S0140-6736(96)12118-8.
2. Cines DB, Blanchette VS. Immune thrombocytopenic purpura. New Engl J Med. 2002;346(13):995–1008. doi:10.1056/NEJMra010501.
3. Olsson B, Andersson PO, Jernas M, Jacobsson S, Carlsson B, Carlsson LM, et al. T-cell-mediated cytotoxicity toward platelets in chronic idiopathic thrombocytopenic purpura. Nat Med. 2003;9(9):1123–4. doi:10.1038/nm921.
4. Gasbarrini A, Franceschi F, Tartaglione R, Landolfi R, Pola P, Gasbarrini G. Regression of autoimmune thrombocytopenia after eradication of *Helicobacter pylori*. Lancet. 1998;352(9131):878. doi:10.1016/S0140-6736(05)60004-9.
5. Suerbaum S, Michetti P. *Helicobacter pylori* infection. New Engl J Med. 2002;347(15):1175–86. doi:10.1056/NEJMra020542.
6. Zentilin P, Savarino V, Garnero A, Accardo S, Seriolo B. Is *Helicobacter pylori* infection a risk factor for disease severity in rheumatoid arthritis? Gastroenterology. 1999;116(2):503–4.
7. de Luis DA, Varela C, de La Calle H, Canton R, de Argila CM, San Roman AL, et al. *Helicobacter pylori* infection is markedly increased in patients with autoimmune atrophic thyroiditis. J Clin Gastroenterol. 1998;26(4):259–63.

8. Radic M. Role of *Helicobacter pylori* infection in autoimmune systemic rheumatic diseases. World J Gastroenterol. 2014;20(36):12839–46. doi:10.3748/wjg.v20.i36.12839.
9. Malfertheiner P, Megraud F, O'Morain CA, Atherton J, Axon AT, Bazzoli F, et al. Management of *Helicobacter pylori* infection—the Maastricht IV/Florence Consensus Report. Gut. 2012;61(5):646–64. doi:10.1136/gutjnl-2012-302084.
10. Fallone CA, Chiba N, van Zanten SV, Fischbach L, Gisbert JP, Hunt RH, et al. The Toronto consensus for the treatment of *Helicobacter pylori* infection in adults. Gastroenterology. 2016;151(1):51–69.e14. doi:10.1053/j.gastro.2016.04.006.
11. Murakami K, Sakurai Y, Shiino M, Funao N, Nishimura A, Asaka M. Vonoprazan, a novel potassium-competitive acid blocker, as a component of first-line and second-line triple therapy for *Helicobacter pylori* eradication: a phase III, randomised, double-blind study. Gut. 2016;65(9):1439–46. doi:10.1136/gutjnl-2015-311304.
12. Emilia G, Longo G, Luppi M, Gandini G, Morselli M, Ferrara L, et al. *Helicobacter pylori* eradication can induce platelet recovery in idiopathic thrombocytopenic purpura. Blood. 2001;97(3):812–4.
13. Veneri D, Franchini M, Gottardi M, D'Adda M, Ambrosetti A, Krampera M, et al. Efficacy of *Helicobacter pylori* eradication in raising platelet count in adult patients with idiopathic thrombocytopenic purpura. Haematologica. 2002;87(11):1177–9.
14. Kohda K, Kuga T, Kogawa K, Kanisawa Y, Koike K, Kuroiwa G, et al. Effect of *Helicobacter pylori* eradication on platelet recovery in Japanese patients with chronic idiopathic thrombocytopenic purpura and secondary autoimmune thrombocytopenic purpura. Br J Haematol. 2002;118(2):584–8.
15. Hashino S, Mori A, Suzuki S, Izumiyama K, Kahata K, Yonezumi M, et al. Platelet recovery in patients with idiopathic thrombocytopenic purpura after eradication of *Helicobacter pylori*. Int J Hematol. 2003;77(2):188–91.
16. Ando K, Shimamoto T, Tauchi T, Ito Y, Kuriyama Y, Gotoh A, et al. Can eradication therapy for *Helicobacter pylori* really improve the thrombocytopenia in idiopathic thrombocytopenic purpura? Our experience and a literature review. Int J Hematol. 2003;77(3):239–44.
17. Takahashi T, Yujiri T, Shinohara K, Inoue Y, Sato Y, Fujii Y, et al. Molecular mimicry by *Helicobacter pylori* CagA protein may be involved in the pathogenesis of H. pylori-associated chronic idiopathic thrombocytopenic purpura. Br J Haematol. 2004;124(1):91–6.
18. Ando T, Tsuzuki T, Mizuno T, Minami M, Ina K, Kusugami K, et al. Characteristics of *Helicobacter pylori*-induced gastritis and the effect of H. pylori eradication in patients with chronic idiopathic thrombocytopenic purpura. Helicobacter. 2004;9(5):443–52. doi:10.1111/j.1083-4389.2004.00261.x.
19. Veneri D, Krampera M, Franchini M. High prevalence of sustained remission of idiopathic thrombocytopenic purpura after *Helicobacter pylori* eradication: a long-term follow-up study. Platelets. 2005;16(2):117–9. doi:10.1080/09537100400015153.
20. Stasi R, Rossi Z, Stipa E, Amadori S, Newland AC, Provan D. *Helicobacter pylori* eradication in the management of patients with idiopathic thrombocytopenic purpura. Am J Med. 2005;118(4):414–9. doi:10.1016/j.amjmed.2004.09.014.
21. Fujimura K, Kuwana M, Kurata Y, Imamura M, Harada H, Sakamaki H, et al. Is eradication therapy useful as the first line of treatment in *Helicobacter pylori*-positive idiopathic thrombocytopenic purpura? Analysis of 207 eradicated chronic ITP cases in Japan. Int J Hematol. 2005;81(2):162–8.
22. Emilia G, Luppi M, Zucchini P, Morselli M, Potenza L, Forghieri F, et al. *Helicobacter pylori* infection and chronic immune thrombocytopenic purpura: long-term results of bacterium eradication and association with bacterium virulence profiles. Blood. 2007;110(12):3833–41. doi:10.1182/blood-2006-12-063222.
23. Asahi A, Nishimoto T, Okazaki Y, Suzuki H, Masaoka T, Kawakami Y, et al. *Helicobacter pylori* eradication shifts monocyte Fcgamma receptor balance toward inhibitory FcgammaRIIB in immune thrombocytopenic purpura patients. J Clin Invest. 2008;118(8):2939–49. doi:10.1172/JCI34496.

24. Jarque I, Andreu R, Llopis I, De la Rubia J, Gomis F, Senent L, et al. Absence of platelet response after eradication of *Helicobacter pylori* infection in patients with chronic idiopathic thrombocytopenic purpura. Br J Haematol. 2001;115(4):1002–3.
25. Michel M, Khellaf M, Desforges L, Lee K, Schaeffer A, Godeau B, et al. Autoimmune thrombocytopenic purpura and *Helicobacter pylori* infection. Arch Intern Med. 2002;162(9):1033–6.
26. Michel M, Cooper N, Jean C, Frissora C, Bussel JB. Does *Helicobacter pylori* initiate or perpetuate immune thrombocytopenic purpura? Blood. 2004;103(3):890–6. doi:10.1182/blood-2003-03-0900.
27. Ahn ER, Tiede MP, Jy W, Bidot CJ, Fontana V, Ahn YS. Platelet activation in *Helicobacter pylori*-associated idiopathic thrombocytopenic purpura: eradication reduces platelet activation but seldom improves platelet counts. Acta Haematol. 2006;116(1):19–24. doi:10.1159/000092343.
28. Payandeh M, Sohrabi N, Zare ME, Kansestani AN, Hashemian AH. Platelet count response to *Helicobacter pylori* eradication in Iranian patients with idiopathic thrombocytopenic purpura. Mediterr J Hematol Infect Dis. 2012;4(1):e2012056. doi:10.4084/MJHID.2012.056.
29. Suvajdzic N, Stankovic B, Artiko V, Cvejic T, Bulat V, Bakrac M, et al. *Helicobacter pylori* eradication can induce platelet recovery in chronic idiopathic thrombocytopenic purpura. Platelets. 2006;17(4):227–30. doi:10.1080/09537100500462487.
30. Sayan O, Akyol Erikci A, Ozturk A. The efficacy of *Helicobacter pylori* eradication in the treatment of idiopathic thrombocytopenic purpura—the first study in Turkey. Acta Haematol. 2006;116(2):146–9. doi:10.1159/000093648.
31. Tsumoto C, Tominaga K, Okazaki H, Tanigawa T, Yamagami H, Watanabe K, et al. Long-term efficacy of *Helicobacter pylori* eradication in patients with idiopathic thrombocytopenic purpura: 7-year follow-up prospective study. Ann Hematol. 2009;88(8):789–93. doi:10.1007/s00277-008-0667-5.
32. Kikuchi T, Kobayashi T, Yamashita T, Ohashi K, Sakamaki H, Akiyama H. Eight-year follow-up of patients with immune thrombocytopenic purpura related to *H. pylori* infection. Platelets. 2011;22(1):61–4. doi:10.3109/09537104.2010.515272.
33. Franchini M, Cruciani M, Mengoli C, Pizzolo G, Veneri D. Effect of *Helicobacter pylori* eradication on platelet count in idiopathic thrombocytopenic purpura: a systematic review and meta-analysis. J Antimicrob Chemother. 2007;60(2):237–46. doi:10.1093/jac/dkm195.
34. Stasi R, Sarpatwari A, Segal JB, Osborn J, Evangelista ML, Cooper N, et al. Effects of eradication of *Helicobacter pylori* infection in patients with immune thrombocytopenic purpura: a systematic review. Blood. 2009;113(6):1231–40. doi:10.1182/blood-2008-07-167155.
35. Arnold DM, Bernotas A, Nazi I, Stasi R, Kuwana M, Liu Y, et al. Platelet count response to *H. pylori* treatment in patients with immune thrombocytopenic purpura with and without *H. pylori* infection: a systematic review. Haematologica. 2009;94(6):850–6. doi:10.3324/haematol.2008.005348.
36. British Committee for Standards in Haematology General Haematology Task Force. Guidelines for the investigation and management of idiopathic thrombocytopenic purpura in adults, children and in pregnancy. Br J Haematol. 2003;120(4):574–96.
37. George JN. Management of patients with refractory immune thrombocytopenic purpura. J Thrombosis Haemost. 2006;4(8):1664–72. doi:10.1111/j.1538-7836.2006.02013.x.
38. Stasi R, Provan D. *Helicobacter pylori* and chronic ITP. Hematology Am Soc Hematol Educ Program. 2008:206–11. doi:10.1182/asheducation-2008.1.206.
39. Neunert C, Lim W, Crowther M, Cohen A, Solberg Jr L, Crowther MA, et al. The American Society of Hematology 2011 evidence-based practice guideline for immune thrombocytopenia. Blood. 2011;117(16):4190–207. doi:10.1182/blood-2010-08-302984.
40. Fujimura K, Miyakawa Y, Kurata Y, Kuwana M, Tomiyama Y, Murata M. Reference guide for management of adult idiopathic thrombocytopenic purpura (ITP) 2012 version. Rinsho Ketsueki. 2012;53(4):433–42.

41. Kuwana M. *Helicobacter pylori*-associated immune thrombocytopenia: clinical features and pathogenic mechanisms. World J Gastroenterol. 2014;20(3):714–23. doi:10.3748/wjg.v20.i3.714.
42. Wu Z, Zhou J, Prsoon P, Wei X, Liu X, Peng B. Low expression of FCGRIIB in macrophages of immune thrombocytopenia-affected individuals. Int J Hematol. 2012;96(5):588–93. doi:10.1007/s12185-012-1187-6.
43. Byrne MF, Kerrigan SW, Corcoran PA, Atherton JC, Murray FE, Fitzgerald DJ, et al. *Helicobacter pylori* binds von Willebrand factor and interacts with GPIb to induce platelet aggregation. Gastroenterology. 2003;124(7):1846–54.
44. Franceschi F, Christodoulides N, Kroll MH, Genta RM. *Helicobacter pylori* and idiopathic thrombocytopenic purpura. Ann Intern Med. 2004;140(9):766–7.
45. Maeda S, Ogura K, Yoshida H, Kanai F, Ikenoue T, Kato N, et al. Major virulence factors, VacA and CagA, are commonly positive in *Helicobacter pylori* isolates in Japan. Gut. 1998;42(3):338–43.
46. Perez-Perez GI, Bhat N, Gaensbauer J, Fraser A, Taylor DN, Kuipers EJ, et al. Country-specific constancy by age in cagA+ proportion of *Helicobacter pylori* infections. Int J Cancer. 1997;72(3):453–6.
47. Van Doorn LJ, Figueiredo C, Megraud F, Pena S, Midolo P, Queiroz DM, et al. Geographic distribution of vacA allelic types of *Helicobacter pylori*. Gastroenterology. 1999;116(4):823–30.
48. Wirth HP, Yang M, Peek Jr RM, Tham KT, Blaser MJ. *Helicobacter pylori* Lewis expression is related to the host Lewis phenotype. Gastroenterology. 1997;113(4):1091–8.
49. Gerhard M, Rad R, Prinz C, Naumann M. Pathogenesis of *Helicobacter pylori* infection. Helicobacter. 2002;7(Suppl 1):17–23.
50. Cines DB. ITP: time to "bug off"? Blood. 2007;110(12):3818–9. doi:10.1182/blood-2007-08-105411.
51. Rodeghiero F, Stasi R, Gernsheimer T, Michel M, Provan D, Arnold DM, et al. Standardization of terminology, definitions and outcome criteria in immune thrombocytopenic purpura of adults and children: report from an international working group. Blood. 2009;113(11):2386–93. doi:10.1182/blood-2008-07-162503.

Steroids

Toshiro Takafuta and Kingo Fujimura

Abstract Since the 1950s, corticosteroids, particularly prednisolone, have been key drugs in the initial treatment of immune thrombocytopenia (ITP). However, issues are associated with the long-term efficacy of prednisolone and its side effects in patients treated for a long period of time. Since the 1990s, HD-DEX has attracted attention because of its faster response, shorter treatment period, higher efficacy rate, and tolerability. A number of trials have recently been performed in order to improve the initial treatment of ITP.

1 Introduction

Immune thrombocytopenia (ITP) is mediated by autoantibodies against platelet-specific antigens including the GPIIb/IIIa and GPIb-IX-V complexes. Platelets coated with autoantibodies are captured and cleared by tissue macrophages through Fcγ receptors in the reticuloendothelial system, which includes the spleen and liver. Macrophages also function as antigen-presenting cells that interact with T cells, which, in turn, activate antibody-producing B cells. Antiplatelet autoantibody production is maintained by this pathogenic loop [1, 2]. Cytotoxic T cells directly affect platelets and megakaryocytes and contribute to the diverse pathobiology of ITP [3, 4].

Since the 1950s, corticosteroids have been used as a key drug to treat ITP and are still the mainstay of treatment for ITP [5]. Treatments using corticosteroids prevent the destruction of autoantibody-coated platelets in the reticuloendothelial system. Corticosteroids have also been reported to impair autoantibody production because they decrease platelet-associated IgG levels [1]. Corticosteroids may also increase

T. Takafuta, M.D., Ph.D. (✉)
Department of Clinical Research, Hiroshima-Nishi Medical Center, Hiroshima, Japan
e-mail: takafuta-th@umin.ac.jp

K. Fujimura, M.D., Ph.D.
Department of Nursing, Yasuda Women's University, Hiroshima, Japan
e-mail: k-fujimu@yasuda-u.ac.jp

Y. Ishida, Y. Tomiyama (eds.), *Autoimmune Thrombocytopenia*,
DOI 10.1007/978-981-10-4142-6_13

the production of platelets from megakaryocytes by impairing the ability of macrophages and cytotoxic T cells to destroy platelets within bone marrow [2]. Additionally, they may also have a direct effect on blood vessels and reduce bleeding independent of increases in the platelet count [6, 7]. However, the adverse effects of corticosteroids have become apparent and create significant complications. The deleterious effects of corticosteroids often exceed their benefits.

In this chapter, we review the use of each corticosteroid in the treatment of ITP and reconsider strategies for the management of ITP patients.

2 Prednisolone (Prednisone)

Prednisolone and prednisone are both artificially synthesized corticosteroids that are used in the treatment of various diseases including inflammatory disorders, autoimmune diseases, and lymphoid malignancies. Prednisone is activated to prednisolone in the liver. Only prednisolone is approved in Japan.

George et al. reviewed the clinical course of adult ITP in 12 case series of 1761 adults between 1928 and 1989. Since the 1950s, most adults have been promptly treated with glucocorticoids, and approximately 25% of all patients treated with glucocorticoids may achieve a complete response [5].

Based on these findings, George et al. proposed glucocorticoid therapy in the initial management of a newly diagnosed ITP patient [5]. Although they indicated that patients with asymptomatic mild or moderate thrombocytopenia may be followed with no treatment, oral prednisone (1 mg/kg/day) was recommended as conventional initial therapy for newly diagnosed patients with more severe thrombocytopenia. Similar initial therapy has since been recommended by other reviews [1, 2].

In 1996, George et al. published practical guidelines for ITP developed by explicit methods for the American Society of Hematology [8]. Other guidelines were subsequently published by various medical societies [8–11]. These guidelines also recommend the use of oral corticosteroids in the initial treatment.

In 2012, a panel for Blood Coagulation Abnormalities in Japan belonging to the Ministry of Health, Labour and Welfare of Japan published a reference guide for the management of adult ITP [12]. Although the reference guide also recommends the use of oral prednisolone as the first-line treatment, similar to the other guidelines, it provides considerations prior to the initiation of treatment. Patient backgrounds, including hypertension, diabetes, active infections, osteoporosis, hyperglycemia, immune suppressive states, and peptic ulcers, need to be considered. The aggravation of these complications and occurrence of unexpected adverse events also need to be taken into account. The recommended dosage of prednisolone is 0.5–1.0 mg/kg/day for 2–4 weeks. In patients with various complications and older patients, the reference guide recommends a starting dose of 0.5 mg/kg/day prednisolone. Even if platelet counts do not increase, the daily dose is slowly tapered to the maintenance dose (less than 10 mg/body/day). If the bleeding tendency deteriorates during the tapering or cessation of prednisolone, increasing the dose administered, the reinitiation of prednisolone, or the initiation of other treatments including intravenous immunoglobulin (IVIG) needs to be considered. The efficacy of oral corticosteroids is noted as follows: the platelet count starts to increase 3–4 days after starting the treatment, and, in rare cases, a response is not observed for 1 week or longer. Response rates range between 50 and more than 75%, depending on the intensity and duration of therapy. The incidence of continuous remission ranges is between 10 and 20% [13, 14]. If initial treatment using corticosteroids is ineffective, a bone marrow examination needs to be planned in consideration of other disorders such as myelodysplastic syndrome.

3 Methylprednisolone

An immediate intervention in the platelet count may be required for some patients needing surgical procedures or active central nervous system, gastrointestinal tract, urological, or gynecological bleeding. Many reviews and guidelines note that emergent treatment needs to include IVIG, high-dose intravenous methylprednisolone (mPSL) (1.0 g/body/day for 2–3 days), and platelet transfusions [2, 9–12]. If the bleeding tendency appears to be critical, platelet transfusions in conjunction with IVIG and mPSL need to be considered.

Previous studies reported the efficacy of intravenous mPSL as the first-line treatment [15–17]. von dem Borne et al. investigated the effects of high-dose intravenous mPSL in the treatment of patients with their first attack of ITP and compared them with those of IVIG and oral prednisolone [15]. Their findings demonstrated that high-dose mPSL (HD mPSL) was as effective as IVIG. However, the effects of HD mPSL were transient in all our patients, similar to IVIG, and maintenance treatment using a low oral dose of prednisolone was necessary.

In 2002, Godeau et al. performed a randomized multicenter trial that compared IVIG and HD mPSL with or without oral prednisone. Their findings indicated that IVIG and oral prednisone were more effective than HD mPSL and oral prednisone in adults with severe ITP; however, the latter treatment was effective and tolerated well.

According to these findings, intravenous mPSL is as effective as IVIG in terms of response frequency with no reported side effects. The response to intravenous mPSL was found to be faster than that to oral corticosteroids, whereas the response to mPSL was transient and low-dose oral corticosteroids were required to maintain the platelet count [15].

4 Dexamethasone

Although prednisolone or mPSL is effective for ITP patients, improvements are often transitory. Patients who require long-term oral prednisolone therapy develop various side effects. Since pulsed high-dose dexamethasone (HD-DEX) is tolerated well and effective in patients with plasma cell neoplasms, Anderson reported efficacy with a similar HD-DEX regimen (six cycles of HD-DEX: 40 mg/day for 4 days every 28 days) in ten refractory ITP patients [18]. All patients had increased platelet counts, and long-term effects were observed for at least 6 months after the last cycle of treatments. No serious side effects were detected. Although the response rate in the study by Anderson was 100%, a similar protocol using HD-DEX was not as effective for ITP patients in other small cohort studies [19–26]. Therefore, based on the findings of these small cohort studies, the efficacy of HD-DEX remains controversial.

In 2003, Cheng et al. reported the effectiveness of HD-DEX as an initial treatment for 125 ITP patients [27]. The initial regimen was a single course of oral DEX (40 mg/body/day for 4 consecutive days). The findings obtained were impressive because the initial response rate was 85%, the relapse rate was 50%, and the sustained response rate was 42%. Moreover, a second therapy course using HD-DEX was effective in all relapsed patients. In 2007, Mazzucconi et al. reported the findings of two different prospective pilot studies: a monocenter study and multicenter study, using HD-DEX in newly diagnosed, untreated ITP patients [28]. In their multicenter study, 95 patients with severe ITP were treated using HD-DEX (oral or intravenous DEX 40 mg/body/day for 4 consecutive days, every 14 days, for 4 cycles). The response rate was 85.6% and relapse-free survival at 15 months was 81%. These findings [27, 28] suggested that it is possible to shorten the duration and reduce the adverse effects of corticosteroid treatment by using HD-DEX. Wei et al. very recently performed a prospective multicenter randomized trial to compare the efficacy and safety of HD-DEX and conventional prednisone for newly diagnosed ITP patients [29]. In this study, 192 patients were randomized to HD-DEX (oral 40 mg/body/day for 4 days, one or two courses) or prednisone (1.0 mg/kg/day for 4 weeks and then tapered). One or two courses of HD-DEX resulted in better outcomes both in overall initial response rates (82.1% vs 67.4%) and complete response rates (50.5% vs 26.8%) than those with prednisone. Moreover, the time to a response with HD-DEX was shorter than that with prednisone.

According to the findings of these recent large cohort studies [27–29], one to four courses of HD-DEX worked more effectively and rapidly than other corticosteroid treatments. A large number of reviews and guidelines have described, but not recommended HD-DEX because supporting evidence has been limited.

5 Combination Therapy with DEX and Rituximab

Rituximab is also recommended for use in the treatment of refractory ITP as a second- [9–11] or third-line treatment [12].

Zaja et al. reported the findings of a randomized, open-label trial using HD-DEX with rituximab to treat ITP [30]. A total of 101 newly diagnosed ITP patients were randomized to receive HD-DEX (40 mg/body/day) for 4 days with or without 375 mg/m^2 rituximab weekly for 4 weeks. The sustained response rate was higher in patients treated with DEX plus rituximab than in those treated with DEX alone (63% vs 36%). However, a higher rate of adverse events was observed in the rituximab arm. Following this study, other trials using HD-DEX plus a regular dose of rituximab (375 mg/m^2) [31, 32] or low dose of rituximab (100 mg/m^2) [33, 34] were performed. Their findings demonstrated that the overall response of the experimental group was similar to that of HD-DEX alone; however, the sustained response was more pronounced in the experimental group. These findings indicate that rituximab more strongly reduced the number of autoantibody-producing B cells than HD-DEX alone and contributed to a longer sustained response. Choi et al. recently described a novel triple therapy for ITP using HD-DEX, low-dose rituximab, and cyclosporine [35]. This trial was a single-arm phase IIb study, and 20 patients including refractory cases were prospectively enrolled to receive HD-DEX (40 mg/body/day for 4 days, oral cyclosporine 2.5–3 mg/kg/day from days 1 to 28, and intravenous low-dose rituximab 100 mg on days 7, 14, 21, and 28). The response rate at 6 months was 60%, and the relapse-free survival rate was 92% at 12 months. By adding cyclosporine to HD-DEX and rituximab, T cells may also be targeted and implicated in sustaining the pathogenic loop. Although adverse events induced by the addition of rituximab to HD-DEX are still problematic, these combination therapies may have the advantage of reducing the treatment period.

6 Conclusions

Novel treatments including thrombopoietin receptor agonists and rituximab have recently been approved for the treatment of ITP. However, all current guidelines recommend the use of corticosteroids as the first-line treatment. In consideration of selecting the type of corticosteroid to be used, various protocols have been attempted and published. HD-DEX has yet to be approved by a systematic review using a meta-analysis and needs to be approved by guidelines in the next revised edition.

References

1. Karpatkin S. Autoimmune (idiopathic) thrombocytopenic purpura. Lancet. 1997;349(9064):1531–6. doi:10.1016/S0140-6736(96)12118-8.
2. Cines DB, Blanchette VS. Immune thrombocytopenic purpura. New Engl J Med. 2002;346(13):995–1008. doi:10.1056/NEJMra010501.
3. Kuwana M, Ikeda Y. The role of autoreactive T-cells in the pathogenesis of idiopathic thrombocytopenic purpura. Int J Hematol. 2005;81(2):106–12.
4. McMillan R, Wang L, Tomer A, Nichol J, Pistillo J. Suppression of in vitro megakaryocyte production by antiplatelet autoantibodies from adult patients with chronic ITP. Blood. 2004;103(4):1364–9. doi:10.1182/blood-2003-08-2672.
5. George JN, el-Harake MA, Raskob GE. Chronic idiopathic thrombocytopenic purpura. New Engl J Med. 1994;331(18):1207–11. doi:10.1056/NEJM199411033311807.
6. Kitchens CS, Weiss L. Ultrastructural changes of endothelium associated with thrombocytopenia. Blood. 1975;46(4):567–78.
7. Kitchens CS. Amelioration of endothelial abnormalities by prednisone in experimental thrombocytopenia in the rabbit. J Clin Invest. 1977;60(5):1129–34. doi:10.1172/JCI108864.

8. George JN, Woolf SH, Raskob GE, Wasser JS, Aledort LM, Ballem PJ, et al. Idiopathic thrombocytopenic purpura: a practice guideline developed by explicit methods for the American Society of Hematology. Blood. 1996;88(1):3–40.
9. British Committee for Standards in Haematology General Haematology Task Force. Guidelines for the investigation and management of idiopathic thrombocytopenic purpura in adults, children and in pregnancy. Br J Haematol. 2003;120(4):574–96.
10. Provan D, Stasi R, Newland AC, Blanchette VS, Bolton-Maggs P, Bussel JB, et al. International consensus report on the investigation and management of primary immune thrombocytopenia. Blood. 2010;115(2):168–86. doi:10.1182/blood-2009-06-225565.
11. Neunert C, Lim W, Crowther M, Cohen A, Solberg Jr L, Crowther MA, et al. The American Society of Hematology 2011 evidence-based practice guideline for immune thrombocytopenia. Blood. 2011;117(16):4190–207. doi:10.1182/blood-2010-08-302984.
12. Fujimura K, Miyakawa Y, Kurata Y, Kuwana M, Tomiyama Y, Murata M. Reference guide for management of adult idiopathic thrombocytopenic purpura (ITP) 2012 version. [Rinsho Ketsueki] Jpn J Clin Hematol. 2012;53(4):433–42.
13. Ben-Yehuda D, Gillis S, Eldor A. Clinical and therapeutic experience in 712 Israeli patients with idiopathic thrombocytopenic purpura. Israeli ITP Study Group. Acta Haematol. 1994;91(1):1–6.
14. Stasi R, Stipa E, Masi M, Cecconi M, Scimo MT, Oliva F, et al. Long-term observation of 208 adults with chronic idiopathic thrombocytopenic purpura. Am J Med. 1995;98(5):436–42.
15. von dem Borne AE, Vos JJ, Pegels JG, Thomas LL, van der L. High dose intravenous methylprednisolone or high dose intravenous gamma globulin for autoimmune thrombocytopenia. Br Med J. 1988;296(6617):249–50.
16. Godeau B, Zini JM, Schaeffer A, Bierling P. High-dose methylprednisolone is an alternative treatment for adults with autoimmune thrombocytopenic purpura refractory to intravenous immunoglobulins and oral corticosteroids. Am J Hematol. 1995;48(4):282–4.
17. Alpdogan O, Budak-Alpdogan T, Ratip S, Firatli-Tuglular T, Tanriverdi S, Karti S, et al. Efficacy of high-dose methylprednisolone as a first-line therapy in adult patients with idiopathic thrombocytopenic purpura. Br J Haematol. 1998;103(4):1061–3.
18. Andersen JC. Response of resistant idiopathic thrombocytopenic purpura to pulsed high-dose dexamethasone therapy. New Engl J Med. 1994;330(22):1560–4. doi:10.1056/NEJM199406023302203.
19. Arruda VR, Annichino-Bizzacchi JM. High-dose dexamethasone therapy in chronic idiopathic thrombocytopenic purpura. Ann Hematol. 1996;73(4):175–7.
20. Caulier MT, Rose C, Roussel MT, Huart C, Bauters F, Fenaux P. Pulsed high-dose dexamethasone in refractory chronic idiopathic thrombocytopenic purpura: a report on 10 cases. Br J Haematol. 1995;91(2):477–9.
21. Warner M, Wasi P, Couban S, Hayward C, Warkentin T, Kelton JG. Failure of pulse high-dose dexamethasone in chronic idiopathic immune thrombocytopenia. Am J Hematol. 1997;54(4):267–70.
22. Stasi R, Brunetti M, Pagano A, Stipa E, Masi M, Amadori S. Pulsed intravenous high-dose dexamethasone in adults with chronic idiopathic thrombocytopenic purpura. Blood Cells Mol Dis. 2000;26(6):582–6. doi:10.1006/bcmd.2000.0336.
23. Borst F, Keuning JJ, van Hulsteijn H, Sinnige H, Vreugdenhil G. High-dose dexamethasone as a first- and second-line treatment of idiopathic thrombocytopenic purpura in adults. Ann Hematol. 2004;83(12):764–8. doi:10.1007/s00277-004-0908-1.
24. Naithani R, Mahapatra M, Kumar R, Mishra P, Saxena R. High dose dexamethasone therapy shows better responses in acute immune thrombocytopenia than in chronic immune thrombocytopenia. Platelets. 2010;21(4):270–3. doi:10.3109/09537101003637257.
25. Nakazaki K, Hosoi M, Hangaishi A, Ichikawa M, Nannya Y, Kurokawa M. Comparison between pulsed high-dose dexamethasone and daily corticosteroid therapy for adult primary immune thrombocytopenia: a retrospective study. Intern Med. 2012;51(8):859–63.
26. Sakamoto K, Nakasone H, Tsurumi S, Sasaki K, Mitani K, Kida M, et al. Prednisone versus high-dose dexamethasone for untreated primary immune thrombocytopenia. A retrospective

study of the Japan Hematology & Oncology Clinical Study Group. J Thromb Thrombolysis. 2014;37(3):279–86. doi:10.1007/s11239-013-0939-3.
27. Cheng Y, Wong RS, Soo YO, Chui CH, Lau FY, Chan NP, et al. Initial treatment of immune thrombocytopenic purpura with high-dose dexamethasone. New Engl J Med. 2003;349(9):831–6. doi:10.1056/NEJMoa030254.
28. Mazzucconi MG, Fazi P, Bernasconi S, De Rossi G, Leone G, Gugliotta L, et al. Therapy with high-dose dexamethasone (HD-DXM) in previously untreated patients affected by idiopathic thrombocytopenic purpura: a GIMEMA experience. Blood. 2007;109(4):1401–7. doi:10.1182/blood-2005-12-015222.
29. Wei Y, Ji XB, Wang YW, Wang JX, Yang EQ, Wang ZC, et al. High-dose dexamethasone vs prednisone for treatment of adult immune thrombocytopenia: a prospective multicenter randomized trial. Blood. 2016;127(3):296–302; quiz 70. doi:10.1182/blood-2015-07-659656.
30. Zaja F, Baccarani M, Mazza P, Bocchia M, Gugliotta L, Zaccaria A, et al. Dexamethasone plus rituximab yields higher sustained response rates than dexamethasone monotherapy in adults with primary immune thrombocytopenia. Blood. 2010;115(14):2755–62. doi:10.1182/blood-2009-07-229815.
31. Gudbrandsdottir S, Birgens HS, Frederiksen H, Jensen BA, Jensen MK, Kjeldsen L, et al. Rituximab and dexamethasone vs dexamethasone monotherapy in newly diagnosed patients with primary immune thrombocytopenia. Blood. 2013;121(11):1976–81. doi:10.1182/blood-2012-09-455691.
32. Bussel JB, Lee CS, Seery C, Imahiyerobo AA, Thompson MV, Catellier D, et al. Rituximab and three dexamethasone cycles provide responses similar to splenectomy in women and those with immune thrombocytopenia of less than two years duration. Haematologica. 2014;99(7):1264–71. doi:10.3324/haematol.2013.103291.
33. Li Z, Mou W, Lu G, Cao J, He X, Pan X, et al. Low-dose rituximab combined with short-term glucocorticoids up-regulates Treg cell levels in patients with immune thrombocytopenia. Int J Hematol. 2011;93(1):91–8. doi:10.1007/s12185-010-0753-z.
34. Gomez-Almaguer D, Tarin-Arzaga L, Moreno-Jaime B, Jaime-Perez JC, Ceballos-Lopez AA, Ruiz-Arguelles GJ, et al. High response rate to low-dose rituximab plus high-dose dexamethasone as frontline therapy in adult patients with primary immune thrombocytopenia. Eur J Haematol. 2013;90(6):494–500. doi:10.1111/ejh.12102.
35. Choi PY, Roncolato F, Badoux X, Ramanathan S, Ho SJ, Chong BH. A novel triple therapy for ITP using high-dose dexamethasone, low-dose rituximab, and cyclosporine (TT4). Blood. 2015;126(4):500–3. doi:10.1182/blood-2015-03-631937.

High-Dose Immunoglobulin

Tatsuo Oyake and Yoji Ishida

Abstract Approximately 70% of the ITP patients responded to high dose of intravenous immunoglobulin. The 2011 ASH guidelines recommend an initial dose of 1 g/kg as a one-time dose. This dosage may be repeated if necessary. The EU recommendations described that adult ITP patients at high risk of bleeding or prior to surgery to correct the platelet count should be indicated for the administration of intravenous immunoglobulin. Adverse events with intravenous immunoglobulin are common, but generally acceptable. High doses of immunoglobulin are thought to be involved in the Fc receptor blockade of macrophages in the reticuloendothelial system. Several other mechanisms were elucidated.

1 Introduction

In 1981, Imbach et al. [1] reported that treatment with high-dose intravenous immunoglobulin (IVIG) (0.4 g (kg day)) for 5 days improved platelet counts in 13 children with idiopathic thrombocytopenic purpura (ITP). All 13 children had initial platelet counts less than 3×10^9/L. This clinical study demonstrated an increase in platelet counts in 12 of the 13 children within 5 days, but a transient increase over the following 10 days. Subsequently, more than 100 clinical studies have confirmed the safety and efficacy of IVIG for the treatment of ITP in children and adults [2–7].

T. Oyake (✉) • Y. Ishida
Division of Hematology and Oncology, Department of Internal Medicine, Iwate Medical University School of Medicine, 19-1 Uchimaru, Morioka, Iwate Prefectire 020-8505, Japan
e-mail: toyake@iwate-med.ac.jp; yoji.ishida@gmail.com

Y. Ishida, Y. Tomiyama (eds.), *Autoimmune Thrombocytopenia*,
DOI 10.1007/978-981-10-4142-6_14

2 Indication and Dose of IVIG

Spontaneous and permanent remission was observed in more than 70% of children with ITP within 1 year of onset [8, 9]. First-line treatment for children newly diagnosed with ITP is IVIG at a total dose of 0.8–1.0 g/kg given on 1 day or over 2 consecutive days (grade IB) [10]. The use of IVIG in children with ITP will be discussed in detail in another chapter.

Spontaneous remission is much less common in adults with ITP. The 2011 ASH guidelines recommend longer courses of corticosteroids over either shorter courses of corticosteroids or IVIG in adults newly diagnosed with ITP. In addition, the guidelines recognize that the majority of clinicians use a platelet count of less than 30×10^9/L as a threshold for treatment [12]. The decision to use IVIG should be based on the patient's severity of bleeding, bleeding risk, activity level, likely side effects of treatment, and patient preference [11]. Take it for example, the indication should be based on the patients with life-threatning bleeding or before surgery or delivery. Cohen et al. [12] described bleeding risk according to age, in which patients older than 60 years of age with a platelet count less than 3×10^9/L had an estimated 5 year fatal bleeding risk of 48% compared with a risk of 2.2% for those younger than 40 years.

When IVIG is chosen, the response is transient and platelet counts usually return to pretreatment levels within 3–4 weeks [13]. The EU recommendations indicate the current IVIG core SPC (core summaries of product characteristics) indication and dosing as follows [14, 15]: for primary immune thrombocytopenia (ITP), in patients at high risk of bleeding or prior to surgery to correct the platelet count, there are two alternative treatment schedules, (1) 0.8–1 g/kg given on day 1 (this dose may be repeated once within 3 days), or (2) 0.4 g/kg given daily for 2–5 days. The treatment can be repeated if relapse occurs.

Though the 2011 ASH guidelines recommend an initial dose of 1 g/kg, this recommendation is based on the results of a small, randomized trial [16]. This dosage may be repeated if necessary (grade 2B). IVIG has been proven to have a rapid onset of action (grade 2B) and should be considered along with corticosteroids (grade 2B) with the aim of rapidly increasing the platelet count.

3 Efficacy

Since the report of Imbach et al. [1], investigators have recognized the effectiveness of IVIG for patients with ITP. In a review of 28 published reports of IVIG in 282 adults, 64% of patients had a peak platelet count >100,000/μL, and 83% had a peak platelet count >50,000/μL after the initial infusion [17]. IVIG is more likely to cause a platelet increase within 24 h at a dose of 1 g/kg (1–2 infusions over 2 days) compared with the previous regimen (0.4 g/(kg day) over 5 days) [18]. A randomized trial to compare the efficacy of 1 g/(kg day) IVIG for 2 days with the conventional dose (0.4 g/(kg day)) for 5 days was performed. This study indicated that the

2-day regimen required shorter hospitalization and corrected thrombocytopenia slightly faster than the 5-day course [18]. Godeau et al. [16] reported the results of a randomized IVIG trial comparing 0.5 and 1 g/kg. In their study, on day 4, the proportion of responses, defined by a platelet count >80 × 10^9/L and at least twice the initial platelet count, was significantly higher in the group receiving 1 g/kg ($P = 0.05$). They concluded that initial treatment with 1 g/kg of IVIG was more effective than 0.5 g/kg in adults with autoimmune thrombocytopenic purpura. The 2011 ASH guidelines recommend that the dose should initially be 1 g/kg as a one-time dose and that this dosage may be repeated if necessary (grade 2B) [11].

Peng et al. [19] reported that the presence of anti-GPIb-IX autoantibodies was a predictor for poor response to IVIG treatment in adults with ITP. Patients with ITP that had anti-GPIb-IX autoantibody present had only a 36.4% response rate compared with an 80.0% response rate for those who were negative for anti-GPIb-IX autoantibodies (relative risk 2.2; 95% confidence interval 1.6–3.1).

Papagianni et al. [20] reported IVIG responsiveness and outcome might be correlated with FcγRIIa and FcγRIIIa polymorphic variants. The high-affinity FcγRIIIa variant 158 V for the Fc portion of the immunoglobulin was implicated in the pathogenesis of ITP, whereas FcγRIIa (131R) and FcγRIIIa (158V) variants, which have low affinity for the Fc portion of immunoglobulin, did not seem to impact the therapeutic efficacy of IVIG.

4 Adverse Events

Adverse events with IVIG are common, but generally acceptable, and include headache, backache, nausea, increase in blood pressure, and fever [21, 22]. In 2007, Bussel et al. [23] evaluated the safety and tolerability of IVIG for patients with ITP when IVIG was infused at rates ranging from 0.08 mL/(kg min) (the standard maximum licensed rate) to 0.14 mL/(kg min). The incidence of infusion-related adverse events was similar for all infusion rates. Headache was the most commonly reported infusion-related adverse event (17%). Urticaria (5.5%), hypertension (5.5%), and other symptoms less than 5% were observed. The majority were mild in severity. No other drug-related, treatment-emergent events were serious.

5 Mechanism

The potential immunomodulatory mechanisms of IgG have been described [24, 25]. High doses of immunoglobulin are thought to be involved in the Fc receptor blockade of macrophages in the reticuloendothelial system [26–28], neutralization of autoantibodies (anti-idiotypes), binding to variable regions of T and B cells (V-connected network) [29], downregulation of T-cell and B-cell function, and upregulation of Treg-cell function [30, 31].

References

1. Imbach P, Barandun S, d'Apuzzo V, Baumgartner C, Hirt A, Morell A, Rossi E, Schoni M, Vest M, Wagner HP. High dose intravenous gamma globulin for idiopathic thrombocytopenic purpura in childhood. Lancet. 1981;1:1228–31.
2. Bussel JB, Kimberly RP, Inman RD, Schulman I, Cunningham-Rundles C, Cheung N, Smithwick EM, O'Malley J, Barandun S, Hilgartner MW. Intravenous gamma globulin treatment of chronic idiopathic thrombocytopenic purpura. Blood. 1983;62:480–6.
3. Warrier I, Lusher JM. Intravenous gamma globulin treatment for chronic idiopathic thrombocytopenic purpura in children. Am J Med. 1984;76:193–8.
4. Carroll RR, Noyes WD, Rosse WF, Kitchen CS. Intravenous immunoglobulin administration in the treatment of severe chronic immune thrombocytopenic purpura. Am J Med. 1984;76: 181–6.
5. Oral A, Nusbacher J, Hill JB, Lewis JH. Intravenous gamma globulin in the treatment of chronic idiopathic thrombocytopenic purpura in adults. Am J Med. 1984;76:187–92.
6. Bussel JB, Pham LC. Intravenous treatment with gammaglobulin in adults with immune thrombocytopenic purpura: review of the literature. Vox Sang. 1987;52:206–11.
7. Bussel JB, Eldor A, Kelton JG, Varon D, Brenner B, Gillis S, Angiolillo A, Kulkarni R, Abshire TC, Kelleher J, IGIV-C in ITP Study Group. IGIV, a novel intravenous immunoglobulin: evaluation of safety, efficacy, mechanisms of action, and impact on quality of life. Thromb Haemost. 2004;91:771–8.
8. Rosthøj S, Hedlund-Treutiger I, Rajantie J, Zeller B, Jonsson OG, Elinder G, Wesenberg F, Henter JI, NOPHO ITP Working Group. Duration and morbidity of newly diagnosed idiopathic thrombocytopenic purpura in children: a prospective nordic study of an unselected cohort. J Pediatr. 2003;143(3):302–7.
9. Kuhne T, Buchanan GR, Zimmerman S, Michaels LA, Kohan R, Berchtold W, Imbach P, Intercontinental Childhood ITP Study Group. A prospective comparative study of 2540 infants and children with newly diagnosed idiopathic thrombocytopenic purpura (ITP) from the Intercontinental Childhood ITP Study Group. J Pediatr. 2003;143(5):605–8.
10. Beck CE, Nathan PC, Parkin PC, Blanchette VS, Macarthur C. Corticosteroids versus intravenous immune globulin for the treatment of acute immune thrombocytopenic purpura in children: a systematic review and meta-analysis of randomized controlled trials. J Pediatr. 2005;147(4):521–7.
11. Neuner C, et al. The American Society of Hematology 2011 evidence-based practice guideline for immune thrombocytopenia. Blood. 2011;117(16):4190–207.
12. Cohen YC, Djuibegovic B, Shamai-Lubovitz O, Mozes B. The bleeding risk and natural history of idiopathic thrombocytopenic purpura in patients with persistent low platelet counts. Arch Intern Med. 2000;160(11):1630–8.
13. Godeau B, Lesage S, Divine M, Wirquin V, Farcet JP, Bierling P. Treatment of adult chronic autoimmune thrombocytopenic purpura with repeated high-dose intravenous immunoglobulin. Blood. 1993;82:1415–21.
14. Kerr J, Quinti I, Eibl M, Chapel H, Spath PJ, Sewell WA, Salama A, van Schaik IN, Kuijpers TW, Peter HH. Is dosing of therapeutic immunoglobulins optimal? A review of a three-decade long debate in Europe. Front Immunol. 2014;5:629.
15. Sewell WA, Kerr J, Behr-Gross ME, Peter HH, Kreuth IG Working Group. European consensus proposal for immunoglobulin therapies. Eur J Immunol. 2014;44(8):2207–14.
16. Godeau B, Caulier MT, Decuypere L, Rose C, Schaeffer A, Bierling P. Intravenous immunoglobulin for adults with autoimmune thrombocytopenic purpura: results of a randomized trial comparing 0.5 and 1 g/kg b.w. Br J Haematol. 1999;107(4):716–9.
17. Bussel J. Intravenous immune serum globulin in immune thrombocytopenia: clinical results and biochemical evaluation. Vox Sang. 1985;49(Suppl 1):44–50.

18. Kurlander R, Coleman RE, Moore J, Gockerman J, Rosse W, Siegal R. Comparison of the efficacy of a two-day and a five-day schedule for infusing intravenous gamma globulin in the treatment of immune thrombocytopenic purpura in adults. Am J Med. 1987;83(Suppl 4A):17–24.
19. Peng J, Ma SH, Liu J, Hou Y, Liu XM, Niu T, Xu RR, Guo CS, Wang XM, Cheng YF, Ni H, Hou M. Association of autoantibody specificity and response to intravenous immunoglobulin G therapy in immune thrombocytopenia: a multicenter cohort study. J Thromb Haemost. 2014; 12(4):497–504.
20. Papagianni A, Economou M, Tragiannidis A, Karatza E, Samarah F, Gombakis N, Athanassiadou-Piperopoulou F, Vavatsi-Christaki N, Athanassiou-Metaxa M. FcγRIIa and FcγRIIIa polymorphisms in childhood primary immune thrombocytopenia: implications for disease pathogenesis and outcome. Blood Coagul Fibrinolysis. 2013;24(1):35–9.
21. Blanchette VS, Luke B, Andrew M, Sommerville-Nielsen S, Bamard D, De Veber B, Gent M. A prospective, randomized trial of high-dose intravenous immune globulin G therapy, oral prednisone therapy, and no therapy in childhood acute immune thrombocytopenic purpura. J Pediatr. 1993;123:989.
22. Duhem C, Dicato MA, Ries F. Side-effects of intravenous immune globulins. Clin Exp Immunol. 1994;97(Suppl 1):79.
23. Bussel JB, Hanna K, IGIV-C in ITP Study Group. Safety and tolerability of a novel chromatography-based intravenous immunoglobulin when administered at a high infusion rate in patients with immune thrombocytopenic purpura. Am J Hematol. 2007;82(3):192–8.
24. Schwab I, Nimmerjahn F. Intravenous immunoglobulin therapy: how does IgG modulate the immune system? Nat Rev Immunol. 2013;13(3):176–89.
25. Bouhlal H, Martinvalet D, Teillaud JL, Fridman C, Kazatchkine MD, Bayry J, Lacroix-Desmazes S, Kaveri SV. Natural autoantibodies to Fcγ receptors in intravenous immunoglobulins. J Clin Immunol. 2014;34(Suppl 1):S4–11.
26. Newland AC. Annotation: the use and mechanisms of action of intravenous immunoglobulin: an update. Br J Haematol. 1989;72:301–5.
27. Saleh M, Court W, Huster W, et al. Effect of commercial immunoglobulin G preparation on human monocyte Fc-receptor dependent binding of antibody coated platelets. Br J Haematol. 1988;68:47–51.
28. Kimberly RP, Salmon JE, Bussel JB, Crow MK, Hilgartner MW. Modulation of mononuclear phagocyte function by intravenous γ-globulin. J Immunol. 1984;132(2):745–50.
29. Rossi F, Dietrich G, Kazatchkine MD. Anti-idiotypes against autoantibodies in normal immunoglobulins: evidence for network regulation of human autoimmune responses. Immunol Rev. 1989;110:135–49.
30. Zhu D, Ravindranath MH, Terasaki PI, Miyazaki T, Pham T, Jucaud V. Suppression of allo-human leucocyte antigen (HLA) antibodies secreted by B memory cells in vitro: intravenous immunoglobulin (IVIG) versus a monoclonal anti-HLA-E IgG that mimics HLA-I reactivities of IVIG. Clin Exp Immunol. 2014;177(2):464–77.
31. Othy S, Hegde P, Topcu S, Sharma M, Maddur MS, Lacroix-Desmazes S, Bayry J, Kaveri SV. Intravenous gammaglobulin inhibits encephalitogenic potential of pathogenic T cells and interferes with their trafficking to the central nervous system, implicating sphingosine-1 phosphate receptor 1-mammalian target of rapamycin axis. J Immunol. 2013;190(9):4535–41.

Splenectomy

Shugo Kowata and Yoji Ishida

Abstract In immune thrombocytopenic purpura (ITP) patients, an interaction between T cells and B cells induces antiplatelet autoantibody production, and macrophages digest the antibody-platelet complex in the spleen. However, splenectomy removes the microenvironment important for the interaction among B cells, T cells, macrophages, and opsonized platelets. Moreover, splenectomy leads to a high frequency of durable responses in adult patients with ITP. Perioperative complications of splenectomy include bleeding, infection, and thrombosis. Additionally, long-term complications include overwhelming sepsis by encapsulated bacteria, vascular/thrombotic events, and cancer. Recent guidelines and expert consensus reports list splenectomy as a second-line therapy for patients who have failed corticosteroid therapy. More recently, there has been a tendency to avoid and defer splenectomy in favor of new treatment options, resulting in a decrease in the use of splenectomy for ITP.

1 Immune Thrombocytopenic Purpura (ITP) and the Spleen

The spleen is a key lymphoid organ for generating B-lymphocyte-mediated humoral immunity. In ITP patients, there is an increase in the number of CD20+ B cells in the red pulp of the spleen [1]. Furthermore, there is an interaction between T-cell- and B-cell-induced antiplatelet autoantibody production, resulting in accelerated platelet destruction and impaired platelet production [2], primarily in the spleen. Splenic macrophages are mainly considered as scavengers for senescent erythrocytes and help control infections by eliminating pathogens and inducing adaptive immunity [3]. In ITP patients, splenic macrophages that digest opsonized platelets via the Fcγ receptor are an indispensable ally to the maintenance of antiplatelet autoantibody production [4].

S. Kowata (✉) • Y. Ishida
Division of Hematology and Oncology, Department of Internal Medicine, Iwate Medical University School of Medicine, Morioka, Japan
e-mail: skowata@iwate-med.ac.jp; yoji.ishida@gmail.com

Y. Ishida, Y. Tomiyama (eds.), *Autoimmune Thrombocytopenia*,
DOI 10.1007/978-981-10-4142-6_15

2 Splenectomy

Splenectomy as treatment for ITP was initially performed in 1916 after the successful treatment of hemolytic anemia with splenectomy in some patients [5]. Splenectomy was subsequently the primary therapy until corticosteroids were introduced in the 1950s. Splenectomy removes the microenvironment important for the interaction among B cells, T cells, macrophages, and opsonized platelets, resulting in a decreased titer of antiplatelet antibody and a decrease in the removal of the macrophages. Previously, the spleen was removed by open surgery via a midline abdominal incision [6]. The current laparoscopic splenectomy technique is associated with significantly reduced procedure-related morbidity and a shorter hospital stay than the open method [7]. More recently, there has been an increasing trend to avoid and defer splenectomy, resulting in a decrease in the rate of splenectomy for ITP from 50–60% to 10–25% [8, 9].

2.1 *Indication*

Recent guidelines and expert consensus reports list splenectomy as a second-line therapy for ITP patients who have failed corticosteroid therapy [6]. However, there has not been a clinical trial to compare splenectomy with other treatments, including no treatment. In addition, splenectomy is irreversible, and there are no preoperative characteristics that can predict response to splenectomy [10]. Thus, it remains unclear which patients should be favorably indicated for splenectomy compared to other second-line therapies, including rituximab, cyclophosphamide, azathioprine, and the newer thrombopoietic agents romiplostim and eltrombopag. Moreover, there is no evidence regarding the optimal timing of splenectomy, because some adult patients may improve spontaneously or over time as a result of treatment [11]. Thus, an international consensus report suggests deferring splenectomy until the chronic phase (>12 months) [12]. In addition, American Society of Hematology (ASH) guidelines suggest treatment with thrombopoietin receptor agonists (TPO-RAs) for patients who have both contraindication to splenectomy and who have failed at least one other therapy before splenectomy [13]. Under these situations, many patients and physicians now prefer to delay or avoid splenectomy when patients relapse after frontline therapy, although the curative potential of splenectomy is superior to that of other available treatments.

2.2 *Response and Relapse*

It has been thought that the curative potential of splenectomy is superior to that of other available second-line treatments. For instance, Kojouri et al. reported a complete response in 1731 (66%) of 2623 adult patients with follow-up for 1–153 months in a large systematic review [10]. Moreover, Vianelli et al. reported that 180 of 206 (77%) achieved complete response, 26 (11%) achieved response, and 68 (33%) responsive patients relapsed. Eventually, 138 (59%) patients maintained response without any long-term treatment in a retrospective analysis of 233 patients with follow-up over 10 years [14]—most relapses occur during the first year [15]. Furthermore, Mikhael et al. showed that the short-term non-response rate was 8.2% and long-term relapse rate was 43.6 per 1000 patient years, resulting in an approximate 5 year failure rate of 28% in a large systematic review. Thus, splenectomy results in higher initial relapse rates, particularly in the first 2 years after surgery, although the relapse rate may decline over time [16].

3 Risk and Complication of Splenectomy

Splenectomy is an invasive treatment associated with short-term complications related to general anesthesia and surgery and long-term complications related to loss of splenic functions. Perioperative complications include bleeding, infection, and thrombosis. Patients with a platelet count of $\leq 20 \times 10^9$/L had a much longer hospital stay, received more blood transfusions, and suffered more complications than those with platelet counts of $>20 \times 10^9$/L [17]. Long-term complications include sepsis by encapsulated bacteria, vascular/thrombotic events, and cancer.

In a systematic review, Kojouri et al. revealed that mortality in ITP patients was 1.0% (48 of 4955 patients) with laparotomy and 0.2% (3 of 1301 patients) with laparoscopy and that the complication rate was 12.9% (318 of 2465) with laparotomy and 9.6% (88 of 921 patients) with laparoscopy [10]. A historical population cohort study in splenectomized patients who have undergone splenectomy for various indications showed a higher relative risk (RR) for death within 90 days post-splenectomy (RR 2.3); however, the RR decreased to 0.5 by day 365 and decreased further to 0.4 at > 365 days postsplenectomy [18]. These data indicate that splenectomized patients may have a reduced long-term risk of death in spite of several short-term complications.

3.1 *Infection*

It has been evident that asplenic patients are at increased risk of life-threatening infections. In addition, most therapies for ITP are immunosuppressive, which may also increase the risk of infection.

In a retrospective analysis of ITP patients, the cumulative incidence of sepsis was 10.1% in non-splenectomized patients and 11.1% in splenectomized patients, with a median follow-up of 56 months. The cumulative incidence of early sepsis after splenectomy (<90 days) was 2.6%, and that of late sepsis (>90 days) was 8.8%, suggesting that the infection rate remained elevated, even with longer-term follow-up. Predictors of sepsis in ITP patients include age > 60 years, presence of comorbidities, male sex, race, and splenectomy [9]. A historical population cohort study conducting splenectomized ITP patients compared to non-splenectomized ITP patients showed a higher RR for hospital contact-initiated infection within 90 days after splenectomy (RR 2.6); however, this decreased to 1.0–1.4 at >90 days postsplenectomy [19].

Pneumococcal infections remain the most important cause of severe sepsis and septic shock following splenectomy [20]. Recent guidelines recommend providing pneumococcal, meningococcal, and *Haemophilus influenzae* vaccination before splenectomy and periodically every 5 years or according to titers [13]. Splenectomized patients should be educated about the risk of postsplenectomy infection and have a home supply of antibiotics for use in case of febrile illness [12].

3.2 Thrombosis

Splenectomy induces deep venous thrombosis as a perioperative complication. A retrospective study showed that patients splenectomized for various indications had an increased risk of deep venous thrombosis and pulmonary embolism (rate ratios = 2.2) compared with that in the general population [21]. The cumulative incidence of abdominal venous thromboembolism in ITP patients after splenectomy was 1.6% compared with 1% in non-splenectomized ITP patients. However, the increased risk was observed during the early phase (<90 days) after splenectomy, suggesting that it was associated with the surgical procedure [9].

ITP patients have a greater risk of deep venous thrombosis. The cumulative incidence of deep venous thrombosis and pulmonary embolism in ITP patients after splenectomy was 4.3% compared with 1.7% in non-splenectomized ITP patients. In addition, there was increased risk of deep venous thrombosis and pulmonary embolism both early and late (≥90 days) after splenectomy [9]. Therefore, an international consensus report recommends that ITP patients should receive appropriate postoperative thromboprophylaxis after splenectomy [12].

3.3 Atherosclerosis

Loss of splenic function may also induce systemic atherosclerosis as a long-term complication. A small series of patients with hereditary spherocytosis who underwent splenectomy had a higher RR for stroke and heart attack (RR 5.9) [22]. In addition, the largest retrospective study also showed that patients splenectomized for various indications had an increased risk of death due to pulmonary embolism, coronary artery disease, and ischemic stroke (rate ratios = 1.4–4.5) at more than 10 years after splenectomy [21]. Although it has been difficult to accurately quantify the risk of atherosclerosis and thrombosis in splenectomized ITP patients, these data strongly indicate that loss of splenic function following splenectomy may induce systemic atherosclerosis and subsequently lead to ischemic heart disease and stroke as long-term complications.

3.4 Cancer

In some epidemiological studies [23, 24], splenectomy for various indications has been associated with an excess risk of developing cancer. The largest retrospective study showed that splenectomized patients, who had no malignancy prior to splenectomy, had an increased risk of certain solid tumors (rate ratios = 1.3–1.9) and hematologic malignancies, including acute myeloid leukemia (rate ratios = 1.8–6.0). They also had an increased risk of death due to any cancer (rate ratios = 1.3–4.7). Many of the observed risks were increased more than 10 years after splenectomy [21].

Accordingly, although it has been difficult to accurately quantify the risk of cancer in splenectomized ITP patients, loss of splenic function by splenectomy may induce cancer as a long-term complication.

References

1. Olsson B, Ridell B, Jernås M, Wadenvik H. Increased number of B-cells in the red pulp of the spleen in ITP. Ann Hematol. 2012;91(2):271–7.
2. Stasi R. Immune thrombocytopenia: pathophysiologic and clinical update. Semin Thromb Hemost. 2012;38(5):454–62.
3. Borges da Silva H, Fonseca R, Pereira RM, Cassado Ados A, Álvarez JM, D'Império Lima MR. Splenic macrophage subsets and their function during blood-borne infections. Front Immunol. 2015;6:480.
4. Kuwana M, Okazaki Y, Ikeda Y. Splenic macrophages maintain the anti-platelet autoimmune response via uptake of opsonized platelets in patients with immune thrombocytopenic purpura. J Thromb Haemost. 2009;7(2):322–9.
5. Yoshida Y. Historical review. The light and shadow of Paul Kaznelson: his life and contribution to hematology. Ann Hematol. 2008;87(11):877–9.
6. Dolan JP, Sheppard BC, DeLoughery TG. Splenectomy for immune thrombocytopenic purpura: surgery for the 21st century. Am J Hematol. 2008;83(2):93–6.
7. Winslow ER, Brunt LM. Perioperative outcomes of laparoscopic versus open splenectomy: a meta-analysis with an emphasis on complications. Surgery 2003;134(4):647–653; discussion 654–5.
8. Rodeghiero F, Ruggeri M. Is splenectomy still the gold standard for the treatment of chronic ITP? Am J Hematol. 2008;83(2):91.
9. Boyle S, White RH, Brunson A, Wun T. Splenectomy and the incidence of venous thromboembolism and sepsis in patients with immune thrombocytopenia. Blood. 2013;121(23):4782–90.
10. Kojouri K, Vesely SK, Terrell DR, George JN. Splenectomy for adult patients with idiopathic thrombocytopenic purpura: a systematic review to assess long-term platelet count responses, prediction of response, and surgical complications. Blood. 2004;104(9):2623–34.
11. Sailer T, Lechner K, Panzer S, Kyrle PA, Pabinger I. The course of severe autoimmune thrombocytopenia in patients not undergoing splenectomy. Haematologica. 2006;91(8):1041–5.

12. Provan D, Stasi R, Newland AC, Blanchette VS, Bolton-Maggs P, Bussel JB, Chong BH, Cines DB, Gernsheimer TB, Godeau B, Grainger J, Greer I, Hunt BJ, Imbach PA, Lyons G, McMillan R, Rodeghiero F, Sanz MA, Tarantino M, Watson S, Young J, Kuter DJ. International consensus report on the investigation and management of primary immune thrombocytopenia. Blood. 2010;115(2):168–86.
13. Neunert C, Lim W, Crowther M, Cohen A, Solberg Jr L, Crowther MA, American Society of Hematology. The American Society of Hematology 2011 evidence-based practice guideline for immune thrombocytopenia. Blood. 2011;117(16):4190–207.
14. Vianelli N, Palandri F, Polverelli N, et al. Splenectomy as a curative treatment for immune thrombocytopenia: a retrospective analysis of 233 patients with a minimum follow up of 10 years. Haematologica. 2013;98(6):875–80.
15. Aleem A. Durability and factors associated with long term response after splenectomy for primary immune thrombocytopenia (ITP) and outcome of relapsed or refractory patients. Platelets. 2011;22(1):1–7.
16. Mikhael J, Northridge K, Lindquist K, Kessler C, Deuson R, Danese M. Short-term and long-term failure of laparoscopic splenectomy in adult immune thrombocytopenic purpura patients: a systematic review. Am J Hematol. 2009;84(11):743–8.
17. Keidar A, Feldman M, Szold A. Analysis of outcome of laparoscopic splenectomy for idiopathic thrombocytopenic purpura by platelet count. Am J Hematol. 2005;80(2):95–100.
18. Yong M, Thomsen RW, Schoonen WM, Farkas DK, Riis A, Fryzek JP, Sørensen HT. Mortality risk in splenectomised patients: a Danish population-based cohort study. Eur J Intern Med. 2010;21(1):12–6.
19. Thomsen RW, Schoonen WM, Farkas DK, Riis A, Jacobsen J, Fryzek JP, Sørensen HT. Risk for hospital contact with infection in patients with splenectomy: a population-based cohort study. Ann Intern Med. 2009;151(8):546–55.
20. Theilacker C, Ludewig K, Serr A, Schimpf J, Held J, Bögelein M, Bahr V, Rusch S, Pohl A, Kogelmann K, Frieseke S, Bogdanski R, Brunkhorst FM, Kern WV, Splenectomy, Pneumococcus, and Fulminant Infection SPLEEN OFF Study Group. Overwhelming postsplenectomy infection: a prospective multicenter cohort study. Clin Infect Dis. 2016;62(7):871–8.
21. Kristinsson SY, Gridley G, Hoover RN, Check D, Landgren O. Long-term risks after splenectomy among 8,149 cancer-free American veterans: a cohort study with up to 27 years follow-up. Haematologica. 2014;99(2):392–8.
22. Schilling RF. Spherocytosis, splenectomy, strokes, and heart attacks. Lancet. 1997;350(9092):1677–8.
23. Linet MS, Nyrén O, Gridley G, Adami HO, Buckland JD, McLaughlin JK, Fraumeni Jr JF. Causes of death among patients surviving at least one year following splenectomy. Am J Surg. 1996;172(4):320–3.
24. Mellemkjoer L, Olsen JH, Linet MS, Gridley G, McLaughlin JK. Cancer risk after splenectomy. Cancer. 1995;75(2):577–83.

Rituximab

Yuji Yamada and Yoshitaka Miyakawa

Abstract Rituximab has recently been shown to be effective for chronic ITP. Though it is still in off-label use, current guidelines recommend rituximab as second- or third-line therapy. At the same time, its toxicity must be taken into account, and all the appropriate precautions should be performed before its use.

1 The Use of Rituximab for ITP

Rituximab is a monoclonal antibody against one of the B-cell surface proteins, CD20. This medication leads to apoptosis of B cells and can reduce the production of antibodies. Therefore, rituximab is estimated to be effective for B cell-related autoimmune diseases [1], including ITP. Rituximab has been approved for the treatment of non-Hodgkin lymphoma and ANCA-associated vasculitis in Japan. In addition to these indications, it is also approved for the treatment of chronic lymphoid leukemia and rheumatoid arthritis in the United States (USA) and Europe. But it is not currently approved for the treatment of ITP. Based on the recent clinical studies, it is expected that rituximab will be approved in the near future, and in fact, rituximab is widely in off-label use for ITP in the United States and Europe.

2 Evidence Behind the Use of Rituximab

The efficacy of rituximab for ITP has been demonstrated in several clinical trials and systematic reviews.

For example, a phase II trial including 60 patients with chronic ITP, who had not received splenectomy, showed a good 1-year response (platelet count above 50,000/

Y. Yamada (✉)
Department of Medicine, Mount Sinai Beth Israel, New York, NY, USA
e-mail: yuyamada@mountsinai.org

Y. Miyakawa
Department of General Internal Medicine, Center for Thrombosis and Hemostasis, Saitama Medical University, Saitama, Japan
e-mail: miyakawa@saitama-med.ac.jp

Y. Ishida, Y. Tomiyama (eds.), *Autoimmune Thrombocytopenia*,
DOI 10.1007/978-981-10-4142-6_16

mL) in 40% of the patients (95% CI, 28–52%) [2]. Moreover, a systematic review of observational studies showed that pooled estimate of overall platelet count response was 62.5% (95% CI, 52.6–72.5%) in 313 patients from 19 eligible reports [3]. However, it is also suggested that the rate of long-term responses in more than 1 year is lower at between 18 and 35% [4].

To compare the efficacy of rituximab with the standard of care, a randomized placebo-controlled trial (the RITP trial) was conducted for corticosteroid unresponsive patients. Although this trial showed no significant difference in the rate of long-term treatment failure which was the primary endpoint, a longer duration of response and numerically higher response rates with rituximab were suggested [5]. Additionally, a meta-analysis of randomized trials was conducted by Chugh et al. [6]. This study included untreated patients as well as those who were previously treated with corticosteroids and compared rituximab with placebo. Both groups received the standard of care. This study showed a better sustained complete response (platelet count above 100,000/mL in median duration of 5 months) rate in rituximab group (47%) than placebo group (33%). A partial response (platelet count above 30,000–50,000/mL) was also superior in rituximab group (58%) compared to placebo group (47%) [6].

Since, the rituximab effects can be delayed, rituximab is frequently administered in combination with other treatments. The combination of rituximab and high-dose dexamethasone has also been shown to be effective in randomized trials. For example, a randomized open-label phase III trial conducted in Denmark showed that for the patients with newly diagnosed ITP, addition of rituximab to dexamethasone yields a higher sustained response rate than dexamethasone alone at 6 months (58 vs. 37%, respectively) [7].

As for Japanese population, an open-label phase III clinical trial was recently conducted by Miyakawa et al. for 26 patients with chronic ITP, who had relapsed and were refractory to conventional therapy. The percentage of patients who had achieved the platelet count $\geq 50 \times 10^9$/L at week 24 was 30.8% (95% CI, 14.3–51.8%), [8] (Fig. 1). Though there are no available data on long-term outcomes of

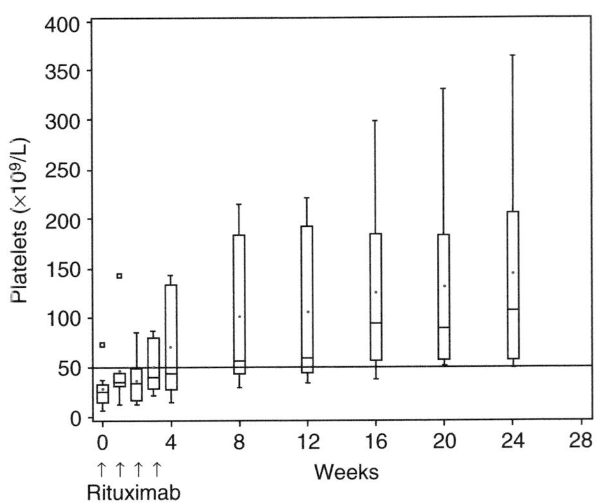

Fig. 1 Phase III trial for Japanese population. Box plots of platelet counts of patients who met primary response are shown in this figure. The time to response is around 4–8 weeks after the administration of rituximab

adults in Japan, those of children have already been reported. A retrospective study showed a 5-year relapse-free rate of 14% (95% CI, 0–27%) [9].

Based on the results in these trials, rituximab is now considered as one of the standard treatment choices for ITP in the guidelines, and medication approval is being processed in Japan.

3 Statements in the National Guidelines

The statement on the use of rituximab for ITP is slightly different between guidelines as below (Table 1).

In an international consensus report published in 2010, rituximab is listed as one of the second-line treatment options [10]. This report shows no preference for a particular therapy in the second-line options. The American Society of Hematology (ASH) evidence-based practice guideline published in 2011 has similar statements, which suggests rituximab be considered for patients at risk of bleeding who have failed one line of therapy such as corticosteroids, IVIG, or splenectomy (grade 2C) [11].

On the other hand, guidelines for ITP issued by the British Committee for Standards in Haematology (BCSH), General Haematology Task Force in 2003, consider rituximab as one of the third-line treatments, and splenectomy is the second-line treatment. The Japanese reference guide for the treatment of ITP published in 2012 also states rituximab is the third-line treatment since rituximab is not approved in Japan [12].

The difference between guidelines is mainly on whether rituximab can be used before the consideration of splenectomy. In fact, there has been no randomized trial to compare the efficacy of splenectomy versus rituximab as a second-line therapy,

Table 1 Comparison of guidelines for ITP

	International consensus report	ASH	BCSH	Japan
First line	Corticosteroids IVIG	Corticosteroids IVIG	Corticosteroids IVIG	Corticosteroids
Second line	Splenectomy	Splenectomy	Splenectomy	Splenectomy
	TPO-R agonists	TPO-R agonists	High-dose steroids	
	Rituximab	**Rituximab**	IVIG	
	Immunosuppressants		Danazol	
	Danazol		Immunosuppressants	
Third line	TPO-R agonists		IFN-α	TPO-R agonists
			Rituximab	Immunosuppressants
			MMF	**Rituximab**
			Plasmapheresis	

and therefore choosing an appropriate option is challenging. The response rates with splenectomy are generally reported to be higher and more durable than with rituximab, while many clinicians and patients prefer to avoid splenectomy since a late spontaneous remission can occur, and splenectomy is relatively invasive. We need to balance the risks and benefits of these options on a case-by-case basis.

4 How to Use Rituximab

Most of the studies explained above administered rituximab doses of 375 mg/m^2 IV weekly for 4 weeks. This is considered as the "standard" dose, though at the current time the best regimen of rituximab for ITP patients is yet unknown. Lower doses (100 mg IV weekly for 4 weeks) may also be effective, although associated with a longer time to response [13]. Due to the potential toxicity and expense of this medication, further studies are required to determine the optimal dose.

5 Rituximab Toxicities

Adverse effects of rituximab include infusion reaction, immunosuppressive effects including hepatitis B reactivation and infection [14], and progressive multifocal leukoencephalopathy (PML) [15]. Khellaf and colleagues evaluated safety outcomes in 248 patients. Overall, 87 adverse events were reported in 44 patients (19%). Thirty-eight patients showed minor intolerance to rituximab infusions (15%); infusions had to be stopped for only three patients. Seven showed infection (3%), with an incidence of 2.3 infections/100 patient-years. Three patients died of infection 12–14 months after rituximab infusions, but the role of rituximab was questionable [14]. Arnold and colleagues also evaluated safety outcomes in 306 patients, of whom 10 (3.3%) had severe or life-threatening complications after rituximab treatment. Nine patients (2.9%) were reported to die, though the association between rituximab administration and the outcome is unclear [3]. PML was not shown in these studies but reported in another case series [15].

In order to prevent the adverse events as much as possible, precautions should be taken prior to rituximab therapy. Infusion reaction can be preventable with use of antipyretic and anti-allergic agents. Patients should be screened for hepatitis B infection prior to the initiation of rituximab. If patients have occult or active hepatitis B, rituximab should be either avoided or used with prophylactic antiviral treatment. Additionally, immunizations should be updated at least 2 weeks prior to the use of rituximab since rituximab has also been reported to interfere with response to immunizations [16].

References

1. Looney RJ. B cell-targeted therapy in diseases other than rheumatoid arthritis. J Rheumatol Suppl 2005;73:25–28; discussion 29–30.
2. Godeau B, Porcher R, Fain O, et al. Rituximab efficacy and safety in adult splenectomy candidates with chronic immune thrombocytopenic purpura: results of a prospective multicenter phase 2 study. Blood. 2008;112(4):999–1004.
3. Arnold DM, Dentali F, Crowther MA, et al. Systematic review: efficacy and safety of rituximab for adults with idiopathic thrombocytopenic purpura. Ann Intern Med. 2007;146(1): 25–33.
4. Medeot M, Zaja F, Vianelli N, et al. Rituximab therapy in adult patients with relapsed or refractory immune thrombocytopenic purpura: long-term follow-up results. Eur J Haematol. 2008;81(3):165–9.
5. Ghanima W, Khelif A, Waage A, et al. Rituximab as second-line treatment for adult immune thrombocytopenia (the RITP trial): a multicentre, randomised, double-blind, placebo-controlled trial. Lancet. 2015;385(9978):1653–61.
6. Chugh S, Darvish-Kazem S, Lim W, et al. Rituximab plus standard of care for treatment of primary immune thrombocytopenia: a systematic review and meta-analysis. Lancet Haematol. 2015;2(2):e75–81.
7. Gudbrandsdottir S, Birgens HS, Frederiksen H, et al. Rituximab and dexamethasone vs dexamethasone monotherapy in newly diagnosed patients with primary immune thrombocytopenia. Blood. 2013;121(11):1976–81.
8. Miyakawa Y, Katsutani S, Yano T, et al. Efficacy and safety of rituximab in Japanese patients with relapsed chronic immune thrombocytopenia refractory to conventional therapy. Int J Hematol. 2015;102(6):654–61.
9. Matsubara K, Takahashi Y, Hayakawa A, et al. Long-term follow-up of children with refractory immune thrombocytopenia treated with rituximab. Int J Hematol. 2014;99(4):429–36.
10. Provan D, Stasi R, Newland AC, et al. International consensus report on the investigation and management of primary immune thrombocytopenia. Blood. 2010;115(2):168–86.
11. Neunert C, Lim W, Crowther M, et al. The American Society of Hematology 2011 evidence-based practice guideline for immune thrombocytopenia. Blood. 2011;117(16):4190–207.
12. Fujimura K, Miyakawa Y, Kurata Y. Reference guide for management of adult idiopathic thrombocytopenic purpura (ITP) 2012 version. Rinsho Ketsueki. 2016;53(4):433–42.
13. Zaja F, Vianelli N, Volpetti S, et al. Low-dose rituximab in adult patients with primary immune thrombocytopenia. Eur J Haematol. 2010;85(4):329–34.
14. Khellaf M, Charles-Nelson A, Fain O, et al. Safety and efficacy of rituximab in adult immune thrombocytopenia: results from a prospective registry including 248 patients. Blood. 2014;124(22):3228–36.
15. Carson KR, Evens AM, Richey EA, et al. Progressive multifocal leukoencephalopathy after rituximab therapy in HIV-negative patients: a report of 57 cases from the Research on Adverse Drug Events and Reports project. Blood. 2009;113(20):4834–40.
16. Nazi I, Kelton JG, Larche M, et al. The effect of rituximab on vaccine responses in patients with immune thrombocytopenia. Blood. 2013;122(11):1946–53.

Thrombopoietin Receptor Agonists

Yoshiaki Tomiyama

Abstract Thrombopoietin receptor agonists (TPO-RAs) should be considered for the treatment of "refractory" autoimmune thrombocytopenia (ITP). In contrast to other medications, TPO-RAs increase platelets via stimulating the production of megakaryocytes/platelets in the bone marrow. This chapter has dealt with the mechanism, efficacy, and safety of TPO-RAs.

1 Introduction

Thrombopoietin (TPO) has been cloned as the ligand for orphan cytokine receptor, c-Mpl, by independent three groups in 1994 [1–3]. TPO is a single 95 kDa glycoprotein consisting of 332-amino acid protein that is the primary regulator of megakaryocyte and platelet development. TPO is synthesized primarily in the liver and is secreted into circulation. Although it has long been thought that hepatic transcription and translation of the TPO gene appear constant, recent study reveals that TPO mRNA and its production can be stimulated, at least in part, by desialylated, senescent platelet clearance via hepatocyte Ashwell-Morrell receptor. Hepatocyte Ashwell-Morrell receptor regulates TPO production via Janus kinase 2 (JAK2)-signal transducer and activator of transcription 3 (STAT3) signaling [4, 5]. Secreted TPO is removed from circulation by binding of the TPO receptor (c-Mpl) on platelets and bone marrow megakaryocytes. Thus, plasma TPO levels usually increase in response to the decreased in platelet/megakaryocyte mass. Actually, plasma TPO levels are markedly increased in patients with hypoplastic thrombocytopenia such as aplastic anemia (AA) or chemotherapy-induced thrombocytopenia (CIT). In sharp contrast, in patients with ITP, plasma TPO levels are within normal range or slightly increased [6–9] (refer to chapters "T-Cell Abnormalities," "ITP in Adults," "Diagnosis in General," "Differential Diagnosis: Secondary ITP," "Differential Diagnosis:

Y. Tomiyama, M.D.
Department of Blood Transfusion, Osaka University Hospital,
2-15 Yamadaoka, Suita, Osaka 565-0871, Japan
e-mail: yoshi@hp-blood.med.osaka-u.ac.jp

Y. Ishida, Y. Tomiyama (eds.), *Autoimmune Thrombocytopenia*,
DOI 10.1007/978-981-10-4142-6_17

Hypoplastic Thrombocytopenia," and "Differential Diagnosis: Congenital Macrothrombocytopenia"). From a view point of plasma TPO levels, ITP appears to be a suitable disease for clinical application of TPO.

2 TPO and Recombinant TPOs

N-terminus of TPO has a receptor-binding domain showing considerable homology to erythropoietin, while C-terminus of TPO is highly glycosylated and contributes protein stability. The TPO receptor, c-Mpl, contains two cytokine receptor homology modules (CRM1 and CRM2), and CRM1 is the distal CRM. TPO exclusively binds to CRM1 (the distal CRM) of c-Mpl in the ratio 1:2 and then activates several transduction pathways such as JAK2 and STAT5 to increase the production of mature megakaryocyte and platelets [10]. Although TPO could stimulate proliferation of stem cells and early progenitor cells of all lineage, its major effect is to stimulate proliferation of early and late stages of megakaryocyte maturation. Recombinant human TPO (rhTPO) and pegylated recombinant human megakaryocyte growth and development factor (PEG-rHuMGDF) were developed soon after its cloning for clinical studies in thrombocytopenic disorders. PEG-rHuMGDF is a truncated form of TPO that contains the first 163 amino acids of endogenous TPO. However, PEG-rHuMGDF paradoxically induced persistent thrombocytopenia in 13 of 325 healthy volunteers. The thrombocytopenia was caused by the antibody to PEG-rHuMGDF that cross-reacted with endogenous TPO and neutralized its biological activity [11]. Although rhTPO did not show such adverse effects, the development of rhTPO as well as PEG-rHuMGDF was regrettably stopped in 1998.

3 TPO Receptor Agonists (TPO-RAs or TPO Mimetics)

To prevent the development of neutralizing antibodies induced by recombinant TPOs, several TPO-RAs that stimulate c-Mpl without inducing neutralizing antibodies have been developed for the treatment of thrombocytopenic disorders. Among them two TPO-RAs are now available in daily clinical practice: romiplostim and eltrombopag. These drugs are obtained by screening of peptide or small nonpeptide libraries for the ability to stimulate the growth or reporter genes such as STAT in TPO-dependent cell lines.

3.1 Structure of TPO-RAs (Fig. 1)

Romiplostim (Nplate®, Romiplate® in Japan, AMG531; Amgen)

Romiplostim is subcutaneously administered once a week for clinical use. Romiplostim is a peptide-based drug with a molecular weight of 59,000 Da and designated as a "peptibody" that is a fusion protein of IgG_1 Fc fragments and TPO mimetic peptides. Active sites of romiplostim are two identical TPO mimetic peptides

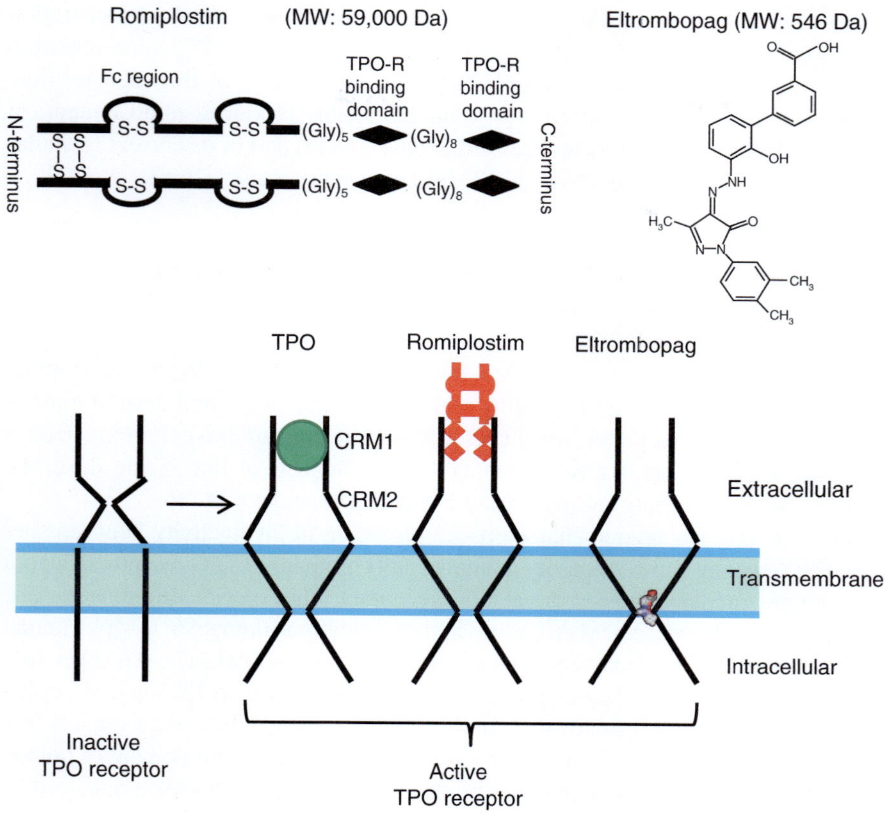

Fig. 1 Structure and binding site of romiplostim and eltrombopag. *Upper panel*: romiplostim is a "peptibody" and TPO receptor-binding domain consists of 14 amino acids (Ile-Glu-Gly-Pro-Thr--Leu-Arg-Gln-Trp-Leu-Ala-Ala-Arg-Ala), and eltrombopag is a nonpeptide compound. *Lower panel*: binding sites for TPO, romiplostim, and eltrombopag on the TPO receptor, c-Mpl. *CRM* cytokine receptor homology module

(Ile-Glu-Gly-Pro-Thr-Leu-Arg-Gln-Trp-Leu-Ala-Ala-Arg-Ala) linked via 8-glycine bridge as a linker [12, 13]. IgG_1 Fc fragments covalently bound with the peptide-containing domain are dimerized via disulfide bonds. The Fc fragments extend the half-life of romiplostim in the circulation, since peptides tend to have poor stability and pharmacokinetic properties. Romiplostim is bound to TPO receptor, and the binding was inhibited by rhTPO, suggesting that romiplostim binds to CRM1 of c-Mpl (Fig. 1).

Romiplostim was active in mice, rats, rabbits, and monkeys and induced dose-dependent increase in platelets in all species, although nonhuman primates were less responsive compared with other tested species. The first human study was conducted in healthy volunteers based on the data obtained from rhesus monkeys. A single intravenous dose of 10 μg/kg was initially investigated in human volunteers, which was anticipated to be a no-effect dose. However, this dose was found to increase platelet count almost sixfold. This distinct effect between humans and rhesus monkeys was probably due to a much higher affinity of romiplostim for human c-Mpl than the monkey c-Mpl. A clinically effective dose that increases platelet count twofold was identified as 1 μg/kg. Intravenous (IV) administration of 1 μg/kg gave a peak of 12,900 pg/mL, while subcutaneous (SC) administration gave undetectable levels of romiplostim concentrations probably due to slow adsorption (less than 18 pg/mL). IV and SC routes produced almost identical effects in healthy volunteers and peaked at days 14–15, and in its current formulation, romiplostim is administered as SC injection every week [10, 13].

Eltrombopag (Promacta® in the United States or Revolade® in EU and Japan, SB497115; Novartis)

Eltrombopag is an orally administered, low molecular weight (546 Da), nonpeptide TPO-RA. In human studies in healthy male volunteers, single oral dose of eltrombopag did not increase platelet count. However, daily oral administration for 10 days increased platelet counts dose dependently. For subjects at the 75 mg dose, the increase in platelet count started on day 6 and peaked at days 14–16.

Eltrombopag has unique characteristics regarding in vivo activity between species. Eltrombopag showed activity in human and chimpanzee TPO receptors, but not cynomolgus monkey, mouse, or rat TPO receptors. This species difference is due mostly to a single amino acid difference in transmembrane domain of c-Mpl. Human and chimpanzee TPO receptors have a histidine at residue 499, whereas other species have a leucine 499. Exchanging of leucine 499 for histidine 499 made the cynomolgus monkey TPO receptor responsive to eltrombopag. These data suggest that the binding site of eltrombopag is not CRM1 but transmembrane domain of human TPO receptor. Thus, the binding sites of eltrombopag and rhTPO seem quite different (Fig. 1) [2].

3.2 Medical Indication and Efficacy of TPO-RAs in ITP Management

For use in adult patients with chronic ITP, both TPO-RAs have been approved in many countries. In the United States, each TPO-RA is only available for patients with "refractory" chronic ITP who have had an insufficient response to corticosteroids, immunoglobulins, or splenectomy and who have an increased risk of bleeding. In EU, indication of TPO-RAs is much more limited, and each drug is only available for splenectomized patients who are refractory to other treatments or may be available for nonsplenectomized patients where surgery is contraindicated [14, 15].

For children with chronic ITP who have had an insufficient response to corticosteroids, immunoglobulins, or splenectomy, eltrombopag has been approved by the US Food and Drug Administration (FDA) in June, 2015, and by the European Commission (EC) in April, 2016 [16, 17]. Efficacy and safety for the treatment of symptomatic children ITP with romiplostim has also been demonstrated [18], and approval for child ITP is now underway.

Therapeutic goal of ITP is not to normalize the platelet count, but to elevate platelet count to a safe range (mostly above $50 \times 10^3/\mu L$) to minimize the risk of bleeding with minimal side effects of drugs such as corticosteroids and TPO-RAs [15]. In this context, patients with ITP were eligible if platelet counts were less than $30 \times 10^3/\mu L$, and they had failed at least one prior treatment in most clinical studies employing either of TPO-RA. Platelet count $>50 \times 10^3/\mu L$ by TPO-RA was considered as platelet response in most studies. These clinical studies have indicated that each drug is very effective in the treatment of chronic ITP as described below.

Romiplostim

Long-term (24 weeks) administration of romiplostim in 63 splenectomized and 62 nonsplenectomized patients with ITP was assessed in two parallel trials both of which are in a double-blind randomized controlled trial conducted in multiple centers internationally [19]. All patients were randomized 2:1 (romiplostim:placebo) to receive a starting dose of 1 μg/kg. Doses of drug were adjusted to maintain platelet count of $50–200 \times 10^3/\mu L$. The primary endpoints were to get a durable platelet response (platelet count $\geq 50 \times 10^3/\mu L$ during 6 or more of the last 8 weeks of treatment) and treatment safety. A durable platelet response was achieved by 16 of 42 (38%) splenectomized patients with romiplostim, while that was achieved by 25 of 41 (61%) nonsplenectomized patients with romiplostim. The overall platelet response including the durable or transient platelet response was 79% (33/42) of splenectomized and 88% (36/41) of nonsplenectomized patients. In the placebo groups, 0/21 splenectomized patients and 3/21 nonsplenectomized patients responded. Mean doses of romiplostim for splenectomized patients were 4–5 μg/kg, while those for nonsplenectomized patients were approximately 3 μg/kg. Twelve of 23 (52%) splenectomized or nonsplenectomized patients with romiplostim discontinued all of their concurrent ITP drugs.

A clinical study with nonsplenectomized ITP patients suggested that as compared with standard of care, romiplostim treatment may induce greater improvement in quality of life [20].

Eltrombopag

In contrast to SC administration of romiplostim, eltrombopag is orally administrated and is absorbed with a peak concentration occurring 2–6 h after oral administration. Eltrombopag pharmacokinetics is altered when the drug is administered with polyvalent cations such as iron, calcium, magnesium, etc. Eltrombopag should be taken at least 4 h before or after any products such as antacids, dairy products or other calcium-containing food products, or mineral supplements containing polyvalent cations. In vitro studies indicate that eltrombopag is metabolized in the liver, and systemic exposure to eltrombopag is increased in patients with mild or moderate to severe hepatic impairment (41 and 80–93% increases in AUC_{∞}, respectively). Thus, administration of eltrombopag to patients with moderate to severe hepatic impairment should be undertaken with caution and should be closely monitored [21].

Six-week administration and 6-month administration (RAISE study) of eltrombopag were assessed in phase III clinical studies in a double-blind randomized controlled trial conducted in multiple centers internationally [22, 23]. The doses for these studies were 50 mg or matching placebo once daily, and patients with platelet count <50 × 10^3/μL on day 22 or after may have had their dose increased to 75 mg. In addition, in RAISE dose decreases to 25 mg once daily were required for patients with platelet count >200 × 10^3/μL. For patients with platelet count of >400 × 10^3/μL, study treatment was interrupted and resumed at the next lowest dose when platelet count fell to <150 × 10^3/μL. The primary endpoints were the odds of achieving platelet count 50–400 × 10^3/μL during the 6-month treatment periods. Seventy-nine percent (106/135) of patients in the eltrombopag group responded at least once, compared with 28% (17/62) of patients in the placebo group. The odds of responding over the 6-month treatment period were greater (odds ratio = 8.2, 99% CI 3.59–18.73; $p < 0.0001$) for eltrombopag group. Fifty-nine percent (37/63) in the eltrombopag group reduced or discontinued baseline treatments compared with 32% (10/31) of patients in the placebo group. Thus, eltrombopag is effective for management of chronic ITP, and starting dose is 50 mg once daily for most patients and could be increased to 75 mg once daily.

Unique Pharmacokinetics of Eltrombopag in East Asian Peoples

Patient ethnicity may affect the pharmacokinetics of eltrombopag. AUC exposure to eltrombopag was approximately twofold greater among Japanese healthy volunteers than among non-Asian (predominantly Caucasian) volunteers and 87% greater among ITP patients of East Asian descent compared to non-East Asian ITP patients. From these data, it has been recommended that for patients of East Asian ancestry (such as Japanese, Korean, Chinese, Taiwanese, etc.), initiate dose of eltrombopag should be reduced to 25 mg once daily. It is noteworthy that a Japanese clinical trial evaluated the efficacy and safety of eltrombopag at a starting dose of 12.5 mg and a maximum dose of 50 mg in the treatment of Japanese patients with previously treated chronic ITP [24]. During the first 3 weeks of treatment with 12.5 mg eltrombopag, 22% (5/23) of Japanese patients responded. Since disease state is in chronic nature and 12.5 mg tablet is only available in Japan so far, it is possible that 25 mg every-other-day administration as a starting dose may be suitable for some chronic ITP patients of East Asian ancestry to prevent overshooting of platelet count.

3.3 Clinical Safety

For romiplostim and eltrombopag long-term extension studies have been being performed, respectively [25, 26]. Both TPO-RAs were generally safe and well tolerated in log-term extension studies. In romiplostim studies, headache was the most commonly

Table 1 Possible adverse effects of TRO receptor agonists

1.	Thrombotic complications
2.	Induction of reticulin formation in bone marrow
3.	Increase in blast cell count
4.	Rebound thrombocytopenia upon stopping treatment

reported adverse event, followed by nasopharyngitis, fatigue, contusion, upper respiratory tract infection, diarrhea, and epistaxis. In eltrombopag studies, headache was also the most common, followed by nasopharyngitis, upper respiratory tract infection, and fatigue. These common events were mostly mild. Eltrombopag may cause hepatotoxicity, and ALT, aspartate aminotransferase (AST), and bilirubin should be monitored during treatment [26].

In terms of the development of neutralizing antibodies against endogenous TPO, no patient developed such antibodies. Although two patients treated with romiplostim developed antibodies that neutralized romiplostim, but resolved after drug withdrawal, the antibodies did not cross-react with TPO or affect platelet count [13].

Since long-term treatment with TPO-RAs would be expected in chronic ITP, one should pay special attention to possible severe complications listed in Table 1.

Thrombotic Complications

It has been suggested that ITP itself may be not only a hemorrhagic disease but also a prothrombotic disease. Population-based studies showed evidence that the risk for venous thrombosis is higher (around two time) in chronic ITP compared with controls. For arterial thrombosis there is a trend for increased risk in patients with chronic ITP, but bot statistically significant [27]. Arterial thrombotic and venous thromboembolic events have been reported for patients with both romiplostim groups and eltrombopag groups, but also in placebo groups. There is no relationship between platelet counts and thrombotic events during the treatment of TPO-RAs. Most of the patients with thromboembolic events were old age and had pre-existing risks for thrombosis (e.g., Factor V Leiden, antiphospholipid syndrome, diabetes mellitus, smoking, etc.) [25, 26]. Although it is still uncertain that TPO-RAs may apparently induce arterial thrombotic/venous thromboembolic events, special attention should be paid for patients having pre-existing risks for thrombosis when starting TPO-RAs.

Induction of Reticulin Formation in Bone Marrow

Interleukin 11, GM-CSF, and TPO agents may increase bone marrow reticulin, possibly through local release of transforming growth factor-β from the increased number of bone marrow megakaryocytes. Prolonged administration of large doses of romiplostim to mice produced bone marrow fibrosis that was reversible within 4 weeks by stopping romiplostim [28]. The presence of or increase in bone marrow reticulin was reported in some patients with long-term treatment with romiplostim, and most of them had reticulin levels of mild to moderate [29, 30]. Because of this possible adverse effect, all patients treated with TPO-RAs continue to be monitored for clinical signs of any progressive bone marrow abnormalities.

Increase in Blast Cell Count

TPO-RAs may stimulate the growth of hematopoietic malignancies or increased progression of myelodysplastic syndrome (MDS). In a recent randomized, double-blind, placebo-controlled study for International Prognostic Scoring System (IPSS) low/int-1 MDS with thrombocytopenia, 750 μg/body of romiplostim was administered. Although platelet count increased in romiplostim group, romiplostim group showed a tendency to increase risk to transform to acute myelogenous leukemia (AML). AML rates through 58 weeks were romiplostim 6.0% and placebo 4.9% (HR 1.20, 95% CI, 0.38–3.84). Study drug was discontinued because of an initial concern of AML risk based on interim data (interim HR, 2.51) [31]. In this context, differential diagnosis between ITP and MDS with thrombocytopenia is very important.

3.4 Recent Topics: Remission Induced by TPO-RAs

TPO-RAs can effectively increase in platelet number in chronic ITP, but long-term treatment may be required to maintain the platelet response. However, recent data suggest that a certain number of chronic ITP patients (3–32%) may achieve sustained remission (platelet counts >50 × 10^3/μL or 100 × 10^3/μL) after discontinuing each of TPO-RAs [32–34]. In a prospective study Newland et al. examined remission rate (platelet counts >50 × 10^3/μL for 24 consecutive weeks with no ITP treatments) after discontinuing romiplostim for ITP patients with a duration of ≤6 months who were treated with romiplostim for ≤12 months. Remission was observed in 24 patients (32%) [34]. The cases of remission seen in this study may also have included spontaneous remission as a natural course of newly diagnosed adult ITP, since in a retrospective study spontaneous remissions occurred in 8 of 87 untreated cases (9%) after observation periods of 6 months or more [35].

There are at least two potential mechanisms of remission. Firstly, TPO-RA-induced platelet increase may restore immune tolerance by increased exposure to platelet autoantigens [34]. Secondarily, it has been suggested that TPO-RA (romiplostim) stimulation may improve regulatory T-cell ($CD4^+$, $CD25^{hi}$) function in patients with ITP [36]. In addition, in a mouse model of ITP in which regulatory T cells were deficient, recombinant TPO administration induced sustained remission of ITP and promotion of peripheral induction of $Foxp3^+$, $CD4^+$, and $CD25^{hi}$ regulatory T cells in conjunction with elevated circulating TGF-β levels [37]. Further studies are necessary to determine the real remission rate induced by TPO-RAs as well as its mechanisms of remission.

4 Summary

Long-term extension studies indicated that each TPO-RA was effective, generally safe, and well tolerated in patients with previously treated chronic ITP. However, one should still pay attention to specific adverse events of TPO-RAs such as thrombotic events and reticulin (or collagen) formation of bone marrow. On the other hand, TPO-RAs may possess additional effects to induce sustained remission even after discontinuation of TPO-RAs in a certain number of ITP patients.

Acknowledgment This work was supported by Grant-in-Aid for Scientific Research from the Ministry of Education, Culture, Sports, Science and Technology in Japan and the Ministry of Health, Labour and Welfare in Japan.

References

1. Bartley TD, Bogenberger J, Hunt P, Li YS, Lu HS, Martin F, et al. Identification and cloning of a megakaryocyte growth and development factor that is a ligand for the cytokine receptor Mpl. Cell. 1994;77:1117–24.
2. Lok S, Kaushansky K, Holly RD, Kuijper JL, Lofton-Day CE, Oort PJ, et al. Cloning and expression of murine thrombopoietin cDNA and stimulation of platelet production in vivo. Nature. 1994;369:565–8.
3. de Sauvage FJ, Hass PE, Spencer SD, Malloy BE, Gurney AL, Spencer SA, et al. Stimulation of megakaryocytopoiesis and thrombopoiesis by the c-Mpl ligand. Nature. 1994;369:533–8.
4. Grozovsky R, Begonja AJ, Liu K, Visner G, Hartwig JH, Falet H, et al. The Ashwell-Morell receptor regulates hepatic thrombopoietin production via JAK2-STAT3 signaling. Nat Med. 2015;21:47–54.
5. Grozovsky R, Giannini S, Falet H, Hoffmeister KM. Regulating billions of blood platelets: glycans and beyond. Blood. 2015;126:1877–84.
6. Kosugi S, Kurata Y, Tomiyama Y, Tahara T, Kato T, Tadokoro S, et al. Circulating thrombopoietin level in chronic immune thrombocytopenic purpura. Br J Haematol. 1996;93:704–6.
7. Emmons RV, Reid DM, Cohen RL, Meng G, Young NS, Dunbar CE, et al. Human thrombopoietin levels are high when thrombocytopenia is due to megakaryocyte deficiency and low when due to increased platelet destruction. Blood. 1996;87:4068–71.
8. Nagata Y, Shozaki Y, Nagahisa H, Nagasawa T, Abe T, Todokoro K. Serum thrombopoietin level is not regulated by transcription but by the total counts of both megakaryocytes and platelets during thrombocytopenia and thrombocytosis. Thromb Hemost. 1997;77:808–14.
9. Schrezenmeier H, Griesshammer M, Hornkohl A, Nichol JL, Hecht T, Heimpel H, et al. Thrombopoietin serum levels in patients with aplastic anaemia: correlation with platelet count and persistent elevation in remission. Br J Haematol. 1998;100:571–6.
10. Kuter DJ. New thrombopoietic growth factors. Blood. 2007;109:4607–16.
11. Li J, Yang C, Xia Y, Bertino A, Glaspy J, Roberts M, et al. Thrombocytopenia caused by the development of antibodies to thrombopoietin. Blood. 2001;98:3241–8.
12. Kuter DJ. Thrombopoietin and thrombopoietin mimetics in the treatment of thrombocytopenia. Annu Rev Med. 2009;60:193–206.
13. Molineux G. The development of romiplostim for patients with immune thrombocytopenia. Ann N Y Acad Sci. 2011;1222:55–63.
14. Provan D, Stasi R, Newland AC, Blanchette VS, Bolton-Maggs P, Bussel JB, et al. International consensus report on the investigation and management of primary immune thrombocytopenia. Blood. 2010;115:168–86.

15. Neunert C, Lim W, Crowther M, Cohen A, Solberg Jr L, Crowther MA, American Society of Hematology. The American Society of Hematology 2011 evidence-based practice guideline for immune thrombocytopenia. Blood. 2011;117:4190–207.
16. Bussel JB, de Miguel PG, Despotovic JM, Grainger JD, Sevilla J, Blanchette VS, et al. Eltrombopag for the treatment of children with persistent and chronic immune thrombocytopenia (PETIT): a randomised, multicentre, placebo-controlled study. Lancet Haematol. 2015;2:e315–25.
17. Grainger JD, Locatelli F, Chotsampancharoen T, Donyush E, Pongtanakul B, Komvilaisak P, et al. Eltrombopag for children with chronic immune thrombocytopenia (PETIT2): a randomised, multicentre, placebo-controlled trial. Lancet. 2015;386:1649–58.
18. Tarantino MD, Bussel JB, Blanchette VS, Despotovic J, Bennett C, Raj A, et al. Romiplostim in children with immune thrombocytopenia: a phase 3, randomised, double-blind, placebo-controlled study. Lancet. 2016;388:45–54.
19. Kuter DJ, Bussel JB, Lyons RM, Pullarkat V, Gernsheimer TB, Senecal FM, et al. Efficacy of romiplostim in patients with chronic immune thrombocytopenic purpura: a double-blind randomised controlled trial. Lancet. 2008;371:395–403.
20. Kuter DJ, Rummel M, Boccia R, Macik BG, Pabinger I, Selleslag D, et al. Romiplostim or standard of care in patients with immune thrombocytopenia. N Engl J Med. 2010;363:1889–99.
21. Nieto M, Calvo G, Hudson I, Feldschreiber P, Brown D, Lee CC, et al. The European Medicines Agency review of eltrombopag (Revolade) for the treatment of adult chronic immune (idiopathic) thrombocytopenic purpura: summary of the scientific assessment of the Committee for Medicinal Products for Human Use. Haematologica. 2011;96:e33–40.
22. Bussel JB, Provan D, Shamsi T, Cheng G, Psaila B, Kovaleva L, et al. Effect of eltrombopag on platelet counts and bleeding during treatment of chronic idiopathic thrombocytopenic purpura: a randomised, double-blind, placebo-controlled trial. Lancet. 2009;373:641–8.
23. Cheng G, Saleh MN, Marcher C, Vasey S, Mayer B, Aivado M, et al. Eltrombopag for management of chronic immune thrombocytopenia (RAISE): a 6-month, randomised, phase 3 study. Lancet. 2011;377:393–402.
24. Tomiyama Y, Miyakawa Y, Okamoto S, Katsutani S, Kimura A, Okoshi Y, et al. A lower starting dose of eltrombopag is efficacious in Japanese patients with previously treated chronic immune thrombocytopenia. J Thromb Haemost. 2012;10:799–806.
25. Kuter DJ, Bussel JB, Newland A, Baker RI, Lyons RM, Wasser J, et al. Long-term treatment with romiplostim in patients with chronic immune thrombocytopenia: safety and efficacy. Br J Haematol. 2013;161:411–23.
26. Saleh MN, Bussel JB, Cheng G, Meyer O, Bailey CK, Arning M, et al. Safety and efficacy of eltrombopag for treatment of chronic immune thrombocytopenia: results of the long-term, open-label EXTEND study. Blood. 2013;121:537–45.
27. Rodeghiero F. Is ITP a thrombophilic disorder? Am J Hematol. 2016;91:39–45.
28. Kuter DJ, Mufti GJ, Bain BJ, Hasserjian RP, Davis W, Rutstein M. Evaluation of bone marrow reticulin formation in chronic immune thrombocytopenia patients treated with romiplostim. Blood. 2009;114:3748–56.
29. Bussel JB, Kuter DJ, Pullarkat V, Lyons RM, Guo M, Nichol JL, et al. Safety and efficacy of long-term treatment with romiplostim in thrombocytopenic patients with chronic ITP. Blood. 2009;113:2161–71.
30. Brynes RK, Orazi A, Theodore D, Burgess P, Bailey CK, Thein MM, et al. Evaluation of bone marrow reticulin in patients with chronic immune thrombocytopenia treated with eltrombopag: data from the EXTEND study. Am J Hematol. 2015;90:598–601.
31. Giagounidis A, Mufti GJ, Fenaux P, Sekeres MA, Szer J, Platzbecker U, et al. Results of a randomized, double-blind study of romiplostim versus placebo in patients with low/intermediate-1-risk myelodysplastic syndrome and thrombocytopenia. Cancer. 2014;120:1838–46.
32. Ghadaki B, Nazi I, Kelton JG, Arnold DM. Sustained remissions of immune thrombocytopenia associated with the use of thrombopoietin receptor agonists. Transfusion. 2013;53:2807–12.

33. González-López TJ, Pascual C, Álvarez-Román MT, Fernández-Fuertes F, Sánchez-González B, Caparrós I, et al. Successful discontinuation of eltrombopag after complete remission in patients with primary immune thrombocytopenia. Am J Hematol. 2015;90:E40–3.
34. Newland A, Godeau B, Priego V, Viallard JF, López Fernández MF, Orejudos A, et al. Remission and platelet responses with romiplostim in primary immune thrombocytopenia: final results from a phase 2 study. Br J Haematol. 2016;172:262–73.
35. Stasi R, Stipa E, Masi M, Cecconi M, Scimò MT, Oliva F, et al. Long-term observation of 208 adults with chronic idiopathic thrombocytopenic purpura. Am J Med. 1995;98:436–42.
36. Bao W, Bussel JB, Heck S, He W, Karpoff M, Boulad N, et al. Improved regulatory T-cell activity in patients with chronic immune thrombocytopenia treated with thrombopoietic agents. Blood. 2010;116:4639–45.
37. Nishimoto T, Numajiri M, Nakazaki H, Okazaki Y, Kuwana M. Induction of immune tolerance to platelet antigen by short-term thrombopoietin treatment in a mouse model of immune thrombocytopenia. Int J Hematol. 2014;100:341–4.

Others (Syk Inhibitor and Other Medications)

Yoji Ishida

Abstract There are several management options for chronic refractory ITP patients. As the chance of inducing a durable remission is low, the objective of the next treatment is the achievement of adequate stable platelet levels while minimizing adverse events. This chapter includes anti-D immunoglobulin, cyclophosphamide, vincristine and vinblastine, danazol, Syk inhibitor, and other drugs (azathioprine, cyclosporine, mycophenolate mofetil, interferon, and ascorbic acid). While in the near future, several new agents might be used clinically for treating refractory ITP.

1 Anti-D Immunoglobulin

Intravenous (IV) Rho(D) immune globulin (anti-D), instead of high-dose immunoglobulin, is used in children and adult patients with idiopathic thrombocytopenic purpura (ITP) [1–3]. Increase in platelet count begins at 2–3 days after the IV anti-D administration, and response rates of 27–63% are usually achieved. The increase in platelets lasts for several weeks and patients respond well to re-treatment. Generally, children respond better than adults do. In addition, nonsplenectomized patients respond better than splenectomized patients do [1–5]. The most common side effect associated with the treatment is slight to moderate anemia, which results from mild hemolysis with decreased haptoglobin, increased lactate dehydrogenase, and increase in indirect bilirubin levels [6]. The mechanism by which the platelet count increases is not clearly understood. However, it is believed that anti-D-coated red blood cells block Fc receptors on macrophages. Other mechanisms that have been reported include reduction in antigen-specific B-cell priming and modulations of Fcγ receptors and inflammatory cytokine levels [7, 8].

Y. Ishida, M.D., Ph.D.
Division of Hematology and Oncology, Department of Internal Medicine, Iwate Medical University School of Medicine, 19-1 Uchimaru, Morioka, Iwate Prefecture 020-8505, Japan
e-mail: yoji.ishida@gmail.com

Y. Ishida, Y. Tomiyama (eds.), *Autoimmune Thrombocytopenia*,
DOI 10.1007/978-981-10-4142-6_18

The anti-D products of Cangene (WinRho SDF) and CSL Behring (Rhophylac) were approved by the FDA in 1995. However, WinRho SDF was voluntarily withdrawn from the European market in August, 2009, because of safety concerns [9].

In the United States of America, corticosteroids, IV immunoglobulin, and anti-D are all considered appropriate frontline treatments for ITP in both adults and children. In 2010, a specific warning was issued by the US Food and Drug Administration, which highlighted the risks of intravascular hemolysis and acute renal failure and disseminated intravascular coagulation after anti-D administration to patients with ITP [10]. However, Despotovic and Neunert [11] revealed that the estimated incidence of an acute hemolytic reaction in such patients was 0.03%. The authors also concluded that there was sufficient evidence to support the use of anti-D as a frontline treatment for ITP in adults and children (grade 2B recommendation). Until the full nature of these adverse effects is assessed, this agent should be used with caution.

2 Cyclophosphamide

Since 1960 [12], a variety of nonsteroidal immunosuppressant agents have been used to treat ITP that is refractory to splenectomy and glucocorticoid treatment. Finch et al. [13] described that the expected success rate of nonsteroidal immunosuppressant therapy in chronic refractory ITP is 15–35% in adults and probably higher in children. Laros and Penner [14] were the first to use cyclophosphamide for the treatment of refractory ITP. In that study, 7 out of the 11 treated patients showed excellent responses to the cyclophosphamide therapy and remained in complete hematologic remission for 10–40 months after therapy discontinuation. Verlin et al. [15] also reported that 15 out of 22 splenectomized patients with refractory ITP responded well to cyclophosphamide treatment, whereas 7 out of 8 unsplenectomized patients with refractory ITP responded well to the treatment.

Reiner et al. [16] reported that out of 20 patients treated with pulse cyclophosphamide therapy, 13 (65%) achieved complete response, 4 (20%) achieved partial response, and 3 (15%) failed to respond. In the aforementioned clinical studies, cyclophosphamide was administered either at a dosage of 50–200 mg/day or intermittently over a 4-h period every 2–3 weeks [15–17]. Furthermore, platelet count usually increased 2–4 weeks after the treatment and reached a maximum increase in 4–6 weeks. This indicates that continuous treatment would be necessary to maintain an effective response to the treatment. The major adverse events recorded were leukopenia, infection, alopecia, hemorrhagic cystitis, and secondary malignancy. Although no randomized large-scale clinical trial has been performed, the use of cyclophosphamide for the treatment of refractory ITP patients is worth considering.

3 Vincristine and Vinblastine

Vincristine and vinblastine [18–21] are vinca alkaloids that were introduced for the treatment of ITP. They may be as effective as cyclophosphamide is; however, they act more rapidly than cyclophosphamide does. Vincristine is usually administered at a dose of 0.025 mg/kg to a maximum dose of 2 mg in adults [21]. On the other hand, vinblastine is usually administered at a dose of 0.125 mg/kg [21]. Platelet count usually increases in 1 week after treatment initiation with the vinca alkaloids. Ahn et al. [22] and Manoharan [23] introduced the administration of the vinca alkaloids by slow infusion. The authors reported that 11 out of 34 treated patients achieved complete remission at 7–10-day intervals with vincristine or vinblastine. However, Simon et al. [24] reported of prolonged complete remission in only 2 out of 12 patients with refractory ITP who were treated with vincristine or vinblastine. The major adverse event from treatment with vinca alkaloids is peripheral neuropathy; however, it is reversible after treatment is discontinued. The mechanism of action of vincristine and vinblastine has been postulated to be via the inhibition of microtubule-dependent events that are required for monocyte-macrophage function [25].

The administration method of vinca alkaloids was modified from a slow infusion of the drugs to a vinca alkaloid-loaded platelet infusion in some studies [26–28]. In one of the studies, after 11 patients with refractory ITP were administered the treatment, six achieved complete remissions, three had partial remissions, and two experienced treatment failure [26]. The platelets were initially incubated with vinca alkaloids in vitro, after which they were infused into the patients. The “vinca alkaloid-loaded platelets” were opsonized with an antiplatelet antibody and phagocytosed by macrophages in the spleen, which resulted in the destruction of the macrophages.

4 Danazol

Danazol is an attenuated androgen that has been reported to be useful for treating ITP that is refractory to corticosteroid therapy and/or splenectomy. For instance, Ahn et al. [29] reported that out of 22 patients who were treated with danazol, 15 benefited from the treatment, and 11 achieved sustained normalization of their platelet counts. Furthermore, Buelli et al. [30] have reported on 14 patients with ITP that was refractory to steroid treatment and/or splenectomy. The patients were treated with danazol for 2 months. After treatment, the authors observed excellent responses (platelet count $>100 \times 10^9$/l) in five patients, good responses (platelet count $>50 \times 10^9$/l) in two patients, and poor responses (no increase in platelet count) in seven patients. The authors concluded that danazol was well tolerated in most of the patients and is therefore better suited for long-term treatment than steroids are. Maloisel et al. [31] have reported on the efficacy and safety of danazol in the treatment of patients with refractory ITP. The study showed that 38 patients experienced partial or complete response to therapy (67%), among whom 27 (46%) remained in remission for a median (± SD) of 119 (± 45) months. In addition, severe adverse events were reported in nine patients (16%). The general adverse events observed were acne, hirsutism, dyslipidemia, amenorrhea, and liver function abnormalities. The postulated mechanism of action of danazol is induction of a reduction in Fc receptor expression on monocytes or macrophages [32].

5 Syk Inhibitors

Syk (spleen tyrosine kinase) is a non-receptor tyrosine kinase that plays an important role in biological functions. For instance, it plays a critical role in intracellular signal transduction of B-cell receptors on B lymphocytes and Fc receptors on macrophages. Taniguchi et al. [33] were the first to identify and succeed in cloning Syk, which is highly expressed in the cells of the hematopoietic system.

It is generally accepted that the ligand-binding receptor chain contains one or more immunoreceptor tyrosine-based activation motifs (ITAMs). Receptor ligation leads to phosphorylation of ITAMs, which primarily occurs in the membrane Src tyrosine kinase [34]. In ITP, platelets that are bound by antiplatelet antibody bind to Fc receptors on macrophages. This is followed by phosphorylation of the tyrosine units of ITAMs by Src tyrosine kinase. The phosphorylated ITAMs then phosphorylate Syk, which results in the autophosphorylation of Syk. The phosphorylated Syk activates PI3 kinase and phospholipase C, which then induce actin polymerization and result in phagocytosis by macrophages. Syk is therefore a critical molecule in phagocytosis.

Fostamatinib disodium (R788) is the oral prodrug of R406, a relatively selective small molecule inhibitor of Syk. It was reported that treatment with R788 effectively prevented antiplatelet antibody-induced thrombocytopenia in mice [35]. Furthermore, a phase II study revealed that treatment with R788 (75–175 mg, twice daily) induced a sustained improvement in platelet count in 50% of 16 patients with refractory ITP [35]. Neutropenia was the common adverse event reported in the phase II study [36]. The most common adverse event that has been observed from R788 treatment in clinical studies is gastrointestinal toxicity, including diarrhea (in up to 45% of the patients) and nausea.

6 Other Drugs

In the past, many patients with refractory ITP required treatment with third-line agents; however, the use of such drugs was limited by modest response rates. Therefore, evidence to support their use in refractory ITP is generally limited to uncontrolled case series [37–39]. Some of the third-line agents are azathioprine [40–42], cyclosporine [43–45], mycophenolate mofetil [46], interferon [47–49], and ascorbic acid [50–52].

In the near future, the following drugs might be used clinically [53] for treating refractory ITP: tocilizumab (IDEC-151) [54]; ruplizumab, an anti-CD40 ligand (hu5c8) [55]; GMA161, a humanized anti-human FcγRIII antibody [56]; rozrolimupab, a human anti-RhD monoclonal antibody [57]; SM101, a soluble FcγRIIB [58]; avatrombopag (E5501), a small molecule thrombopoietin receptor agonist [59]; 23A11, a murine anti-VPAC1 monoclonal immunoglobulin G1 antibody [60]; amifostine, a cytoprotective agent that improves thrombopoiesis [61]; and oseltamivir phosphate, a sialidase inhibitor [62].

References

1. Salama A, Kiefel V, Amberg R, Mueller-Eckhardt C. Treatment of autoimmune thrombocytopenic purpura with rhesus antibodies anti-Rh. (D). Blut. 1984;49:29–35.
2. Baglin TP, Smith MP, Boughton BJ. Rapid and complete response of immune thrombocytopenic purpura to a single injection of rhesus anti-D immunoglobulin. Lancet. 1986;1(8493):1329–30.
3. Bussel JB, Graziano JN, Kimberly RP, Pahwa S, Aledort LM. Intravenous anti-D treatment of immune thrombocytopenic purpura: analysis of efficacy, toxicity, and mechanism of effect. Blood. 1991;77(9):1884–93.
4. Cooper N, Woloski BM, Fodero EM, et al. Does treatment with intermittent infusions of intravenous anti-D allow a proportion of adults with recently diagnosed immune thrombocytopenic purpura to avoid splenectomy? Blood. 2002;99(6):1922–7.
5. Hill QA. How does dapsone work in immune thrombocytopenia? Implications for dosing. Blood. 2015;125(23):3666–8.
6. Andrew M, Blanchette VS, Adams M, Ali K, Barnard D, Chan KW, DeVeber LB, Esseltine D, Israels S, Korbrinsky N, et al. A multicenter study of the treatment of childhood chronic idiopathic thrombocytopenic purpura with anti-D. J Pediatr. 1992;120:522–7.
7. Scaradavou A, Woo B, Woloski BM, Cunningham-Rundles S, Ettinger LJ, Aledort LM, Bussel JB. Intravenous anti-D treatment of immune thrombocytopenic purpura: experience in 272 patients. Blood. 1997;89(8):2689–700.
8. Pizzuto J, Ambriz R. Therapeutic experience on 934 adults with idiopathic thrombocytopenic purpura: multicentric trial of the Cooperative Latin American Group on Hemostasis and Thrombosis. Blood. 1984;64:1179–83.
9. WinRho SDF was voluntarily withdrawn from the European market in August, 2009 because of safety concerns. http://www.mhra.gov.uk/Safetyinformation/Safetywarningsalertsandrecalls/Safetywarningsandmessagesformedicines/Monthlylistsofinformationforhealthcareprofessionalsonthesafetyofmedicines/CON057078
10. US Food and Drug Administration. WinRho SDF (Rho(D) immune globulin intravenous (human): risk of intravascular hemolysis. http://www.fda.gov/Safety/MedWatch/SafetyInformation/SafetyAlertsforHumanMedicalProducts/ucm203739.htm. Accessed 26 Sept 2013.
11. Despotovic JM, Neunert CE. Is anti-D immunoglobulin still a frontline treatment option for immune thrombocytopenia? Hematology Am Soc Hematol Educ Program. 2013;2013:283–5.
12. Dameshek W, Schwartz R. Treatment of certain "autoimmune" diseases with antimetabolites: a preliminary report. Trans Assoc Am Phys. 1960;73:113–27.
13. Finch SC, Castro O, Cooper M, Covey W, Erichson R, McPhedran P. Immunosuppressive therapy of chronic idiopathic thrombocytopenic purpura. Am J Med. 1974;56(1):4–12.
14. Laros RK, Penner JA. "Refractory" thrombocytopenia purpura treated successfully with cyclophosphamide. J Am Med Assoc. 1971;215:445–9.
15. Verlin M, Laros RK, Penner JA. Treatment of refractory thrombocytopenic purpura with cyclophosphamide. Am J Hematol. 1976;1:97–104.
16. Reiner A, Gernsheimer T, Slichter SJ. Pulse cyclophosphamide therapy for refractory autoimmune thrombocytopenic purpura. Blood. 1995;85:351–8.
17. Weinerman B, Maxwell L, Hryniuk W. Intermittent cyclophosphamide treatment of autoimmune thrombocytopenia. Can Med Assoc J. 1974;16:1100–2.
18. Sultan Y, Delobel J, Jeanneau C, Caen JP. Effect of periwinkle alkaloids in idiopathic thrombocytopenic purpura. Lancet. 1971;1(7697):496–7.
19. Marmont AM, Damasio EE, Gori E. Vinblastine sulphate in idiopathic thrombocytopenic purpura. Lancet. 1971;2(7715):94.
20. Marmont AM, Damasio EE. Clinical experiences with cytotoxic immunosuppressive treatment of idiopathic thrombocytopenic purpura. Acta Haematol. 1971;46(2):72–91.
21. Ahn YS, Harrington WJ, Seelman RC, Eytel CS. Vincristine therapy of idiopathic and secondary thrombocytopenias. N Engl J Med. 1974;291(8):376–80.

22. Ahn YS, Harrington WJ, Mylvaganam R, Allen LM, Pall LM. Slow infusion of vinca alkaloids in the treatment of idiopathic thrombocytopenic purpura. Ann Intern Med. 1984;100(2):192–6.
23. Manoharan A. Slow infusion of vincristine in the treatment of idiopathic thrombocytopenic purpura. Am J Hematol. 1986;21(2):135–8.
24. Simon M, Jouet JP, Fenaux P, Pollet JP, Walter MP, Bauters F. The treatment of adult idiopathic thrombocytopenic purpura. Infusion of vinblastine in ITP. Eur J Haematol. 1987;39(3):193–6.
25. Paulson JC, McClure WO. Inhibition of axoplasmic transport by colchicine, podophyllotoxin, and vinblastine: an effect on microtubules. Ann N Y Acad Sci. 1975;253:517–27.
26. Ahn YS, Byrnes JJ, Harrington WJ, Cayer ML, Smith DS, Brunskill DE, Pall LM. The treatment of idiopathic thrombocytopenia with vinblastine-loaded platelets. N EngI J Med. 1978;298:1101–7.
27. Shvidel L. Vincristine-loaded platelet infusion for treatment of refractory autoimmune hemolytic anemia and chronic immune thrombocytopenia: rethinking old cures. Am J Hematol. 2006;81(6):423–5.
28. Weigert O. Successful salvage treatment of chronic refractory immune thrombocytopenia using a simplified method to generate vincristine-loaded platelets. Thromb Haemost. 2008;100(4):705–7.
29. Ahn YS, Harrington WJ, Simon SR, Mylvaganam R, Pall LM, So AG. Danazol for the treatment of idiopathic thrombocytopenic purpura. N Engl J Med. 1983;308(23):1396–9.
30. Buelli M, Cortelazzo S, Viero P, Minetti B, Comotti B, Bassan R, Barbui T. Danazol for the treatment of idiopathic thrombocytopenic purpura. Acta Haematol. 1985;74(2):97–8.
31. Maloisel F, Andres E, Zimmer J, Noel E, Zamfir A, Koumarianou A, Dufour P. Danazol therapy in patients with chronic idiopathic thrombocytopenic purpura: long-term results. Am J Med. 2004;116(9):590–4.
32. Schreiber AD, Chien P, Tomaski A, Cines DB. Effect of danazol in immune thrombocytopenic purpura. N Engl J Med. 1987;316(9):503–8.
33. Taniguchi T, Kobayashi T, Kondo J, Takahashi K, Nakamura H, Suzuki J, Nagai K, Yamada T, Nakamura S, Yamamura H. Molecular cloning of a porcine gene Syk that encodes a 72-kDa protein-tyrosine kinase showing high susceptibility to proteolysis. J Biol Chem. 1991;266(24):15790–6.
34. Mocsai A, Ruland J, Tybulewicz VL. The Syk tyrosine kinase: a crucial player in diverse biological functions. Nat Rev Immunol. 2010;10(69):387–402.
35. Podolanczuk A, Lazarus AH, Crow AR, Grossbard E, Bussel JB. Of mice and men: an open-label pilot study for treatment of immune thrombocytopenic purpura by an inhibitor of Syk. Blood. 2009;113(14):3154–60.
36. Weinblatt ME, Kavanaugh A, Burgos-Vargas R, Dikranian AH, Medrano-Ramirez G, Morales-Torres JL, Murphy FT, Musser TK, Straniero N, Vicente-Gonzales AV, Grossbard E. Treatment of rheumatoid arthritis with a Syk kinase inhibitor: a twelve-week, randomized, placebo-controlled trial. Arthritis Rheum. 2008;58(11):3309–18.
37. Vesely SK, Perdue JJ, Rizvi MA, Terrell DR, George JN. Management of adult patients with persistent idiopathic thrombocytopenic purpura following splenectomy: a systematic review. Ann Intern Med. 2004;115:29–31.
38. Arnold DM, Nazi I, Santos A, Chan H, Heddle NM, Warkentin TE, Kelton JG. Combination immunosuppressant therapy for patients with chronic refractory immune thrombocytopenic purpura. Blood. 2010;115:29–31.
39. Lakshmanan S, Cuker A. Contemporary management of primary immune thrombocytopenia in adults. J Thromb Haemost. 2012;10(10):1988–98.
40. Bouroncle BA, Doan CA. Refractory idiopathic thrombocytopenic purpura treated with azathioprine. N Engl J Med. 1966;275(12):630–6.
41. Sussman LN. Azathioprine in refractory idiopathic thrombocytopenic purpura. JAMA. 1967;202(4):259–63.
42. Bouroncle BA, Doan CA. Treatment of refractory idiopathic thrombocytopenic purpura. JAMA. 1969;207(11):2049–52.

43. Emilia G, Messora C, Longo G, Bertesi M. Long-term salvage treatment by cyclosporin in refractory autoimmune haematological disorders. Br J Haematol. 1996;93:341–4.
44. Kappers-Klunne MC, van't Veer MB. Cyclosporin A for the treatment of patients with chronic idiopathic thrombocytopenic purpura refractory to corticosteroids or splenectomy. Br J Haematol. 2001;114:121–5.
45. Emilia G, Morselli M, Luppi M, Longo G, Marasca R, Gandini G, et al. Long-term salvage therapy with cyclosporin A in refractory idiopathic thrombocytopenic purpura. Blood. 2002;99:1482–5.
46. Hou M, Peng J, Shi Y, Zhang C, Qin P, Zhao C, et al. Mycophenolate mofetil (MMF) for the treatment of steroid-resistant idiopathic thrombocytopenic purpura. Eur J Haematol. 2003;70:353–7.
47. Proctor SJ. alpha Interferon therapy in the treatment of idiopathic thrombocytopenic purpura. Eur J Cancer. 1991;27(Suppl 4):S63–8.
48. Ishii H, Oh H, Uchida Y, Nakamura H, Endo N, Asai T, et al. Effect of interferon (IFN) on refractory idiopathic thrombocytopenic purpura: administration of 6 million units of recombinant IFN alpha-2b. Intern Med. 1992;31:1343–7.
49. Vianelli N, Tazzari PL, Baravelli S, Ricci F, Valdre L, Tura S. Interferon-alpha 2b is not effective in the treatment of refractory immune thrombocytopenic purpura [Letter]. Haematologica. 1998;83:761–3.
50. Brox AG, Howson-Jan K, Fauser AA. Treatment of idiopathic thrombocytopenic purpura with ascorbate. Br J Haematol. 1988;70:341–4.
51. Vianelli N, Gugliotta L, Gianni L, Belmonte MM, Catani L, Tura S. Ascorbic acid for the treatment of chronic refractory idiopathic thrombocytopenic purpura (ITP). Haematologica. 1992;77:92–3.
52. Jubelirer SJ. Pilot study of ascorbic acid for the treatment of refractory immune thrombocytopenic purpura. Am J Hematol. 1992;43:44–6.
53. Shih A, Nazi I, Kelton JG, Arnold DM. Novel treatments for immune thrombocytopenia. Presse Med. 2014;43(4 Pt 2):e87–95.
54. Kuwana M, Nomura S, Fujimura K, Nagasawa T, Muto Y, Kurata Y, et al. Effect of a single injection of humanized anti-CD154 monoclonal antibody on the platelet-specific autoimmune response in patients with immune thrombocytopenic purpura. Blood. 2004;103:1229–36.
55. Patel VL, Schwartz J, Bussel JB. The effect of anti-CD40 ligand in immune thrombocytopenic purpura. Br J Haematol. 2008;141:545–8.
56. Flaherty MM, MacLachlan TK, Troutt M, Magee T, Tuaillon N, Johnson S, et al. Nonclinical evaluation of GMA161—an anti-human CD16 (FcgammaRIII) monoclonal antibody for treatment of autoimmune disorders in CD16 transgenic mice. Toxicol Sci. 2012;125:299–309.
57. Robak T, Windyga J, Trelinski J, von Depka PM, Giagounidis A, Doyen C, et al. Rozrolimupab, a mixture of 25 recombinant human monoclonal RhD antibodies, in the treatment of primary immune thrombocytopenia. Blood. 2012;120:3670–6.
58. Konstaninova TS, Leonidovna IV, Hellmann A, et al. Interim results from a phase Ib/IIa clinical trial with the soluble Fc-Gamma IIb receptor SM101 for the treatment of primary immune thrombocytopenia. Blood. 2012;120: Abstract 3388.
59. Bussel J, Zhang Y, Tang S, McIntosh J, Kuter D. A phase II 6-month extension study of the efficacy, safety, and tolerability of E5501 (AKR501) in subjects with chronic immune thrombocytopenia (CITP). Haematologica. 2011;96: Abstract 0221.
60. Peeters K, Loyen S, Van Kerckhoven S, Stoffels K, Hoylaerts MF, Van Geet C, et al. Thrombopoietic effect of VPAC1 inhibition during megakaryopoiesis. Br J Haematol. 2010;151:54–61.
61. Fan H, Zhu HL, Li SX, Lu XC, Zhai B, Guo B, et al. Efficacy of amifostine in treating patients with idiopathic thrombocytopenia purpura. Cell Biochem Biophys. 2011;59:7–12.
62. Shao L, Wu Y, Zhou H, Qin P, Ni H, Peng J, Hou M. Successful treatment with oseltamivir phosphate in a patient with chronic immune thrombocytopenia positive for anti-GPIb/IX autoantibody. Platelets. 2015;26(5):495–7.

Transfusion

Takaaki Hato

Abstract The efficacy of platelet transfusion in the management of ITP remains obscure. In patients with hematologic disorders undergoing myelosuppressive chemotherapy or hematopoietic stem cell transplantation, platelets are widely transfused prophylactically, and a platelet transfusion threshold of 10,000/μL has been recommended to be safe and effective. In ITP, however, prophylactic platelet transfusion is not recommended because the rise in platelet counts following platelet transfusion is not seen because of rapid destruction of transfused platelets. In ITP patients with severe active bleeding, anecdotal evidence suggests successful treatment of platelet transfusion alone or in combination with intravenous immunoglobulin. Platelet transfusion may be also considered before splenectomy in ITP patients. Recent studies suggest that laparoscopic splenectomy can be a safe and feasible procedure in ITP patients with platelet count less than 10×10^3/μL without platelet transfusion.

1 Introduction

Platelets are primary mediators of hemostasis at the vascular injury sites and play a crucial role on hemostatic plug formation. The history of platelet transfusion demonstrates that platelet transfusion has contributed to a reduction in fetal hemorrhage in thrombocytopenic patients with acute leukemia [1]. In spite of obvious beneficial effect of platelet transfusion on hemostatic management, the role of platelet transfusion on management of ITP patients remains largely undefined and underexplored. Evidence regarding platelet transfusion have been mainly provided from studies with thrombocytopenic patients with hematological malignancies. This chapter will discuss evidence regarding the clinical indications for platelet transfusion in thrombocytopenic patients with hematological malignancies and ITP.

T. Hato
Division of Blood Transfusion and Cell Therapy, Ehime University Hospital,
Toon, Ehime 791-0295, Japan
e-mail: takahato@m.ehime-u.ac.jp

Y. Ishida, Y. Tomiyama (eds.), *Autoimmune Thrombocytopenia*,
DOI 10.1007/978-981-10-4142-6_19

2 Platelet Counts Required for Hemostasis

It is well known that thrombocytopenia is a hemorrhagic risk factor. However, it is not entirely clear how low platelet numbers causes the inability of hemostasis. Platelets are required to maintain vascular integrity which are regulated by interaction of substances released from platelets with intercellular endothelial junctions [2]. A previous study showed that approximately 7100/μL/day of platelets is required for maintaining vascular integrity [3]. If this amount of platelets is supplied from bone marrow or platelet transfusion, it would be theoretically assumed that vascular integrity is maintained to prevent thrombocytopenic patients from spontaneous bleeding. Recently, an animal experiment, in which tail bleeding time was measured in mice with different degree of thrombocytopenia, showed that mice with platelet counts from 2.5 to 20% of control mice (equivalent with 5000–40,000/μL in humans) arrested bleeding although the mean bleeding times were significantly prolonged compared with the control [4]. In sharp contrast, mice with platelet counts less than 2.5% of control were not able to arrest bleeding. A human study, in which radiolabeled autologous red cells were infused into patients with aplastic anemia, revealed that fecal blood loss was markedly elevated in all patients with platelet counts of less than 5000/μL [5]. A recent PLADO study reflecting modern medical health care showed the significantly increased bleeding at platelet counts less than 5000/μL [6]. These findings suggest that platelet counts required to maintain hemostasis in humans is greater than 5000/μL.

3 Triggers for Platelet Transfusion

Platelets are widely transfused prophylactically in patients with hematological disorders undergoing myelosuppressive chemotherapy or hematopoietic stem cell transplantation. In such patients, it was the standard practice to transfuse platelets at platelet counts below 20,000/μL until the early 1990s. In the late 1990s, four randomized controlled trials were conducted to investigate the different platelet count thresholds to be transfused prophylactically to reduce the bleeding risk [7–10]. All studies demonstrated no difference in major bleeding between patient groups with 10,000/μL and 20,000–30,000/μL threshold, suggesting that a platelet transfusion threshold of 10,000/μL is safe and effective. However, the protocols of these trials allowed patients with fever, fresh bleeding episode, or invasive procedures to be transfused irrespective of platelet counts because of patient safety. In the largest study with 255 patients, 22.6% of platelet transfusion in the 10,000/μL arm were given above the threshold of 10,000/μL, and the protocol violations were 5.4% in the 10,000/μL arm, implying that a total of 28% of the patients with the 10,000/μL arm received platelet transfusion above the 10,000/μL [9]. Moreover, a critical question has been raised as to whether these trials have sufficient statistical power to demonstrate equivalence in terms of the safety of the 10,000/μL transfusion trigger [11]. A recent Cochrane review evaluated these trials regarding platelet transfusion threshold as low quality of evidence [12]. However, without further evidence, Cochrane review concluded that it is reasonable to continue with current practice of administrating prophylactic platelet transfusions using the 10,000/μL threshold in the absence of other risk factors for bleeding such as fever and invasive procedures.

4 Risk Factors for Bleeding

The bleeding risk in thrombocytopenic patients cannot be determined by platelet count alone. Many factors influence the bleeding risk (Table 1) [13–18]. A recent animal study demonstrated that the combination of inflammation with thrombocytopenia rapidly induces bleeding manifestations whereas thrombocytopenia alone did not [19]. This finding may explain why fever and infection are risk factors for bleeding in thrombocytopenic patients. This may be also the case in ITP. However, further studies are required to determine the effect of infection on bleeding risk in ITP patients because infection often induces a cytokine-mediated increase in platelet count in ITP patients.

Hematocrit may affect the risk for bleeding in thrombocytopenic patients. There is evidence that the higher hematocrit reduces the bleeding risk in thrombocytopenic patients [20, 21]. Red cells displace platelets toward the endothelial surface where they can more effectively respond to vascular injury [22, 23]. This effect of red blood cells on platelets may be responsible for reduction of bleeding risk. Although ITP patients usually have a normal range of hematocrit, red blood cell transfusion may promote effective hemostasis in ITP patients with low hematocrit due to massive bleeding.

Table 1 Bleeding risks identified in patients with hematological malignancies

Bleeding risk	Reference
Fever (38.5 °C<)	[13]
Infection	[13]
Anticoagulant drugs	[14]
Amphotericin use	[10, 15]
Hypoalbuminemia	[16]
Uremia	[16]
Recent bleeding episodes	[16]
Recent bone marrow transplantation	[16]
Acute GVHD	[10, 15, 17]
Veno-occlusive disease	[10, 15, 17]
Poor risk disease	[18]

5 Prophylactic Versus Therapeutic Platelet Transfusion

As mentioned above, many bleeding risk factors other than thrombocytopenia have been identified, and no relationship between platelet counts and bleeding risk was demonstrated in a large retrospective study [11, 16]. These findings raised a question as to whether a platelet count threshold-defined prophylactic platelet transfusion is appropriate as a standard clinical practice. Recently, two large randomized controlled studies were conducted to compare the benefit of prophylactic platelet transfusion using a trigger of 10,000/μL with therapeutic platelet transfusion (platelets were transfused only when significant bleeding occurred) in patients with intensive chemotherapy for acute myeloid leukemia and hematopoietic stem cell transplantation [24, 25]. Both studies showed that patients with therapeutic platelet transfusion had a higher risk for bleeding than patients with prophylactic platelet transfusion. These studies suggest that platelet count-defined prophylactic platelet transfusion is justified as an effective supportive care for patients with hematologic malignancies. Patients who received prophylactic platelet transfusion at 10,000/μL threshold can maintain vascular integrity necessary to prevent spontaneous bleeding because the minimum platelet count requirement for vascular integrity is assumed to be around 5000/μL, as described above (see Sect. 2. in this chapter). This may explain the efficacy of platelet count-based prophylactic platelet transfusion strategy. However, in ITP patients, the rise in platelet counts following platelet transfusion is not seen because of rapid destruction of transfused platelets. Prophylactic platelet transfusion should not be applied to ITP patients and therapeutic platelet transfusion can be used for selected patients (see below).

6 Dose of Platelet Transfusion

The appropriate number of platelets in prophylactic platelet transfusion has been assessed in two randomized controlled trials. The PRADO trial compared three different doses (low: $1.1 \times 10^{11}/m^2$, medium: $2.2 \times 10^{11}/m^2$, high: $4.4 \times 10^{11}/m^2$) of platelets with the risk of WHO grade 2 bleeding [6]. This study demonstrated that there was no significant difference in the incidence of major bleeding among three-dose groups, while the number of platelet transfusions given was significantly higher in the low-dose group. This finding suggests that higher doses do not result in higher preventive effect on bleeding; however, it reduces the number of platelet transfusion, which has the advantage of longer intervals between transfusions and of reduced chance of transfusion-associated adverse effects. Another trial, STOP study, evaluated two different doses (low: $1.5–2.9 \times 10^{11}$ platelets/product, high: $3.0–6.0 \times 10^{11}$) of platelet transfusion in patients with chemotherapy-induced thrombocytopenia [26]. Even though the numbers of patients with grade 2 or higher bleeding was comparable in the two groups, the trial was stopped early when 5% of the patients with low dose had grade 4 bleeding. In ITP, there is no study comparing different platelet doses.

7 Platelet Transfusion During Treatment for ITP

The efficacy of platelet transfusion in the management of ITP remains obscure. Transfused platelets have a shortened survival in ITP, and it is thus questionable whether transfused platelets effectively contribute to hemostatic plug formation at the bleeding site [27, 28]. On the other hand, successful treatment of platelet transfusion alone or in combination with intravenous immunoglobulin (IVIG) has been reported [29–32]. Salama et al. [30] reported that ten patients with refractory ITP and bleeding or a high bleeding risk received platelet transfusion, resulting in an increase in the platelet count to $84–157 \times 10^3/\mu L$ and the cessation of bleeding in all patients without any serious adverse effects. Spahr and Rodgers [31] reported that 40 patients were treated with prolonged infusions of IVIG (1 g/kg by continuous infusion over 24 h) and concurrent platelets (1 apheresis unit every 8 h), resulting in an increase in the platelet count >50,000/μL in 62.7% of patients and clinical improvement in bleeding. These studies suggest that platelet transfusion may have clinical benefit for ITP patients with severe active bleeding or surgical procedures. However, there is no randomized controlled study of platelet transfusion in ITP. In a nationwide survey in the United States, 25.8% of inpatients with ITP received platelet transfusion [33]. Although the efficacy of platelet transfusion in these patients was not reported, this survey demonstrated no adverse thrombotic event associated with platelet transfusion in ITP. Platelet transfusion can be thus used as therapeutic transfusion in ITP patients with life-threatening bleeding or emergent surgical procedures. However, prophylactic platelet transfusion to ITP patients with severe thrombocytopenia but no major active bleeding should not be recommended.

Platelet transfusion may be considered before splenectomy in ITP patients refractory to steroids and IVIG. In ITP patients with platelet counts $<10–20 \times 10^3/\mu L$ who underwent laparoscopic splenectomy, retrospective analysis of operative outcomes including blood loss and operative time between patients with and without platelet transfusion showed no significant difference between the two groups [34, 35]. The main cause of the increase in intraoperative blood loss was unexpected bleeding from splenic capsular tears during manipulation or from venous branches near the hilum [34]. In addition, platelet count may increase rapidly to a safe level. Based on these findings, laparoscopic splenectomy can be a safe and feasible procedure in ITP patients with platelet count less than $10 \times 10^3/\mu L$ without platelet transfusion.

References

1. Slichter SJ. Controversies in platelet transfusion therapy. Annu Rev Med. 1980;31:509–40.
2. Nachman RL, Rafii S. Platelets, petechiae, and preservation of the vascular wall. N Engl J Med. 2008;359:1261–70.
3. Hanson SR, Slichter SJ. Platelet kinetics in patients with bone marrow hypoplasia: evidence for a fixed platelet requirement. Blood. 1985;66:1105–9.
4. Morowski M, Vogtle T, Kraft P, et al. Only severe thrombocytopenia results in bleeding and defective thrombus formation in mice. Blood. 2013;121:4938–47.

5. Slichter SJ, Harker LA. Thrombocytopenia: mechanisms and management of defects in platelet production. Clin Haematol. 1978;7:523–39.
6. Slichter SJ, Kaufman RM, Assmann SF, et al. Dose of prophylactic platelet transfusions and prevention of hemorrhage. N Engl J Med. 2010;362:600–13.
7. Diedrich B, Remberger M, Shanwell A, et al. A prospective randomized trial of a prophylactic platelet transfusion trigger of 10 × 10(9) per L versus 30 × 10(9) per L in allogeneic hematopoietic progenitor cell transplant recipients. Transfusion. 2005;45:1064–72.
8. Heckman KD, Weiner GJ, Davis CS, et al. Randomized study of prophylactic platelet transfusion threshold during induction therapy for adult acute leukemia: 10,000/μL versus 20,000/μL. J Clin Oncol. 1997;15:1143–9.
9. Rebulla P, Finazzi G, Marangoni F, et al. The threshold for prophylactic platelet transfusions in adults with acute myeloid leukemia. N Engl J Med. 1997;337:1870–5.
10. Zumberg MS, del Rosario ML, Nejame CF, et al. A prospective randomized trial of prophylactic platelet transfusion and bleeding incidence in hematopoietic stem cell transplant recipients: 10,000/L versus 20,000/microL trigger. Biol Blood Marrow Transplant. 2002;8:569–76.
11. Estcourt LJ, Stanworth SJ, Murphy MF. Platelet transfusions for patients with haematological malignancies: who needs them? Br J Haematol. 2011;154:425–40.
12. Estcourt LJ, Stanworth SJ, Doree C, et al. Comparison of different platelet count thresholds to guide administration of prophylactic platelet transfusion for preventing bleeding in people with haematological disorders after myelosuppressive chemotherapy or stem cell transplantation. Cochrane Database Syst Rev. 2015;11:CD010983.
13. Webert K, Cook RJ, Sigouin CS, et al. The risk of bleeding in thrombocytopenic patients with acute myeloid leukemia. Haematologica. 2006;91:1530–7.
14. Gerber DE, Segal JB, Levy MY, et al. The incidence of and risk factors for venous thromboembolism (VTE) and bleeding among 1514 patients undergoing hematopoietic stem cell transplantation: implications for VTE prevention. Blood. 2008;112:504–10.
15. Lawrence JB, Yomtovian RA, Hammons T, et al. Lowering the prophylactic platelet transfusion threshold: a prospective analysis. Leuk Lymphoma. 2001;41:67–76.
16. Friedmann AM, Sengul H, Lehmann H, et al. Do basic laboratory tests or clinical observations predict bleeding in thrombocytopenic oncology patients? A reevaluation of prophylactic platelet transfusions. Transfus Med Rev. 2002;16:34–45.
17. Najima Y, Ohashi K, Miyazawa M, et al. Intracranial hemorrhage following allogeneic hematopoietic stem cell transplantation. Am J Hematol. 2009;84:298–301.
18. Nevo S, Fuller AK, Hartley E, et al. Acute bleeding complications in patients after hematopoietic stem cell transplantation with prophylactic platelet transfusion triggers of 10 × 10(9) and 20 × 10(9) per L. Transfusion. 2007;47:801–12.
19. Goerge T, Ho-Tin-Noe B, Carbo C, et al. Inflammation induces hemorrhage in thrombocytopenia. Blood. 2008;111:4958–64.
20. Valeri CR, Khuri S, Ragno G. Nonsurgical bleeding diathesis in anemic thrombocytopenic patients: role of temperature, red blood cells, platelets, and plasma-clotting proteins. Transfusion. 2007;47:206S–48S.
21. Eugster M, Reinhart WH. The influence of the haematocrit on primary haemostasis in vitro. Thromb Haemost. 2005;94:1213–8.
22. Turitto VT, Weiss HJ. Red blood cells: their dual role in thrombus formation. Science. 1980;207:541–3.
23. Uijttewaal WS, Nijhof EJ, Bronkhorst PJ, et al. Near-wall excess of platelets induced by lateral migration of erythrocytes in flowing blood. Am J Physiol. 1993;264:H1239–44.
24. Wandt H, Schaefer-Eckart K, Wendelin K, et al. Therapeutic platelet transfusion versus routine prophylactic transfusion in patients with haematological malignancies: an open-label, multicentre, randomised study. Lancet. 2012;380:1309–16.
25. Stanworth SJ, Estcourt LJ, Powter G, et al. A no-prophylaxis platelet-transfusion strategy for hematologic cancers. N Engl J Med. 2013;368:1771–80.

26. Heddle NM, Cook RJ, Tinmouth A, et al. A randomized controlled trial comparing standard- and low-dose strategies for transfusion of platelets (SToP) to patients with thrombocytopenia. Blood. 2009;113:1564–73.
27. Buchanan GR, Scher CS, Button LN, et al. Use of homologous platelet survival in differential diagnoses of chronic thrombocytopenia in childhood. Pediatrics. 1977;59:45–54.
28. Stoll D, Cines DB, Aster RH, et al. Platelet kinetics in patients with idiopathic thrombocytopenic purpura and moderate thrombocytopenia. Blood. 1985;65:584–8.
29. Carr JM, Kruskall MS, Kaye JA, et al. Efficacy of platelet transfusions in immune thrombocytopenia. Am J Med. 1986;80:1051–4.
30. Salama A, Kiesewetter H, Kalus U, et al. Massive platelet transfusion is a rapidly effective emergency treatment in patients with refractory autoimmune thrombocytopenia. Thromb Haemost. 2008;100:762–5.
31. Spahr JE, Rodgers GM. Treatment of immune-mediated thrombocytopenia purpura with concurrent intravenous immunoglobulin and platelet transfusion: a retrospective review of 40 patients. Am J Hematol. 2008;83:122–5.
32. Danese MD, Lindquist K, Gleeson M, et al. Cost and mortality associated with hospitalizations in patients with immune thrombocytopenic purpura. Am J Hematol. 2009;84:631–5.
33. Goel R, Ness PM, Takemoto CM, et al. Platelet transfusions in platelet consumptive disorders are associated with arterial thrombosis and in-hospital mortality. Blood. 2015;125:1470–6.
34. Chen X, Peng B, Cai Y, et al. Laparoscopic splenectomy for patients with immune thrombocytopenia and very low platelet count: is platelet transfusion necessary? J Surg Res. 2011;170:e225–32.
35. Wu Z, Zhou J, Li J, et al. The feasibility of laparoscopic splenectomy for ITP patients without preoperative platelet transfusion. Hepatogastroenterology. 2012;59:81–5.

Therapy in Pregnancy

Yuji Yamada and Yoshitaka Miyakawa

Abstract Glucocorticoids and intravenous immunoglobulins are widely accepted and recommended in guidelines for the treatment in pregnancy. On the other hand, the safety profile of the other options during pregnancy is not well known. Since ITP affects not only pregnant women but also neonates, the effective communication among hematologists, obstetricians, and pediatricians should be established for efficient management.

1 Background

ITP occurs in approximately 1 in 1000 to 1 in 10,000 pregnant women [1, 2], but prospective clinical trials have not been conducted for this population because of its low prevalence and ethical issues. It is relatively difficult to pursue evidence-based medicine, but several international and local guidelines are available and suggest the appropriate management and goal of treatment. The management in pregnancy is generally similar to that of nonpregnant patients. Last but certainly not least, the management in pregnancy requires collaboration of the obstetrician, the hematologist, and the neonatologist.

2 Indications for Treatment

Pregnant patients with no bleeding and platelet counts above 30,000/μl do not require any treatment until 36 weeks gestation if delivery is not imminent [3]. In other words, patients with clinically relevant bleeding need to be treated. In the absence of bleeding, treatment is also indicated for patients with a platelet count

Y. Yamada (✉)
Department of Medicine, Mount Sinai Beth Israel, New York, NY, USA
e-mail: yuyamada@mountsinai.org

Y. Miyakawa
Department of General Internal Medicine, Center for Thrombosis and Hemostasis, Saitama Medical University, Saitama, Japan
e-mail: miyakawa@saitama-med.ac.jp

Y. Ishida, Y. Tomiyama (eds.), *Autoimmune Thrombocytopenia*,
DOI 10.1007/978-981-10-4142-6_20

below 30,000/μl [3] (which can be 20,000/μl according to the BSCH guideline and the international consensus report [2, 4]). Furthermore, if a patient has other risk factors of bleeding, such as the use of anticoagulants, treatment may be indicated even at a higher platelet count, but the target platelet count should be individualized [3].

3 Treatment Options for Pregnant Patients (Table 1)

There are only two treatment options, which have been considered as relatively safe for pregnant women, either glucocorticoids or intravenous immune globulin (IVIG) [2, 3]. These two options are widely accepted and recommended for pregnant women in guidelines. There are no comparative studies between these two options and decision must be made by clinical factors, patient's preference, medication cost, and risks of each therapy.

As far as the choice of corticosteroids is concerned, prednisone or prednisolone is preferred to dexamethasone, which crosses the placenta more readily [3]. While the ASH guideline recommends a starting dose of prednisone 1 mg/kg daily, there is no evidence that a higher starting dose is better than a lower dose [3]. Therefore, other

Table 1 Comparison of guideline recommendations

	International consensus report	ASH	BSCH	Japan
First-line	Prednisone/ prednisolone (10–20 mg/day) IVIG (dose not specified) IV anti-D	Prednisone/ prednisolone (1 mg/kg/day) IVIG (1 g/kg for 2 days)	Prednisone/ prednisolone (1 mg/kg/day) IVIG (0.4 g/kg/day for 5 days or 1 g/kg/day for 2 days)	Prednisolone (10–20 mg/day) * 0.5–1 mg/kg/day can be also considered for severe cases. IVIG (0.4 g/kg/day for 3–5 days)
Second-line	High-dose IV methyl-prednisolone (1000 mg) ± IVIG or azathioprine Splenectomy (second trimester)	Corticosteroids and IVIG Splenectomy (second trimester)	High-dose IV methylprednisolone (1000 mg) ± IVIG Azathioprine Splenectomy (second trimester)	Splenectomy should be avoided
Third-line		Cyclosporine, dapsone, TPO-R agonists, rituximab (not recommended but use in pregnancy described)		

The recommendations are generally similar but statements on splenectomy and azathioprine are different between guidelines experts recommend a starting dose of 0.25–0.5 mg/kg daily. In fact, the Japanese consensus report recommends 10–20 mg/day as a starting dose [5] since a Japanese nationwide study revealed that prednisolone dose of 15 mg/day or more might be associated with premature delivery, preeclampsia, or congenital abnormalities [6]. The international consensus report also recommends this lower starting dose [2].

The conventional dose of IVIG is 0.4 g/kg/day for 5 days, which is recommended in Japanese consensus report [5]. Alternatively, 1 g/kg/day for 2 days can be considered according to ASH and BSCH guidelines [3, 4]. The duration of response to IVIG is usually 2–3 weeks [2], and therefore after an initial response, repeat infusions might be required to prevent bleeding symptoms and keep an adequate platelet count if the patient should be managed only with IVIG.

Besides these two options, laparoscopic splenectomy during the second trimester is suggested as one of the second-line treatments for refractory cases [2–4]. This is because splenectomy during the first trimester may increase the risk of fetal death and premature labor, and the surgery during the third trimester is technically challenging due to uterine enlargement [3]. In Japanese consensus report, consideration of splenectomy prior to pregnancy is recommended for severe cases or patients who suffer from treatment side effects [5] rather than the operation during the second trimester.

The use of azathioprine is also suggested for refractory cases in two of the guidelines [2, 4], based on the safety data in SLE and inflammatory bowel disease [7, 8], though response is usually slow. Otherwise, the safety of rituximab or TPO-R agonists is yet unknown, and most immunosuppressants should not be used because of possible teratogenicity.

4 Management of Delivery

The mode of delivery should be determined based on obstetric indications since there is no evidence indicating that cesarian section can reduce the risk of neonatal cerebral hemorrhage. The current guidelines suggest the target platelet count be 50,000/μl or more for normal delivery and 75,000–80,000/μl for cesarean section with regional anesthesia [2, 3, 5]. However, there are no data to support a minimum required platelet count, and therefore each case must be individually considered, with the risk of the procedure balanced against benefits [2]. If an adequate platelet count has not been achieved and delivery is emergent, platelet transfusion in conjunction with IVIG can be considered [3]. If not emergent, adjustment of corticosteroids dose and planned IVIG generally works to achieve the goal.

5 Neonatal Management

The prevalence of platelet counts below 50,000/μl and 20,000/μl in neonates has been reported to occur in approximately 10 and 5 percent, respectively, in pregnancies with ITP [1]. It is essential for the hematologist and the obstetrician to have good communication with the pediatrician even before the delivery. After the delivery, infant platelet counts can keep decreasing for several days. Therefore, monitoring platelet counts on a daily basis is important for infants born to mothers with ITP [1].

References

1. Gill KK, Kelton JG. Management of idiopathic thrombocytopenic purpura in pregnancy. Semin Hematol. 2000;37(3):275–89.
2. Provan D, Stasi R, Newland AC, et al. International consensus report on the investigation and management of primary immune thrombocytopenia. Blood. 2010;115(2):168–86.
3. Neunert C, Lim W, Crowther M, et al. The American Society of Hematology 2011 evidence-based practice guideline for immune thrombocytopenia. Blood. 2011;117(16):4190–207.
4. British Committee for Standards in Haematology General Haematology Task Force. Guidelines for the investigation and management of idiopathic thrombocytopenic purpura in adults, children and in pregnancy. Br J Haematol. 2003;120(4):574–96.
5. Miyakawa Y. [Consensus report on the management of immune thrombocytopenia in pregnancy]. Rinsho Ketsueki 2015; 56(10):2086–91.
6. Fujimura K, Harada Y, Fujimoto T, et al. Nationwide study of idiopathic thrombocytopenic purpura in pregnant women and the clinical influence on neonates. Int J Hematol. 2002;75(4):426–33.
7. Erkman J, Blythe JG. Azathioprine therapy complicated by pregnancy. Obstet Gynecol. 1972;40(5):708–10.
8. Alstead EM, Ritchie JK, Lennard-Jones JE, Farthing MJ, Clark ML. Safety of azathioprine in pregnancy in inflammatory bowel disease. Gastroenterology. 1990;99(2):443–6.

Part VIII
Child ITP

Clinical Manifestations of ITP in Children

Yukihiro Takahashi

Abstract Most cases of idiopathic thrombocytopenic immune thrombocytopenia purpura (ITP) in children occur before 5 years old, show spontaneous remission under careful observation, and resolve with the use of first-line treatments such as steroids or high-dose immunoglobulin. ITP often develops after viral or bacterial infection, or after vaccination. Severe bleeding symptoms and severe thrombocytopenia ($<20 \times 10^9$/L) are rare but often become refractory. Second-line treatments such as rituximab and thrombopoietin receptor agonists have recently been used for ITP in children, in place of splenectomy. An objective ITP-bleeding assessment score seems necessary for management guidelines and selection of objective treatment in the future.

1 Introduction

Platelets, also known as thrombocytes, play an important role in primary hemostasis. Decreased platelet levels, or thrombocytopenia, causes bleeding tendencies. Acquired thrombocytopenia induced by abnormality of the platelet immune system [1, 2] is referred to as immune thrombocytopenic purpura (ITP). The abbreviation "ITP" was originally an acronym for "idiopathic thrombocytopenic purpura" [3], but the terms "immune thrombocytopenic purpura" [4] or "immune thrombocytopenia" [5, 6] are now used. ITP can be classified as primary or secondary. Primary ITP occurs in the absence of any inciting cause, whereas secondary ITP is caused by an underlying disease or drug exposure [4].

ITP in children is a relatively well-known disease and develops viral or bacterial infection, or after vaccination. Most pediatric cases of ITP show recovery within 6–12 months, differing from ITP in adults, which is typically more prolonged and refractory [7, 8].

Y. Takahashi
Nara Medical University, 840-Shijo-Cho, Kashihara 634-8522, Nara, Japan

Japanese Red Cross Nara Blood Center, 600-1 TsuTsui-Cho,
Yamato Koriyama 639-1123, Nara, Japan
e-mail: nicuyuki@naramed-u.ac.jp; y-takahashi@nara.bc.jrc.or.jp

Y. Ishida, Y. Tomiyama (eds.), *Autoimmune Thrombocytopenia*,
DOI 10.1007/978-981-10-4142-6_21

Many treatments for ITP in adults have recently been developed and have been applied to ITP in children [9–16]. In this chapter, recent advances in the treatment of pediatric ITP are reviewed.

2 Immune Abnormalities in ITP

ITP involves accelerated platelet consumption and reduced platelet production due to antiplatelet autoantibodies [17]. In 1951, Harrington and coworkers revealed the existence of a serum antiplatelet factor in ITP patients. They infused plasma from ITP patients into healthy volunteers, resulting in transient thrombocytopenia [1]. The target antigens of antiplatelet autoantibodies are now known to be against a variety of platelet membrane glycoproteins (GPs), including GPIIb/IIIa and GPIb/IX, or thrombopoietin (TPO) receptor [8, 18, 19], causing the destruction of circulating platelets and suppressing megakaryocyte differentiation and platelet production.

3 Definition of Thrombocytopenia

Thrombocytopenia is technically defined as a platelet count below 150×10^9/L [20], but ITP now uses a platelet count less than 100×10^9/L [4], because of uncertainty over both the boundary platelet count between normal populations and ITP patients, and the clinical significance of platelet counts.

4 Incidence of ITP in Children

The annual incidence of pediatric ITP is estimated to be about 2.2–5.3 cases per 10,000 children [21]. However, this incidence was thought to represent an underestimation, because cases of mild or unrecognized thrombocytopenia might have been missed.

5 Classification of ITP Phase

ITP has been classified into acute and chronic phases, based on recovery before or from 6 months after the onset of thrombocytopenia. However, the expert international working group (IWG) of the European Hematology Association Scientific Working Group on Thrombocytopenia and the Intercontinental Childhood ITP Study (ICIS) group recently proposed the standardization of terminology, definitions, and outcome criteria for ITP in adults and children [4]. ITP phases are now classified into three categories of newly diagnosed ITP, persistent ITP, and chronic ITP (Table 1).

Table 1 Classification of ITP in adults and children as recommended by IWG (EHASWGT/ICIS) in 2009 [4]

Newly diagnosed ITP	Resolution within 3 months of diagnosis
Persistent ITP	Resolution 3–12 months from diagnosis; includes patients not reaching spontaneous remission or not maintaining complete response off therapy
Chronic ITP	Lasting more than 12 months

However, in Japan, ITP in children has adopted the original two-phase classification to avoid confusion with annual transition. Pediatric ITP often occurs around 2 weeks after a viral infection, and most children with ITP recover within 6 weeks. ITP is acute in 70–80% of children and chronic in 20–30%. Recent Japanese data from 2009 to 2011 showed acute-, chronic-, and unclassified-phase ITP children in 64.2, 29.9, and 5.9%, respectively. However, ITP in adults increases with age and is often chronic.

6 Onset of ITP Children

ITP can develop at all ages in children. In newborns, thrombocytopenia developing from antiplatelet antibodies transferred through the placenta from a mother with ITP to the fetus is called passive ITP [22]. ITP in children mainly occurs after viral or bacterial infection or vaccination [23, 24].

7 Clinical and Laboratory Characteristics

Bleeding symptoms are mainly bruising and mucocutaneous bleedings such as petechiae (diameter of 0.5–3 mm, no blanching under pressure, not palpable) or ecchymosis (flat, rounded, or irregular red, blue, purplish, or yellow-green patch larger than petechiae), oral or nasal bleeding, hematuria, or hypermenorrhea. Rarely, organ bleeding such as gastrointestinal or intracranial bleeding occurs [25]. Patients are often noticed incidentally during laboratory examinations performed for unrelated diseases. ITP in children is more frequent in males, whereas adult ITP more involves females. Severe bleeding is rare and is found in children with a platelet count less than 20×10^9/L [4, 26, 27]. Predictors of bleeding due to ITP in children include female sex, older age at presentation (age $\geq$11 years), absence of preceding infection or vaccination, insidious onset, higher platelet count at presentation, presence of antinuclear antibodies, and treatment with a combination of methylprednisolone and intravenous immunoglobulin. Furthermore, children with mucosal bleeding at diagnosis or treatment with intravenous immunoglobulin alone develop chronic ITP less often [7].

8 Bleeding Assessment Tools (BATs) for ITP in Children

The bleeding risk and severity of ITP have usually been evaluated based on peripheral platelet counts and bleeding symptoms. However, objective evaluation of the degree or severity of bleeding symptoms is not easy. Various BATs have been proposed for ITP in children and adults [25, 28–32]. More recently, a new standard in bleeding assessment for ITP in children and adults (ITP-BAT bleeding scale, version 1.0) has been reported from the IWG.

The ITP-BAT bleeding scale is made up of three major bleeding domains of the skin (S), visible mucosae (M), and organs (O), with a gradation of severity (SMOG index). The gradation of severity for each domain is further classified on the site of bleeding with gradings ranging from 0 to 3 or 4 according to the spread of the hemorrhagic area, need for medical intervention and red blood cell transfusion, and reductions in levels of blood hemoglobin. For example, a SMOG index of S2 M2 O3 could represent findings of subcutaneous hematoma (S2), epistaxis (M2), and menorrhagia (O3). Considering the lifelong potential functional impairment caused by intracranial bleeding, the IWG recommends that all cases of intracranial bleeding be reported, irrespective of grade, such as S grade 2 M grade 2 O grade 3 (intracranial grade 2; post trauma, requiring hospitalization). However, the value of summing up the worst grades for all manifestations in each domain is currently uncertain, and interpretation remains ambiguous [25].

9 Diagnosis of ITP in Children

Information about the family and medical history before onset are important. The characteristics of bleeding symptoms and physical and laboratory examinations are crucial for differential diagnosis. The Japanese Society of Pediatric Hematology/Oncology proposed diagnostic criteria for pediatric ITP (Table 2) [33]. However, no gold standards exist for ITP diagnosis, and exclusion of other thrombocytopenic disorders remains central to the diagnosis. Bone marrow examination is usually unnecessary in children and adolescents with typical features of ITP, but when abnormal physical symptoms (such as abnormal rash, recurrent fever, or joint pain), lymphadenopathy, splenomegaly, abnormal cell counts, abnormal morphology of red or white blood cells, and poor response to medical treatments such as immunoglobulin and corticosteroids are present, bone marrow evaluation may be needed to rule out other disorders. In recent years, measurement of plasma levels of TPO, TPO receptor protein, and immature platelets (reticulo-platelets), which may indicate platelet production in the bone marrow, has been developed as complementary inspection methods [8].

Table 2 Diagnostic criteria for ITP children according to the Committee on Platelets of the Society of Japanese Pediatric Hematology/Oncology

1. Bleeding symptoms present
Bleeding symptoms as mainly purpura (petechia or ecchymosis) and also oral bleeding, epistaxis, melena, hematuria, hypermenorrhagia
Joint bleeding does not usually occur. Although patient would be unaware of a bleeding symptom, patient is admitted to clinic after identification of thrombocytopenia
2. Laboratory findings
a. Peripheral blood examinations • Decreased platelets: <100 × 10^9/L. It should be noted that attention to false thrombocytopenia is required when performing automatic blood cell counting • Numbers and morphological features of both red and white blood cells are normal. However, as for bleeding tendency or iron-deficiency anemia, a mild increase or decrease of white blood cells may also be observed.
b. Bone marrow • Numbers of megakaryocytes are normal or increased: Many megakaryocytes lack platelet production • Numbers or morphological features of both red blood cells and granulocyte lineages are normal: Granulocyte/erythroid (G/E) ratio overall; production of both lineages is present Bone marrow examination is not routinely conducted for diagnosis of ITP Bone marrow examination is considered at the presence of abnormal numbers and morphological feature of red and/or white blood cells, at disputable diagnosis of ITP, with the considerable use of corticosteroids or absence of desirable response to administration of large amounts of gamma globulin
3. Exclusion of various diseases that can cause thrombocytopenia[a]
4. ITP diagnosis can be made if the characteristic features of points 1–3 are present[b]
5. Criteria of ITP phase
a. Acute phase: Recovery from thrombocytopenia within 6 months from estimated onset or diagnosis b. Chronic phase: Thrombocytopenia prolonged for 6 months or more from estimated onset or diagnosis preceding virus infection often indicates acute-phase ITP

[a]Major diseases resulting in thrombocytopenia in childhood

[b]Measurement of specific antiplatelet antibody is useful for ITP diagnosis, but no laboratory system is available in Japan

Primary decrease of platelet production: Drug- or radiation-associated thrombocytopenia, aplastic anemia, leukemia, myelodysmorphic syndrome, bone metastasis of cancer, etc.

Primary increase in platelet destruction: Systemic lupus erythematosus, and related diseases, antiphospholipid antibody syndrome, disseminated intravascular syndrome, hemolytic uremic syndrome (HUS), thrombotic thrombocytic purpura (TTP), hemophagocytic syndrome, HIV infection, Kasabach-Merritte syndrome, etc.

Both decreased platelet production and platelet destruction, such as severe infectious disease, etc.

Congenital thrombopenia: Bernard-Soulier syndrome, Wiskott-Aldrich syndrome, X-linked thrombocytopenia, May-Hegglin syndrome, Epstein syndrome, gray platelet syndrome, von Willebrand disease (type "B" and platelet type), amegakaryocytic thrombocytopenia, etc.

10 Differential Diagnoses

A diagnosis of ITP is reached by excluding underlying disorders with thrombocytopenia caused by platelet destruction and/or production and congenital thrombocytopenia. Diagnosis of congenital thrombocytopenia is not easy and is usually achieved based on platelet size and morphology in peripheral blood specimens, clinical manifestations of hemorrhagic and nonhemorrhagic symptoms, and results of platelet-function tests such as platelet aggregation tests using three different inducers adenine diphosphate (*ADP*), *collagen and ristocetin*, platelet-membrane glycoprotein analysis, flow-cytometric analysis with specific-labeled antiplatelet antibodies, electron microscopic analysis, or genetic analysis. A recent distinction algorithm using platelet size for congenital thrombocytopenia is shown in Table 3 [34, 35].

Table 3 Classification of congenital thrombocytopenia by platelet size

Platelet size	Mode of inheritance	Gene	Remarks
Small (MPV: <5 fL[a])			
Wiskott-Aldrich syndrome[a]	X, AR	*WAS*, *WIPF1*	Immunodeficiency, eczema, thrombocytopenia
X-linked thrombocytopenia	X	*WAS*	Thrombocytopenia (mild eczema, susceptibility to infection)
Normal (MPV: 7.2–11.7 fL, 3–4 μm in diameter[b])			
Congenital amegakaryocytic thrombocytopenia	XR	*MPL*	Reduced megakaryocytes, transition to bone marrow failure
Congenital thrombocytopenia with radioulnar synostosis	XD	*HOXA11*	Radioulnar fusion, transition to bone marrow failure
Thrombocytopenia with absent radii syndrome	XR	*RBM8A*	Radial defect, normalization of platelet count with age
Familial platelet disorder with propensity to myeloid malignancy	XD	*RUNX1* (*AML1*)	Transition to AML/MDS
Autosomal-dominant thrombocytopenia, thrombocytopenia 2	XD	*ANKRD26*	Reduction of GP1a and α granules, transition to acute leukemia
Cytochrome C mutation	XD	*CYCS* (*G41S mutation*)	Apoptosis of megakaryocytes
Large (more than twice normal platelets, ≥8 μm in diameter)			
MYH9 disorders	AD	*MYH-9*	
May-Hegglin syndrome			Clear white blood cell inclusions
Sebastian syndrome			Somewhat ambiguous white blood cell inclusion bodies
Fechtner syndrome			Combined with glomerulonephritis and deafness[c]

Table 3 (continued)

Platelet size	Mode of inheritance	Gene	Remarks
Epstein syndrome			Combined with glomerulonephritis and deafness, leukocyte inclusion bodies difficult to recognize
Bernard-Soulier syndrome	AR	*GP1BA*, *GP1BB*, *GP9*	Lack of ristocetin-induced platelet aggregation
DiGeorge/velocardiofacial syndrome	AD	*22q 11.2 del* (*GP1BB*)	Contiguous gene syndrome
α-Actinin abnormality	AD	*ACTN1*	
GPIIb/IIIa mutation	AD	*ITGA2B*, *ITGA3*	Constitutively activated GPIIb/IIIa receptor
Type 2B von Willebrand disease	AD	*VWF*	Increased ristocetin-induced platelet aggregation
Gray platelet syndrome	AR	*NBEAL2*	Low staining (gray) platelets
Paris-Trousseau/Jacobsen syndrome	AD	*11q23 del* (*FLT1*)	Contiguous gene syndrome large alpha granules, mental retardation/neurological symptoms, cardiac malformation
X-linked macrothrombocytopenia	X	*GATA1*	Combined erythrocyte hematopoiesis
β1-Tubulin abnormality	AD	*TUBB1*	Microtubule dysplasia
Periventricular heterotopia	X	*FLNA*	Cortical dysplasia mental retardation/neurological symptoms

MPV mean platelet volume, *X* X-linked inheritance, *AR* autosomal recessive inheritance, *AD* autosomal-dominant inheritance, *WAS* Wiskott-Aldrich syndrome, *WIPF1* WAS/WASL interacting protein family member 1, *MPL* myeloproliferative leukemia virus, *HOXA11* homeobox protein Hox-A11, *RBM8A* RNA-binding motif protein 8A, *RUNX-1* Runt-related transcription factor 1, *VWF* von Willebrand factor, *ANKRD26* ankyrin repeat domain-containing protein 26, *NBEAL2* neurobeachin-like 2, *FLNA* filamin A

[a]Baharin MF et al. A rare case of Wiskott-Aldrich syndrome with normal platelet size: a case report. *J Med Case Rep* 2016;10:188

[b]Demirin H et al. Normal range of mean platelet volume in healthy subjects: insight from a large epidemiologic study. *Thromb Res* 2011;128:358–60

[c]Kunishima S et al. Advances in the understanding of MYH9 disorders. *Curr Opin Hematol* 2010;17:405–10

11 Long-Term Outcomes of ITP in Children

Long-term outcomes of ITP in children have reported that many children who achieve spontaneous remission and serious bleeding are rare [26, 36, 37]. Among those reports, an ICIS group reported on 1,345 subjects from a prospective study focusing on natural history, bleeding manifestations, and management [26]. Remission occurred in 37% of patients between 28 days and 6 months, in 16% between 6 and

12 months, and in 24% between 12 and 24 months. No cases of intracranial hemorrhage were reported, and the most common site of bleeding was the skin, followed by epistaxis. That study concluded that ITP is a benign condition for most affected children and that major hemorrhage, even with severe thrombocytopenia, is rare. However, intracranial bleeding in ITP in children has been reported, albeit rarely [10, 23, 27]. Intracranial bleeding obviously increases the risk of mortality and morbidity. In the case of severe thrombocytopenia, careful follow-up is always necessary.

12 Treatments for ITP in Children

Most cases of ITP in children represent acute-type ITP in which remission can be achieved by watchful waiting or administration of immunoglobulin or steroid [5, 26, 30, 31, 33, 38]. However, the therapeutic strategy for chronic-type ITP in children is not yet well established, and alternative second-line treatments are needed. Current second-line therapies include splenectomy and administration of rituximab [9–11] or TPO receptor agonist [12–16], eradiation therapy of *Helicobacter pylori* in children with chronic immune thrombocytopenia induced by this bacterium [39, 40], and other immunosuppressive or immunomodulatory therapies [41, 42].

Appendix

Member of the Committee on Platelets of the Japanese Society of Pediatric Hematology/Oncology.

Yukihiro Takahashi, Akira Ishiguro, Shinji, Kunishima, Naoaki Kobayashi, Masamune Higashikawa, Naoko Maeda, Youji Sasahara, Masue Imaizumi, Observers, Fumio Bessho, Akira Shirahata, Hisaya Nakadate

Conflict of Interest

The author has no conflicts of interest to declare.

References

1. Harrington WJ, Minnich V, Hollingsworth JW, Moore CV. Demonstration of a thrombocytopenic factor in the blood of patients with thrombocytopenic purpura. J Lab Clin Med. 1951;38:1–10.
2. Cines DB, Blanchette VS. Immune thrombocytopenic purpura. N Engl J Med. 2002;346:995–1008.
3. Ruggeri M, Fortuna S, Rodeghiero F. Heterogeneity of terminology and clinical definition in adult idiopathic thrombocytopenic purpura: a critical appraisal from a systemic review of the literature. Haematologica. 2008;93:98–103.

4. Rodeghiero F, Stasi R, Germheimer T, Michel M, Provan D, Arnold DM, Bussel JB, Cines DB, Chong BH, Cooper N, Godeau B, Lechner K, Mazzucconi MG, McMillan R, Sanz MA, Imbach P, Blanchette V, Kuhne T, Ruggeri M, George JN. Standardization of terminology, definitions and outcome criteria in immune thrombocytopenic purpura of adults and children: report from an international working group. Blood. 2009;113:2386–93.
5. Provan D, Stasi R, Newland AC, Blanchette VS, Bolton-Maggs P, Bussel JB, Chong BH, Cines DB, Gernsheimer TB, Godeau B, Grainger J, Greer I, Hunt BJ, Imbach PA, Lyons G, McMillan R, Rodeghiero F, Sanz MA, Tarantino M, Watson S, Young J, Kuter DJ. International consensus report on the investigation and management of primary immune thrombocytopenia. Blood. 2010;115:168–86.
6. Neunert C, Lim W, Crowther M, Cohen A, Solberg Jr L, Crowther MA, American Society of Hematology. The American Society of Hematology 2011 evidence-based practice guideline for immune thrombocytopenia. Blood. 2011;117:4190–207.
7. Heitink-Polle KMJ, Nijsten J, Boonacker CWB, de Haas M, Bruin MCA. Clinical and laboratory predictors of chronic immune thrombocytopenia in children: a systematic review and meta-analysis. Blood. 2014;124:3295–307.
8. Nomura S. Advances in diagnosis and treatments for immune thrombocytopenia. Clin Med Insights Blood Disord. 2016;9:15–21.
9. Parodi E, Nobili B, Perrotta S, Rosaria Matarese SM, Russo G, Licciardello M, Zecca M, Locatelli F, Cesaro S, Bisogno G, Giordano P, De Mattia D, Ramenghia U. Rituximab (anti-CD20 monoclonal antibody) in children with chronic refractory symptomatic immune thrombocytopenic purpura: efficacy and safety of treatment. Int J Hematol. 2006;84:48–53.
10. Matsubara K, Takahashi Y, Hayakawa A, Tanaka F, Nakadate H, Sakai M, Maeda N, Oka T, Ishii E, Besso F, Morimoto T, Goto H, Hashii Y, Hatakeyama N, Shirahata A, Imaizumi M. Long-term follow-up of children with refractory immune thrombocytopenia treated with rituximab. Int J Hematol. 2014;99:429–36.
11. Ay Y, Karapinar TH, Oymak Y, Toret E, Demirag B, Ince D, Ozcan E, Moueminoglou N, Koker SA, Vergin C. Retrospective analysis of rituximab therapy and splenectomy in childhood chronic and refractory immune thrombocytopenic purpura. Blood Coagul Fibrinolysis. 2016;27:431–5.
12. Bussel JB, Buchanan GR, Nugent DJ, Gnarra DJ, Bomgaars LR, Blanchette VS, Wang YM, Nie K, Jun S. A randomized, double-blind study of romiplostim to determine its safety and efficacy in children with immune thrombocytopenia. Blood. 2011;118:28–36.
13. Garzon AM, Mitchell WB. Use of thrombopoietin receptor agonists in children immune thrombocytopenia. Front Pediatr. 2015; doi:10.3389/fped.2015.00070.
14. Burness CB, Keating GM, Garnock-Jones KP. Eltrombopag: a review in paediatric chronic immune thrombocytopenia. Drugs. 2016;76:869–78.
15. Elgebaly AS, Ashal GE, Elfil M, Menshawy A. Tolerability and efficacy of eltrombopag in chronic immune thrombocytopenia: meta-analysis of randomized controlled trials. Clin Appl Thromb Hemost. 2016; pii: 1076029616663849. [Epub ahead of print].
16. Neunert C, Despotovic J, Haley K, Lambert MP, Nottage K, Shimano K, Bennett C, Klaassen R, Stine K, Thompson A, Pastore Y, Brown T, Forbes PW, Grace RF, Pediatric ITP Consortium of North America (ICON). Thrombopoietin receptor agonist use in children: data from the Pediatric ITP Consortium of North America ICON2 study. Pediatr Blood Cancer. 2016;63:1407–13.
17. McMillan R. Autoantibodies and autoantigens in chronic immune thrombocytopenic purpura. Semin Hematol. 2000;37:239–48.
18. Talaat RM, Elmaghraby AM, Barakat SS, El-Shahat M. Alterations in immune cell subjects and their cytokine secretion profile in childhood idiopathic thrombocytopenic purpura (ITP). Clin Exp Immunol. 2014;176:291–300.
19. Kuwana M, Okazaki Y, Kajihara M, Kaburaki J, Miyazaki H, Kawakami Y, Ikeda Y. Autoantibody to c-Mpl (thrombopoietin receptor) in systemic lupus erythematosus: relationship to thrombocytopenia with megakaryocytic hypoplasia. Arthritis Rheum. 2002;46:2148–59.
20. Nujum ZT, Thomas A, Vijayakumar K, Nair RR, Pillai MR, Indu PS, Sundar S, Gopakumar S, Mohan D, Sudheeshkumar TK. Comparative performance of the probable case definitions

of dengue by WHO (2009) and the WHO-SEAR expert group (2011). Pathog Glob Health. 2014;108:103–10.
21. Terrell DR, Beebe LA, Vesely SK, Neas BR, Segal JB, George JN. The incidence of immune thrombocytopenic purpura in children and adults: a critical review of published reports. Am J Hematol. 2010;85:174–80.
22. Yamada H, Kato EH, Kobashi G, Kishida T, Ebina Y, Kaneuchi M, Suzuki S, Fujimoto S. Passive immune thrombocytopenia in neonates of mothers with idiopathic thrombocytopenic purpura: incidence and risk factors. Semin Thromb Hemost. 1999;25:491–6.
23. Miura T, Mimaya J, Ishii E, Fujisawa K, Ohta S, Taki M, Imaizumi M, Oka T, Kajiwara M, Kitazawa J, Kubota Y, Takahashi Y, Bessho F, Shirahata A. A nationwide survey of childhood idiopathic thrombocytopenic purpura in 2006. J Pediatr Hematol Oncol. 2008;22:378–81. (in Japanese)
24. Kitazawa J, Miura T, Shirahata A, Takahashi Y, Ishii E, Imaizumi M, Ohta S, Oka T, Kajiwara M, Kubota Y, Taki M, Fujisawa K, Bessho R, Mimaya J. Idiopathic thrombocytopenic purpura following vaccinations. J Pediatr Hematol Oncol. 2008;22:382–4. (in Japanese)
25. Rodeghiero F, Michel M, Gernsheimer T, Ruggeri M, Blanchette V, Bussel JB, Cines DB, Cooper N, Godeau B, Greinacher A, Imbach P, Khellaf M, Klaassen RJ, Kühne T, Liebman H, Mazzucconi MG, Newland A, Pabinger I, Tosetto A, Stasi R. Standardization of bleeding assessment in immune thrombocytopenia: report from the International Working Group. Blood. 2013;121:2596–606.
26. Neunert CE, Buchanan GR, Imbach P, Bolton-Mggs PB, Bennet CM, Neufeld E, Vesely SK, Adix L, Blanchette VS, Kuhne T, for the Intercontinental Cooperative ITP Study Group Registry II Participants. Bleeding manifestations and management of children with persistent and chronic immune thrombocytopenia: data from Intercontinental Cooperative ITP Study Group (ICIS). Blood. 2013;121:4457–62.
27. Psaila B, Petrovic A, Page LK, Menell J, Schonholz M, Bussel JB. Intracranial hemorrhage (ICH) in children with immune thrombocytopenia (ITP): study of 40 cases. Blood. 2009;114:4777–83.
28. Buchanan GR, Holtkamp CA. Prednisone therapy for children with newly diagnosed idiopathic thrombocytopenic purpura. A randomized clinical trial. Am J Pediatr Hematol Oncol. 1984;6:355–61.
29. Buchanan GR, Adix L. Grading of hemorrhage in children with idiopathic thrombocytopenic purpura. J Pediatr. 2002;141:683–8.
30. Blanchette VS, Luke B, Andrew M, Sommerville-Nielsen S, Barnard D, de Veber B, Gent M. A prospective, randomized trial of high-dose intravenous immune globulin G therapy, oral prednisone therapy, and no therapy in childhood acute immune thrombocytopenic purpura. J Pediatr. 1993;123:989–95.
31. Bolton-Maggs PH, Moon I. Assessment of UK practice for management of acute childhood idiopathic thrombocytopenic purpura against published guidelines. Lancet. 1997;350(9078): 620–3.
32. Koreth R, Weinert C, Weidorf DJ, Key NS. Measurement of bleeding severity: a critical review. Transfusion. 2004;44(4):605–17.
33. Shirahata A, Ishii E, Eguchi H, Okawa H, Ohta S, Kaneko T, Konishi S, Sako M, Sekine I, Takahashi Y, Taki M, Tsuchiya S, Fujisawa K, Bessho F, Horikoshi Y, Mimaya J, Akatsuka J, Miyazaki S, ITP Committee of the Japanese Society of Pediatric Hematology. Consensus guideline for diagnosis and treatment of childhood idiopathic thrombocytopenic purpura. Int J Hematol. 2006;83:29–38.
34. Sasahara Y, Ouchi M, Imaizumi M. Recent advances in the diagnosis and molecular pathogenesis of congenital thrombocytopenia with small or normal-size platelets. JJPHO. 2013;50:186–91. (in Japanese)
35. Kunishima S. Differential diagnosis of congenital thrombocytopenia with large-side platelets. JJPHO. 2013;50:186–91. (in Japanese)
36. Medeiros D, Buchanan GR. Major hemorrhage in children with idiopathic thrombocytopenic purpura: immediate response to therapy and long-term outcome. J Pediatr. 1998;133:334–9.

37. Kühne T, Imbach P, Bolton-Maggs PH, et al. Newly diagnosed idiopathic thrombocytopenic purpura in childhood: an observational study. Lancet. 2001;358:2122–5.
38. Fujisawa K, Iyori H, Ohkawa H, Konishi S, Bessho F, Shirahata A, Miyazaki S, Akatsuka J, Japanese Study Group on Childhood ITP. A prospective, randomized trial of conventional, dose-accelerated corticosteroids and intravenous immunoglobulin in children with newly diagnosed idiopathic thrombocytopenic purpura. Int J Hematol. 2000;72:376–83.
39. Brito HS, Braga JA, Loggetto SR, Machado RS, Granato CF, Kawakami E. *Helicobacter pylori* infection & immune thrombocytopenic purpura in children and adolescents: a randomized controlled trial. Platelets. 2015;26:336–41.
40. Russo G, Miraglia V, Branciforte F, Matarese SM, Zecca M, Bisogno G, Parodi E, Amendola G, Giordano P, Jankovic M, Corti A, Nardi M, Farruggia P, Battisti L, Baronci C, Palazzi G, Tucci F, Ceppi S, Nobili B, Ramenghi U, De Mattia D, Notarangelo L, AIEOP-ITP Study Group. Effect of eradication of *Helicobacter pylori* in children with chronic immune thrombocytopenia: a prospective, controlled, multicenter study. Pediatr Blood Cancer. 2011;56:273–8.
41. Yamazaki T, Shibuya A, Ishii S, Miura N, Ohtake A, Sasaki N, Araki R, Ota Y, Fujiwara M, Miyajima Y, Uetake K, Hamahata K, Kato K, Kawakami K, Toyoda H, Moriguchi N, Okada M, Nishi M, Ogata Y, Takimoto T, Ohga S, Ohta S, Amemiya S. High-dose Cepharanthine for pediatric chronic immune thrombocytopenia in Japan. Pediatr Int. 2016; doi:10.1111/ped.13151 [Epub ahead of print].
42. Provan D, Newland AC. Current management of primary immune thrombocytopenia. Adv Ther. 2015;32:875–87.

Management and Treatment of Primary Immune Thrombocytopenia in Children

Masue Imaizumi

Abstract Primary immune thrombocytopenic purpura (ITP), the most common isolated thrombocytopenia of childhood, is involved in immunological mechanisms. ITP has shown heterogeneous pathophysiology, clinical features, and response to treatment. Most children with primary ITP recover within 6–12 months, but some patients who develop refractory or chronic ITP require especially careful medical management. To date, most conventional treatments consist of immunosuppressive or immune-modulating drugs. The International Consensus Report on the management of primary ITP has stated the goal for ITP management as achieving a safe level of platelet counts to avoid severe bleeding and minimizing therapy-related adverse effects. More recently, a new class of drugs, rituximab and thrombopoietin receptor (TPO-R) agonists, have been developed for the use in treating patients with ITP including children. The increasing clinical usage of these agents might improve therapeutic approaches and managements for children with ITP.

1 Introduction

Primary immune thrombocytopenic purpura (ITP), the most common isolated thrombocytopenia in children, is characterized by increased platelet destruction in the spleen and by impaired platelet production in the bone marrow [1, 2]. Today, ITP is regarded not as a single disease but collectively as various thrombocytopenic diseases that are commonly involved by immunological mechanisms [1, 3], although its diagnosis yet needs exclusion of any definite disease.

Since the publication of the International Consensus Report [3] and revised American Society of Hematology guidelines [4], the attitude in which pediatrician manage ITP has begun to change. Patients are treated based on symptoms and signs rather than a mere platelet count. The goal of this management is to maintain a safe

M. Imaizumi
Department of Hematology and Oncology, Miyagi Children's Hospital,
4-3-17 Ochiai, Aoba-ku, Sendai 989-3126, Japan
e-mail: imaizumi@miyagi-children.or.jp

Y. Ishida, Y. Tomiyama (eds.), *Autoimmune Thrombocytopenia*,
DOI 10.1007/978-981-10-4142-6_22

platelet count to a level that will minimize or stop bleeding and to lessen the therapy-related adverse effects of importance for children [5]. More recently, in addition to conventional drugs for ITP, the clinical application of newly developed agents, such as rituximab and thrombopoietin receptor (TPO-R) agonists, has demonstrated the efficacy and safety of these agents for children with refractory or chronic ITP.

This review provides a brief summary of treatment for childhood ITP in the first half and, in the second half, emphasizes the clinical studies of rituximab and TPO-R agonists for primary ITP in children.

2 Management of Children with ITP

In 2009, new terminology for ITP was adopted based on the duration: "newly diagnosed" from diagnosis until 3 months, "persistent" from 3 to 12 months, and "chronic ITP" lasting for longer than12 months [6].

The International Consensus Report [3] has stated on the management of patients with primary ITP. Bleeding of children with newly diagnosed ITP most commonly shows mucocutaneous symptom (petechiae, ecchymosis, or epistaxis), but only 3% of cases have significant bleeding such as severe epistaxis or gastrointestinal bleeding. In particular, the incidence of intracranial hemorrhage (ICH) is rare (0.1–0.5%), but its prediction is difficult in a practical sense [7]. Severe bleeding is more likely with platelet counts of less than 10×10^9/L, whereas major bleeding is rarely seen with platelet counts of more than 30×10^9/L. Most cases of children with newly diagnosed ITP without severe bleeding can be managed using a "watch-and-wait" policy under close observation and with consent of parents. Children with ITP showing significant bleeding must consider hospital admission and treatment if accompanied by marked thrombocytopenia (lower than 20×10^9/L). The management of children with persistent ITP is fundamentally the same as that for those with newly diagnosed ITP.

The goal of treatment for children with persistent/refractory or chronic ITP is to maintain platelet counts at higher than safety levels and to minimize the therapy-related side effects, especially those associated with long-term administration of corticosteroids. The main first-line treatments include corticosteroids and intravenous immunoglobulin (IVIG) as described below.

In Japan, the guideline previously proposed by the Japanese Society of Pediatric Hematology/Oncology had been used widely for management of childhood ITP [8]. Recently, however, the new consensus of terminology and standardization as well as clinical application of new drugs has engendered an increased need for a revised guideline for children with ITP in Japan.

3 Conventional Treatments [4, 8]

Conventional treatments for ITP include immunosuppressive therapies that primarily aim to reduce platelet destruction (e.g., corticosteroids, azathioprine, cyclosporine, cyclophosphamide, mycophenolate mofetil, rituximab, and vinca alkaloids), immune-modulating agents that prevent macrophage destruction of antibody-coated platelets (e.g., intravenous immunoglobulin and intravenous anti-D), and surgical therapy that prevents platelet sequestration (i.e., splenectomy). However, patients with ITP do not always respond to conventional "immunosuppressive" treatments.

3.1 First-Line Treatments

Corticosteroids and intravenous immunoglobulin (IVIG) are two major conventional drugs used in the first-line therapy for children with ITP in Japan. Children with newly diagnosed ITP presenting with bleeding symptom and $<20 \times 10^9$/L of platelet counts are treated with prednisolone or prednisone (1–2 mg/kg), which may be effective to induce a response in children within 2–7 days until response. Because of side effects associated with prolonged administration of corticosteroids, they should be used for a maximum of 2 weeks. In a standard way, IVIG is administered at doses of 0.4 g/kg/day (2–5 days) or 0.8–1 g/kg (single day). A rapid increase of platelet is induced in more than 80% of patients usually with a shorter durable response than corticosteroids. With these first-line treatments, approximately 70–80% of children with newly diagnosed ITP are likely to have a complete response within 6–12 months after diagnosis.

However, patients who are severe/refractory or chronic ITP with insufficient response to first-line treatments need careful medical care, in addition to second-line treatments if necessary. Conventional second-line treatments include immunosuppressive agents such as cyclosporine, azathioprine, or mycophenolate. Although splenectomy is another reliable second-line therapy with 70–80% of efficacy at initial response, its application to children has become less frequent because of post-operative risk of infection and, more recently, because of the introduction of new agents such as rituximab and TPO-R agonists in clinical areas.

3.2 Choice of the First-Line Therapy and Chronicity of ITP

When physicians start to treat children with newly diagnosed ITP, the choice of corticosteroids or IVIG might be made dependent on clinical expertise, patient preference, or urgent need to increase platelet counts (generally more rapid response to IVIG than to corticosteroids), rather than on the predictive property for preventing chronic ITP development.

Although the individual course of a child with ITP is difficult to predict, Heitink-Polle et al. assessed therapeutic predictors of chronic ITP using a meta-analysis that revealed significantly fewer chronic ITP patients treated with IVIG (odd ratio: 0.71) than those with other treatments [9]. Moreover, a significantly higher risk for chronic ITP was found for patients treated with a combination therapy of IVIG and standard-dose methylprednisolone (SDMP) than with other treatments (odd ratio: 2.67). Although this meta-analysis might be useful in clinical practice, these data must be verified with more precise evaluation using with multivariate, not univariate, analysis or prospective clinical trials.

4 Rituximab

Rituximab is a chimeric monoclonal antibody that targets CD20 antigen on the B-cell surface. Rituximab was used at first for treatment of B-cell lymphoma. Then, its target diseases were expanded to autoimmune diseases. Previous reports of rituximab used for children with ITP are shown in Table 1 [10–16], in which only few data are available with regard to the long-term efficacy of rituximab for childhood ITP. Recently, a retrospective study in Japan reported the long-term effects of rituximab for 22 children with refractory ITP, for whom the initial CR rate was as high as 41% (9/22), decreased gradually to a 14% (3/22) relapse-free CR rate at 5 years after the first rituximab therapy [16]. Results of this study also suggest that repeated rituximab administration is a promising therapy because patients who had received multiple courses of rituximab after relapse responded each time without adverse effects. They achieved remission during long-term observation.

As shown in Fig. 1, the downward tendency of relapse-free survival (RFS) after initial response is one of major concerns to therapeutic effectiveness of rituximab [15, 16]. From a long-term follow-up conducted for more than 5 years, Patel et al. showed that 52% (34/66) of initial responders subsequently relapsed. Actually, 28 relapsed within 1 year and 6 relapsed during 1–2 years, but none relapsed after 2 years, suggesting that observation for at least 2 years is necessary to assess the long-term efficacy of rituximab for children with chronic ITP [17].

A recent meta-analysis including 324 pediatric patients showed that a pooled CR (platelet count $>100 \times 10^9$/L) rate and an overall response (platelet count $>30 \times 10^9$/L) rate were 39 and 68%, respectively [18]. Rituximab therapy might be promising for refractory ITP patients, and, therefore, it might offer relief from bleeding symptoms and allow for avoidance of splenectomy. However, infection is a major concern, and there have been reports in children of pneumonia, varicella, and reactivation of hepatitis C [4, 18–20].

The relationship of clinical variables with response of rituximab and relapse-free factors has been studied [15, 17, 21]. Patel et al. [17] reported that patients showing a higher degree of response continued to remain in remission for a long-term period compared to those with a lesser degree of response (relapse rate within 1 year; 7% (2/28) in CR vs. 40% (4/10) in PR). Nor were significant predictors of splenectomy, gender, or age for response of rituximab and relapse-free factors. Although the efficacy of rituximab was not high, Matsubara et al. indicated that the initial responders to rituximab achieved remission at significantly higher rate, even after relapse than nonresponders did. Consequently, in clinical practice, the initial response is a useful indicator of the subsequent remission rate.

Table 1 Rituximab for children with chronic ITP

Study	No. of patients	Age at ITP diagnosis (year)	Duration before rituximab (month)	Age at rituximab treatment (year)	Times of injection	Duration of observation (month)	Rate of initial response (CR + PR)	Rate of complete response	Relapsed patients after initial response (%)	Duration until relapse	Patients with severe infection	Patients with serum sickness	Reference
1	24		24 (6–120)	NA	4	9	19 (79)	15 (63)	8 (42)	7.5 (3–18)	0	3	[10]
2	22	5.8 (2.5–15.2)	44 (2–27)	NA	1	NA	13 (59)	7 (47)	5 (38)	9 (4–24)	0	0	[11]
4	36	NA	NA (7–145)	11.2 (2.6–18.3)	4	>12	11 (30)	NA	3 (27)	9 (8–11)	0	2	[12, 13]
3	19	NA (3–18)	NA (1–48)	NA	4–6	18	15 (79)	10 (67)	1 (7)	NA	0	0	[14]
5	49	7.4 (0.7–17.6)	21 (1–175)	10.7 (1.2–17.7)	4–6	39.5	34 (69)	26 (53)	13 (38)	4 (1–8)	0	0	[15]
6	22	4.2 (0.3–11.6)	18.5 (2–120)	5 (0.5–20)	1–4	76.8 (62.4–85.2)	11 (50)	9 (41)	8 (72)	(2–26)	0	1	[16]

NA not assessed
Rituximab: 375 mg/m^2/dose

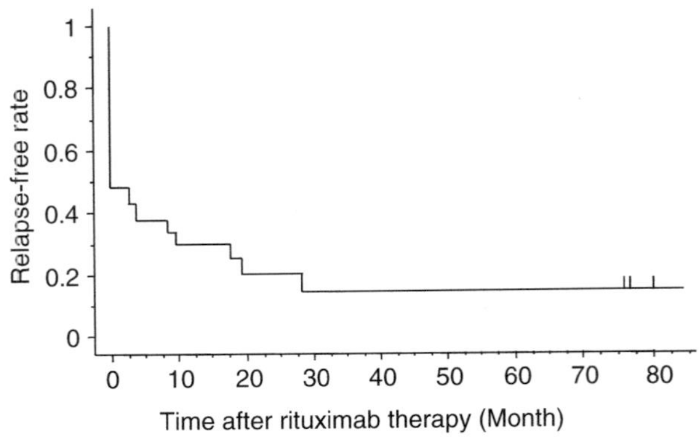

Fig. 1 Relapse-free survival rate of subjects who keep continuing first response to the first course of rituximab during long-term follow-up. The *gray-shaded area* of the initial 4 weeks indicates the evaluation period of the initial response to rituximab [16]

Moreover, the rituximab treatment regimen is not necessarily consistent among ITP patients. A recent systematic review pointed that there is no "standard" dose for rituximab treatment in children [18].

4.1 Development of TPO-R Agents

For refractory or chronic children with ITP whose risk of severe bleeding would grow even with the second-line treatments, a strong desire has persisted for therapeutic agents with distinct action mechanisms. The discovery and development of a human recombinant TPO (rh-TPO, the first generation of TPO) proved that the activation of TPO receptor can increase thrombopoiesis of megakaryocytes, facilitating TPO-based therapies as treatment for ITP [22–24].

However, the initial clinical trials demonstrated that healthy volunteers who received rh-TPO became severely thrombocytopenic because of cross-reactivity between autoantibodies to rh-TPO and endogenous TPO. This result led to the development of new agents that stimulate TPO receptor but led to little immunogenic adverse effect. The newly developed TPO-R agonists (the second generation of TPO) belong to either TPO non-peptide mimetics (eltrombopag) or TPO peptide mimetics (romiplostim) that increase platelet production by promoting the maturation of BM megakaryocytes through activation of TPO receptor signaling.

The properties of eltrombopag (daily p.o. medicine) and romiplostim (weekly SC injection) are presented in Table 2. The approved administration of eltrombopag is 50 mg/day initial dose and 75 mg/day maximum in Europe and the United States, but for the East Asian patients, the applied dosage was reduced to 12.5 mg/day initial and 50 mg/day maximum because of ethnic difference of drug responsiveness [25].

In the prospective and randomized studies for adult with chronic ITP, 109 of 135 patients (79%) showed significant increases of platelet counts, decreases of concurrent drugs, and lower demand of rescue therapies [26]. Therapeutic effects were not significantly influenced by prior treatments, previous splenectomy, or pretreatment platelet counts (Fig. 2).

Table 2 Comparative study of hemorrhagic manifestations between pediatric and adult patients with ITP

	Eltrombopag	Romiplostim
Compound	• A low-molecular compound activating TPO receptor	• An Fc peptide fusion peptibody binding to TPO receptor
Indication	• Adult ITP to which pretreatment is ineffective	• Adult ITP to which pretreatment is ineffective
Dose and effects	• Initial dose: 50 mg/day[a] • Maximum dose: 75 mg/day • Oral administration (daily) • PLT > $50 \times 10^3/\mu L$ (6 week): 60–81% • Thrombocytopenia after discontinuation • Reduction of combined drugs	• Initial dose: 1 mg/kg/week • Maximum dose: 10 mg/kg/week • SC administration (weekly) • PLT > $50 \times 10^3/\mu L$ (6 week): 63–88% • Thrombocytopenia after discontinuation • Reduction of combined drugs
Affecting factors	• No conclusion on children or long-term administration • Little effects of platelet counts, pretreatments, concurrent drug, or splenectomy	• No conclusion on children or long-term administration • Little effects of splenectomy
Adverse effects	• Headache, nasopharyngitis, liver dysfunction • Myelofibrosis • Thrombosis	• Headache • Myelofibrosis • Thrombosis
Antibody	• No induction of TPO-inhibiting antibody	• Possible neutralizing antibody, but no cross reactivity to TPO

Patients aged 1–5 years: 1.2 mg/kg/day (0.8 mg/kg/day for East Asian patients)
[a]Patients weighing less than 27 kg: 37.5 mg/day (25 mg/day for East Asian patients, 12.5 mg/day for Japanese patients)

For romiplostim, the initial dose is 5 μg/kg/week SC and adjusted up to 10 μg/kg/week at maximum with no marked racial difference of drug responsiveness. Similarly to eltrombopag, the efficacy of romiplostim was approximately 80% for adult with chronic ITP. In a randomized and double-blinded clinical trial for 125 patients [27], the percentage of patients who attained reduction or discontinuation of concurrent drugs was 87% for the romiplostim cohort and 38% for the placebo cohort. Moreover, a randomized clinical trial for patients who were refractory ITP without splenectomy, the subsequent execution rate of splenectomy was 9% for the romiplostim cohort and 36% for the standard therapy cohort, suggesting the possible avoidance of splenectomy by incorporating TPO-R agonists to treatment for refractory ITP [28].

The most common adverse effects of TPO-R agonists were headache, although nasopharyngitis and liver dysfunction were also observed for eltrombopag [26, 27, 29–31]. Thrombosis was reported to have a low rate of incidence, but its causal relation remains unclear [28, 31]. As long-term adverse effects, major concerns are the development of myelofibrosis, depletion of hematopoietic stem cells, and induction of other bone marrow abnormalities including malignant diseases. Further investigation of those areas of concern is expected to lead to better understanding.

a

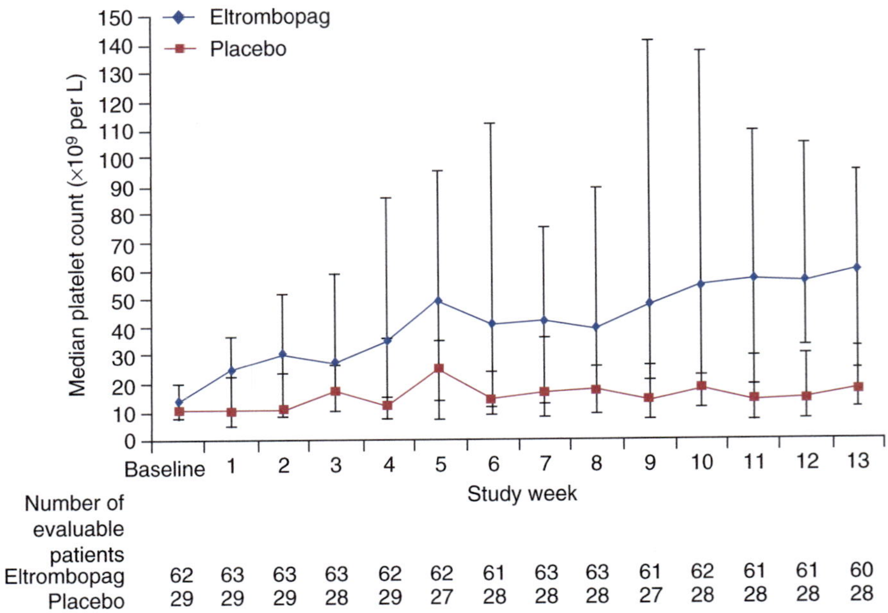

b

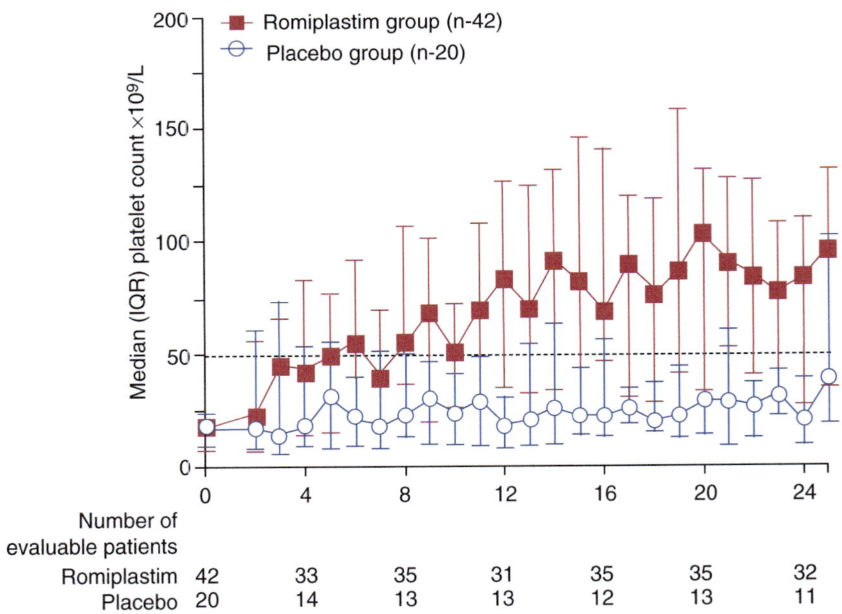

Fig. 2 Prospective randomized clinical trials for children with chronic ITP: (**a**) the result of study with eltrombopag [37]; (**b**) the results of study with romiplostim [38]

4.2 Clinical Studies of TPO-R Agonists for Children

Recently, many reports have described the efficacy and safety of TPO-R agonists for children with chronic ITP who had been treated unsuccessfully with the first-line treatments (Table 3) [32–38]. Patients included children (1–17 years old) with chronic/refractory ITP who received romiplostim or eltrombopag at doses adjusted to less than the maximum dose to maintain platelet counts at least $>50 \times 10^9$/L. In 2011, the first randomized clinical trials with romiplostim were reported: short-term observation (12 weeks) for 18 and 22 patients for whom the respective pretreatment duration was 2.4 and 2.5 years [32, 33]. These studies showed that the efficacy to maintain $>50 \times 10^9$/L of platelet counts without rescue medication was 83.5–88% for patients with romiplostim, as compared to 0% for those with placebo. Nevertheless, the small number of patients and the short-term duration of treatment of these studies might limit the generalization of their conclusions. More recently, a larger study of 62 children (romiplostim, 42; placebo, 20) during 24 weeks of treatment duration revealed that the efficacy of romiplostim was 52% for the romiplostim group as compared to 10% for the placebo group [38]. Another randomized double-blinded and subsequent open-labeled study with eltrombopag has demonstrated its efficacy as 40% for the eltrombopag group, compared to 3% for those of placebo [37]. The efficacy of eltrombopag increased further to 80% (70/87 patients) of efficacy during the following 24 weeks of the open-labeled period. These two recent studies confirmed that both romiplostim and eltrombopag TPO-R agonists are effective for chronic/refractory ITP in children. For these periods, no drug resistance or autoantibody against intrinsic TPO was detected.

Few therapy-associated severe adverse effects leading to forced discontinuation or lethalness have been observed, including headache, epistaxis, local pain, cough and vomiting commonly for both drugs, and liver dysfunction for eltrombopag. Although TPO-R agonists are effective and safe for short-term treatment, a retrospective study of children receiving TPO-R agonists for up to 53 months showed that one of 24 patients developed myelofibrosis in grade 2 [35]. The guideline of the American Society of Hematology continues to advise a cautious attitude related to TPO-R agonists for children with ITP [3].

4.3 Long-Term Safety and Discontinuation of TPO-R Agonists

It has been shown that some adult patients remain CR without treatment after discontinuation [39]. Approximately, 30% of adult patients who received these drugs might be able to maintain a safe or normal platelet count after stopping them [5]. Therefore, it remains to clarify whether TPO-R agonists could shorten the period until recovery or facilitate spontaneous cure in a subset of patients with refractory or chronic ITP.

Table 3 Clinical trials of TPO-R agonists for children with ITP

Study	No. of patient	Duration since ITP diagnosis (years)	Age at TPO-R agonist start (year)	PLT count ($\times 10^9$/L)	Splenectomy prior to treatment	Treatment duration (week or month)	Dose (average or range) (romiplostim: μg/kg/week; eltrombopag: mg/day)	Efficacy (PLT > 50×10^9/L)	Treatment-related serious adverse events	Common adverse events	Discontinuation of romiplostim	Reference
Prospective, randomized	22 (romiplostim, 17; placebo, 5)	2.4 (0.6–14)	10 (1–17)	13 (2–29)	8 (36%)	12 week	Romiplostim: 5	Romiplostim: 88%; placebo: 0%	no	Headache, epistaxis	no	[32]
Prospective, randomized	18 (romiplostim, 12; placebo, 6)	2.5 (1.2–7.0)	8.5 (2–16)	10.5	0	12 week	Romiplostim: 2	Romiplostim: 83.5%; placebo: 0%	no	Headache, epistaxis, cough, vomiting	For 3 weeks after discontinuation, 50% remained in CR	[33]
Retrospective	10	1.9 (0.8–15)	8.5 (2–19)	n.a.	20%	9 month (3–36)	Romiplostim: 4–10	50%	no	Headache, local pain, mood disorder	Three remained in CR	[34]
Retrospective	33 (romiplostim, 21; eltrombopag, 12)	Romiplostim: 4.0; eltrombopag: 5.0	Romiplostim: 11.4 (1.6–19); eltrombopag: 14.5 (3–19)	Romiplostim: 20; eltrombopag: 25	Romiplostim: 2 (9%); eltrombopag: 1 (8%)	Romiplostim: 6–44 month; eltrombopag: 23–53 month	Romiplostim: 8.1; eltrombopag: 66.7	82%	no	Rash, headache, nausea, epistaxis	7 (21%) remained CR after discontinuation	[35]
Prospective	24	2.4 y (1–14)	10 (1–17)	13 (2–29)	8 (36.4%)	167 week (12–242)	Romiplostim: 6.0 (3.1–9.7)	84.6%	no	Headache, respiratory infection, pyrexia	Several patients	[36]

Prospective, ramdom-ized	92 (eltrom-bopag, 63; placebo, 29)	Eltrom-bopag: 2.8; placebo: 3.4	Eltrom-bopag: 9.4 (8.2–10.5); placebo: 9.8 (8.3–11.3)	<30 × 10^9/L	Eltrom-bopag: 4 (6%); placebo: 0 (0%)	Double-blinded: 12 week; open-labeled: 24 week	Eltrom-bopag: 42.8–67.7 (East Asians: 37.2–58.9)	Eltrombopag: 40% (open-labeled: 80%); placebo: 3%	Eltrom-bopag: 8%; pla-cebo: 14%	Nasophar-yngitis, rhinitis, epistasis, cough, headache, liver dys-function	n.a.	[37]
Prospective, randomized	62 (romip-lostim, 4 2; placebo, 20)	Romiplos-tim: 1.9 (1.0–4.2); placebo: 2.2 (1.5–3.7)	Romiplos-tim: 10 (6–14); placebo: 7.5 (6.5–13.5)	<30 × 10^9/L	Romiplos-tim: 1 (2%); placebo: 1 (5%)	25 week	Romiplos-tim: 3.9 (2.4–7.3)	Romiplostim: 52%; placebo: 10%	Romip-lostim: 1 (head-ache, throm-bosis)	Contusion, epistasis, headache, thrombo-cytosis	n.a.	[38]

n.a. not available

5 Conclusion

In these years, with advances in understanding of pathophysiology of ITP and development of new therapeutic agents for ITP, there have been dynamic changes in the management and therapeutic approaches for children with ITP. However, from the viewpoint of children in the process of hematological and immunological development, further investigation needs to clarify their therapeutic role and long-term safety of those new agents for children with primary ITP.

References

1. Nugent DJ. Immune thrombocytopenic purpura of childhood. Hematology Am Soc Hematol Educ Program. 2006:97–103.
2. Cines DB, Bussel JB, Liebman HA, et al. The ITP syndrome: pathogenic and clinical diversity. Blood. 2009;113:6511–21.
3. Provan D, Stasi R, Newland AC, et al. International consensus report on the investigation and management of primary immune thrombocytopenia. Blood. 2010;115:168–86.
4. Neunert C, Lim W, Crowther M, et al. The American Society of Hematology 2011 evidence-based practice guideline for immune thrombocytopenia. Blood. 2011;117:4190–207.
5. Provan D, Newland AC. Current management of primary immune thrombocytopenia. Adv Ther. 2015;32:875–87.
6. Rodeghiero F, Stasi R, Gernsheimer T, et al. Standardization of terminology, definitions and outcome criteria in immune thrombocytopenic purpura of adults and children: report from an international working group. Blood. 2009;113:2386–93.
7. Imbach P, Kuhne T, Muller D, et al. Childhood ITP: 12 months follow-up data from the prospective registry I of the Intercontinental Childhood ITP Study Group (ICIS). Pediatr Blood Cancer. 2006;46:351–6.
8. Shirahata A, Ishii E, Eguchi H, et al. Consensus guideline for diagnosis and treatment of childhood idiopathic thrombocytopenic purpura. Int J Hematol. 2006;83:29–38.
9. Heitink-Poll K, Nijsten J, Boonacker C, et al. Clinical and laboratory predictors of chronic immune thrombocytopenia in children: a systematic review and meta-analysis. Blood. 2014;124:3295–307.
10. Wang J, Wiley JM, Luddy R, et al. Chronic immune thrombocytopenic purpura in children: assessment of rituximab treatment. J Pediatr. 2005;146:217–21.
11. Taube T, Schmid H, Reinhard H, et al. Effect of a single dose of rituximab in chronic immune thrombocytopenic purpura in childhood. Haematologica. 2005;90:281–3.
12. Bennett CM, Rogers ZR, Kinnamon DD, et al. Prospective phase 1/2 study of rituximab in childhood and adolescent chronic immune thrombocytopenic purpura. Blood. 2006;107:2639–42.
13. Rao A, Kelly M, Musselman M, et al. Safety, efficacy, and immune reconstitution after rituximab therapy in pediatric patients with chronic or refractory hematologic autoimmune cytopenias. Pediatr Blood Cancer. 2008;50:822–5.
14. Mueller BU, Bennett CM, Feldman HA, et al., Pediatric Rituximab/ITP Study Group; Glaser Pediatric Research Network. One year follow-up of children and adolescents with chronic immune thrombocytopenic purpura (ITP) treated with rituximab. Pediatr Blood Cancer. 2009;52:259–62.
15. Parodi E, Rivetti E, Amendola G, et al. Long-term follow-up analysis after rituximab therapy in children with refractory symptomatic ITP: identification of factors predictive of a sustained response. Br J Haematol. 2009;144:552–8.
16. Matsubara K, Takahashi Y, Hayakawa A, et al. Long-term follow-up of children with refractory immune thrombocytopenia treated with rituximab. Int J Hematol. 2014;99:429–36.

17. Patel VL, Mahévas M, Lee SY, et al. Outcome at 5 years following response to rituximab therapy in children and adults with immune thrombocytopenia. Blood. 2012;119:5989–95.
18. Ling Y, Zhang L, Gao J, et al. Rituximab for children with immune thrombocytopenia: a systematic review. PLoS One. 2012;7:e36698.
19. Ng PC, Lee KK, Lo AF, et al. Anti B cell targeted immunotherapy for treatment of refractory autoimmune haemolytic anaemia in a young infant. Arch Dis Child. 2003;88:337–9.
20. Goto S, Goto H, Tanoshima R, et al. Serum sickness with an elevated level of human anti-chimeric antibody following treatment with rituximab in a child with chronic immune thrombocytopenic purpura. Int J Hematol. 2009;89:305–9.
21. Grace RF, Bennett CM, Ritchey AK, et al. Response to steroids predicts responses to rituximab in pediatric chronic immune thrombocytopenia. Pediatr Blood Cancer. 2012;58:221–5.
22. Fox JE. Platelet activation: new aspects. Haemostasis. 1996;26(Suppl 4):102–31.
23. Machlus KR, Italiano Jr JE. The incredible journey: from megakaryocyte development to platelet formation. J Cell Biol. 2013;201:785–96.
24. Kaushansky K. Thrombopoietin: the primary regulator of platelet production. Blood. 1995;86:419–31.
25. Tomiyama Y, Miyakawa Y, Okamoto S, et al. A lower starting dose of eltrombopag is efficacious in Japanese patients with previously treated chronic immune thrombocytopenia. J Thromb Haemost. 2012;10:799–806.
26. Cheng G, Saleh MN, Marcher C, et al. Eltrombopag for management of chronic immune thrombocytopenia (RAISE): a 6-month, randomized, phase 3 study. Lancet. 2011;377:393–402.
27. Kuter DJ, Bussel JB, Lyons RM, et al. Efficacy of romiplostim in patients with chronic immune thrombocytopenic purpura: a double-blind randomised controlled trial. Lancet. 2008;371:395–403.
28. Kuter DJ, Rummel M, Boccia R, et al. Romiplostim or standard of care in patients with immune thrombocytopenia. N Engl J Med. 2010;363:1889–99.
29. Bussel JB, Provan D, Shamsi T, et al. Effect of eltrombopag on platelet counts and bleeding during treatment of chronic idiopathic thrombocytopenic purpura: a randomised, double-blind, placebo-controlled trial. Lancet. 2009;373:641–8.
30. Bussel JB, Kuter DJ, George JN, et al. AMG531, a thrombopoiesis-stimulating protein, for chronic ITP. N Engl J Med. 2006;355:1672–81.
31. Bussel JB, Kuter DJ, Pullarkat V, et al. Safety and efficacy of long-term treatment with romiplostim in thrombocytopenic patients with chronic ITP. Blood. 2009;113:2161–71.
32. Bussel JB, Buchanan GR, Nugent DJ, et al. A randomized, double-blind study of romiplostim to determine its safety and efficacy in children with immune thrombocytopenia. Blood. 2011;118:28–36.
33. Elalfy MS, Abdelmaksoud AA, Eltonbary KY. Romiplostim in children with chronic refractory ITP: randomized placebo controlled study. Ann Hematol. 2011;90:1341–4.
34. Pasquet M, Aladjidi N, Guiton C, et al. Romiplostim in children with chronic immune thrombocytopenia (ITP): the French experience. Br J Haematol. 2014;164:266–71.
35. Ramaswamy K, Hsieh L, Leven E, et al. Thrombopoietic agents for the treatment of persistent and chronic immune thrombocytopenia in children. J Pediatr. 2014;165:600–5.
36. Bussel JB, Hsieh L, Buchanan GR, et al. Long-term use of the thrombopoietin-mimetic romiplostim in children with severe chronic immune thrombocytopenia (ITP). Pediatr Blood Cancer. 2015;62:208–13.
37. Grainger JD, Locatelli F, Chotsampancharoen T, et al. Eltrombopag for children with chronic immune thrombocytopenia (PETIT2): a randomised, multicentre, placebo-controlled trial. Lancet. 2015;386:1649–358.
38. Tarantino MD, Bussel JB, Blanchette VS, et al. Romiplostim in children with immune thrombocytopenia: a phase 3, randomised, double-blind, placebo-controlled study. Lancet. 2016;388:45–54.
39. Katsutani S, Tomiyama Y, Kimura A, et al. Oral eltrombopag for up to three years is safe and well-tolerated in Japanese patients with previously treated chronic immune thrombocytopenia: an open-label, extension study. Int J Hematol. 2013;98:323–30.